Essentials of Sports Medicine

D0920709

This book is dedicated to my father
... for even his failings lean'd to Virtue's side

Essentials of Sports Medicine

EDITED BY

Greg R. McLatchie MB ChB FRCS

Consultant in General and Peripheral Vascular Surgery, The General Hospital,
Hartlepool; Visiting Professor, School of Health Sciences, University of
Sunderland; Director, National Sports Medicine Institute, St Bartholomew's
Medical College, London, UK

FOREWORD BY

John E. Davies MRCS LRCP DPhysMed

Hon. Physician to the Welsh Rugby Union; Consultant Physician in Sports
Medicine, Guy's Hospital, and Harley Street Sports Clinic, London, UK

SECOND EDITION

CHURCHILL LIVINGSTONE
EDINBURGH LONDON MADRID MELBOURNE NEW YORK AND
TOKYO 1993

LIBRARY
COLBY-SAWYER COLLEGE
NEW LONDON, NH 03257

RC
1210
.E78
1993
C.1

#28028359

CHURCHILL LIVINGSTONE
Medical Division of Longman Group UK Limited

Distributed in the United States of America by
Churchill Livingstone Inc., 650 Avenue of the Americas, New York,
N.Y. 10011, and by associated companies, branches and
representatives throughout the world.

© Longman Group UK Limited 1993

All rights reserved; no part of this publication
may be reproduced, stored in a retrieval system,
or transmitted in any form or by any means,
electronic, mechanical, photocopying, recording
or otherwise, without either the prior written permission of the
Publishers (Churchill Livingstone, Robert Stevenson
House, 1–3 Baxter's Place, Leith Walk,
Edinburgh EH1 3AF), or a license permitting restricted copying in the
United Kingdom issued by the Copyright Licensing Agency Ltd, 90
Tottenham Court Road, London, W1P 9HE.

First edition 1966
Second edition 1993
  Reprinted 1993

ISBN 0–443–04541–0

British Library Cataloguing in Publication Data
A catalogue record for this book is available from the British Library

Library of Congress Cataloging in Publication Data is available

The
publisher's
policy is to use
**paper manufactured
from sustainable forests**

Typeset by BP Integraphics Ltd, Bath, Avon
Printed in Great Britain by Redwood Books, Trowbridge

Contents

Contributors   vii

Foreword   ix

Preface   xi

Acknowledgements   xii

1. Sport, society and law
   I. N. Steele and A. Dewar   1

2. Sport and exercise in the prevention and treatment of disease
   G. R. McLatchie   21

3. Organization and teaching of sports medicine
   D. A. D. MacLeod and G. R. McLatchie   32

4. Women in sport
   M. O'Brien   46

5. Principles of training
   P. Radford   54

6. Laboratory assessment of performance
   P. A. Butlin   67

7. Diet in sport
   G. R. McLatchie and J. E. Davies   79

8. The value and limitations of protective equipment
   G. R. McLatchie   93

9. General medical problems in sport
   N. A. Dunn and C. Clark   103

10. Infection in sport
    J. C. M. Sharp   112

11. Physiotherapy and strapping in injury management
    T. Donnelly   126

12. Injury in sport
    G. R. McLatchie   140

13. Sudden death and injury in selected sports
    G. R. McLatchie   157

14. Cold injury
    E. L. Lloyd   182

15. Immediate care of the injured
    J. Lloyd Parry   199

16. General principles of investigation
    G. R. McLatchie   222

17. Injuries to the face, teeth and jaws
    D. C. Crawford   229

18. Injuries to the eye and orbit
    C. J. MacEwen   239

19. Head injuries
    G. R. McLatchie   255

20. Injuries to the neck and spine
    G. R. McLatchie   265

21. Injuries to the thorax and abdomen
    G. R. McLatchie   276

22. The assessment of the acutely injured joint
    J. Graham   283

23. Injuries to the upper limbs
    J. Graham   293

24. Injuries to the pelvis, hip and thigh
    J. Graham   308

25. Injuries to the knee and leg
    J. Graham   318

26. Injuries to the ankle and foot
    J. Graham   338

Index   347

Contributors

P. A. Butlin ADV Dip PE MA HE
Principal Lecturer, School of Pharmacology and Health Services,
University of Sunderland, Sunderland, UK

Christopher Clark MD MRCP
Consultant Physician, Hairmyres Hospital, East Kilbride,
Lanarkshire, Scotland

David C. Crawford BDS FDS
Associate Specialist in Dental Surgery, The Dental Hospital,
Glasgow, UK

John E. Davies MRCS LRCP DPhysMed
Hon. Physician to the Welsh Rugby Union; Consultant Physician
in Sports Medicine, Guy's Hospital and Harley Street Sports
Clinic, London, UK

Andrew Dewar CA LlB
Solicitor, Glasgow, UK

Thomas Donnelly MCSP
Physiotherapist, Department of Rehabilitation, Southern General
Hospital, Glasgow, UK

Nigel A. Dunn MRCP
Consultant Physician, Hartlepool General Hospital, Cleveland,
UK

James Graham FRCS
Consultant Orthopaedic Surgeon, The Western Infirmary,
Glasgow, UK

Evan Lloyd FFARCS
Consultant Anaesthetist, Princess Margaret Rose Orthopaedic
Hospital, Edinburgh, UK

Moira O'Brien MB FRCPI
Professor of Anatomy, Trinity College, Dublin, Republic of Ireland

John Lloyd Parry MA MB BChir General Practitioner
Hon. Medical Adviser to the Fédération Equestre Internationale, and the Governing Body of The British Horse Society Horse Trials (Eventing)

Caroline J. MacEwen MBChB FRCS
Consultant Ophthalmic Surgeon, Ninewells Hospital, Dundee, UK

Donald A. D. MacLeod MB ChB FRCS
Consultant Surgeon, St John's Hospital at Hawden, West Lothian, UK. Hon. Surgeon to the Scottish Rugby Union

Peter Radford BSc PhD
Professor of Sports Science, University of Glasgow, Glasgow, UK

J. Clarkson M. Sharp MRCP(Glas) FFPHM
Consultant Epidemiologist, Communicable Diseases Unit (Scotland), Ruchill Hospital, Glasgow, UK

Ian N. Steele LlB NP
Solicitor, Kirkcudbright, Scotland

Foreword

'To have been invited to write the foreword to Greg McLatchie's *Essentials of Sports Medicine* gives me the greatest pleasure, not only as a sports physician, but as a personal friend. Having travelled and had the privilege to lecture with the author over many years, I have never ceased to be amazed at the extensive knowledge which he has imparted to medical and paramedical audiences worldwide. This manifests itself in the book which has a wealth of practical and useful information for its medical readers, irrespective of their disciplines.

Greg McLatchie has probably, in recent years, produced more research bibliography in sports medicine than any other practising physician or surgeon, and his practical involvement and contribution to the martial arts in particular has been immense. Always aware of the need to identify and isolate risk factors in certain sports he has also been instrumental in persuading governing bodies to take note and amend the rules of their particular sports, or effecting a change in protective clothing to achieve the same end'.

The above two paragraphs were written and produced in the first edition of *Essentials of Sports Medicine*, and the Editor, Greg McLatchie, continues to pioneer both the academic and clinical involvement of sports medicine within the UK.

As the first appointed Professor in Sports Medicine and Surgical Sciences in Great Britain, he has attained academic heights with the acknowledgement of his peers. His government appointment as the Director of the National Sports Medicine Institute sees his vision become reality, and his wisdom will ensure the rapid and smooth development of education, research and clinical services in sports medicine. With the Royal Colleges in Scotland now holding a post graduate Diploma in Sports Medicine, the success of the first edition mirrors both the advances in sports medicine and the Editor's recent appointments.

London 1992   J.E.D.

Preface

Since the publication of the first edition of this book in 1986 there have been two major initiatives in establishing sports medicine as a medical speciality in the UK; the Diploma in Sports Medicine of the Scottish Royal Medical Colleges and the National Sports Medicine Institute supported by the Sports Council. One of the aims of the Institute is to encourage regional development of Centres of Sports Medicine throughout the UK by linking in with existing, mainly NHS, facilities. Each unit will have human performance laboratories and ties with local universities to establish measurement and audit as well as continuing medical education.

The philosophy of the text remains unchanged. Sport and the exercise habit have a significant bearing on the 'Health of the Nation'; that the Government now recognizes this is indeed welcome. However, as a profession, we need to be more proactive in the prevention of disease as well as reactive to its occurrence. We have a much better baseline than in 1986 and again should not miss our opportunities.

I am grateful to my friends and colleagues who have assisted me with this book, those who have contributed chapters and who have refereed or criticized and corrected others. In particular, Sam Galbraith, James Graham, Donald Macleod, Andrew Dewar, Ian Steele, Peter Radford, Moira O'Brien, Christopher Clark, Thomas Donnelly, David Crawford, Douglas Hutchinson, Caroline MacEwan, Nigel Dunn, John Davies, Evan Lloyd and John Lloyd Parry deserve a special mention. I am also grateful for help received from the Sports Council and I am indebted to Mr K. Davies, George Outram Newspapers and the Department of Medical Illustration at the Southern General Hospital, Glasgow, for providing the illustrations. Acknowledgements should also go to my secretary, Vera Spalding, and to Kate McLatchie for preparing the manuscripts.

Hartlepool, 1992   G. R. McL

Acknowledgements

I would like to acknowledge with thanks, Cook Critical Care, Laerdal and Lederle Laboratories for their support with the text and illustrations, and also George Outram Newspapers and Mr Dirk van der Werff of the Hartlepool Mail for illustrations (black and white photographs).

G. R. McL

1. Sport, society and law

INTRODUCTION

Physical prowess and ability in sport have been highly prized attributes throughout history. Although early games involved survival skills, usually against opponents or animals, these have become less evident in modern sport. Even in combat sports, with the exception of boxing, intentional injury is against the rules. Yet the sense of excitement is maintained. The quest for adventure is inherent in all activities. It is a need which sport satisfies for both participants and spectators alike.

In 1986 more that 46% of the adult population took part in at least one sporting activity reflecting an increase in 7% over the decade 1977–1986 (Fig. 1.1). Although many more men than women participate there is some evidence that the gap is closing marginally. Up to 1980 an increased trend in participation rather than spectating was observed (Figs 1.2, 1.3, 1.4, 1.5). The reasons were an awareness that regular exercise may be related to good health partly due to a direct effect but also because it engenders a healthy lifestyle. Living standards are improving generally and increasing leisure time means that sport has become accessible to more people. The 'Sport for All' concept has been widely accepted. Contests are now available for everyone from children to the elderly. More importantly perhaps it seems no longer necessary to be excellent at one's chosen sport, a fact which encourages the not so skilled 'athlete' to take part.

The popularity of sport is reflected in the number participating. In 1977, in England, almost 14 000 000 people took part in sport compared to well over 17 000 000 in 1986. Most of the increased participation was observed in women (an extra 1 900 000 compared to 1 500 000 men). These figures represent an 8% and 5.8% change in the rate of participation. Similar increases in the next decade would mean that almost one third of the population would take part in some sort of regular activity.

By 1986 more people were taking part in outdoor sports but for women participation in indoor sports had more than doubled compared to the number of men participating indicating that women seemed less attracted to outdoor sports.

In individual activities those associated with the promotion of a healthy lifestyle proved most popular. Walking regularly, indoor

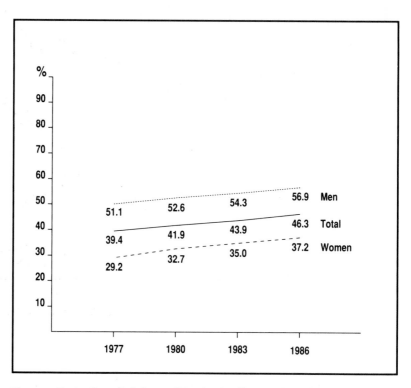

Fig. 1.1 Proportion of adults participating in all sport, Great Britain 1977–1986 (Reproduced by kind permission of the Sports Council)

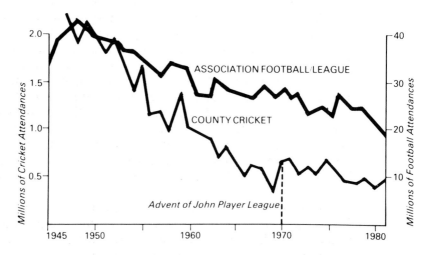

Fig. 1.2 Trends in spectator sport 1945–1981 (Reproduced by kind permission of the Sports Council)

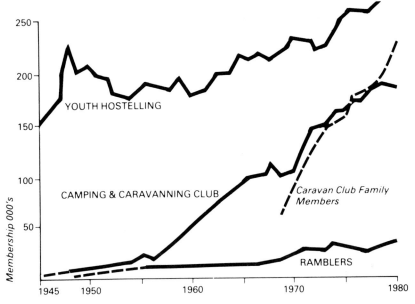

Fig. 1.3   Trends in informal recreation 1945–1980 (Reproduced by kind permission of the Sports Council)

swimming, cycling, gymnastics, jogging and indoor athletics were undertaken on average more than twice per week. Demand fell in camping and caravanning perhaps influenced by the lack of facilities available and inclement weather conditions.

Participation is also strongly influenced by age, social class and geographical region. Not surprisingly activity declined with age but the trends in all age groups were upwards compared to 1977. Social class influences still remain strong. Professional people have a threefold increase in sports activity compared to unskilled or manual workers (Fig. 1.6) and most sporting activity takes place in the South-East of England, perhaps reflecting the greater prosperity of that region in general compared to the rest of the country. There was also a greater gap in participation between the sexes in the North of England than in the South, perhaps a further aspect of the North–South divide (Sports Council 1990).

In parallel with its benefits, risks also exist in sport. If a logical decision is to be made regarding participation, people should be aware of the risks and gains involved in each activity. Because of a continuing experience of injuries sustained and risk situations involved, professional medical, paramedical and sports science

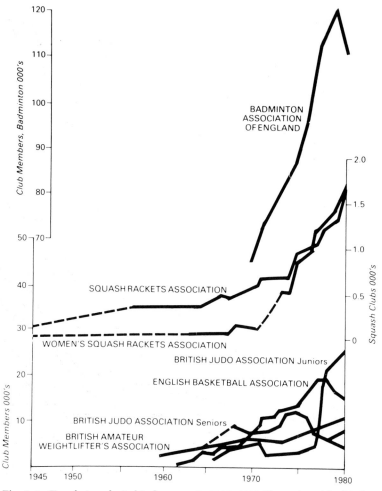

Fig. 1.4   Trends in selected indoor sports 1945–1980 (Reproduced by kind permission of the Sports Council)

bodies have increased in number, their aim being to educate and enlighten the public.

In essence, sports have evolved towards games without physical violence, for the satisfaction both of the competitor and of the spectator. The human requirement can therefore be examined on two levels: firstly the requirement of the participant and secondly that of the spectator.

The participant or competitor requires to prove him or herself. This not only takes the form of acquiring the necessary physical

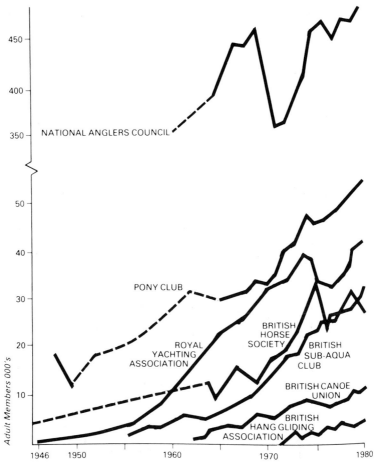

Fig. 1.5 Trends in selected outdoor sports 1946–1980 (Reproduced by kind permission of the Sports Council)

fitness and mental attitude but also allows him or her a break from the routine of everyday life and enables him or her to develop associations—a sense of belonging through being part of a club or society. The spectator has a similar experience with regard to social mingling and belonging, but in addition obtains satisfaction from watching. He can watch others attain levels to which he could not aspire. He can also be involved in violent activity without himself running the risk of injury. However, because many major spectator sports involve violence in some form, this is liable to extend to the spectators themselves. There is growing anxiety that violence is increasing both in sport and around sport. Could

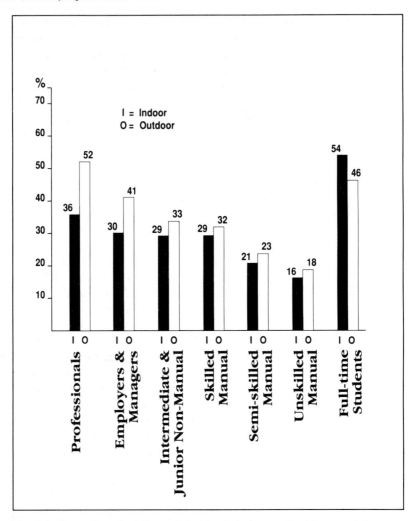

Fig. 1.6 Proportion of adults participating in indoor and outdoor sport, by socio-economic group, Great Britain, 1986 (Reproduced by kind permission of the Sports Council)

this be a reflection of the violent period in which we live, with the sports arena acting as a convenient battleground immune from the normal restraints of society?

CONSENT AND THE POSSIBILITY OF INJURY

In law, any person who is voluntarily involved in sports in which violence and the risk of injury are inherent is taken to be aware of this and thus, by participating, to give his or her implied consent to the possibility of injury. Therefore, someone who takes part in boxing consents to being punched, although such a gesture is not acceptable on the street, where it would constitute a criminal assault. For this reason, injuries sustained in a boxing ring, for example, are considered to be acceptable, if they occur within the rules and generally accepted standards of the sport, and legal remedies for civil damages or under the criminal law could not be sought.

Similarly, spectators consent to the risk of injury while observing. An example is motor sport, where a car could well career from the track during a race. This has indeed sometimes happened, but since consent to such risks is implicit in attendance at the race as a spectator, bystanders are barred from complaining about any injuries incurred, unless there has been some departure from recognized safety standards.[1]

This concept of implicit acceptance of the risk of injury is embodied in the legal maxim *volenti non fit injuria* ('no wrong is done to one who consents'). Such acceptance can only be assumed in connection with risks known to exist within the proper standards applicable to a given activity. Thus in rugby an accident may occur entirely within the rules of the game which gives rise to a serious injury without this resulting in either a criminal charge or an actionable civil wrong. However, a rugby player is not held to have consented to being punched, or kicked in the rucks, and an assault, i.e. a deliberate foul, may lead to civil remedies for any injury sustained, or even (in very serious and blatant cases) to a criminal prosecution.[2]

In any case, spectators, competitors and organizers of all sports meetings are held to owe duties to each other in law. In the context of criminal law either under common law or statute law (which might impose duties on organizers, e.g. in relation to safety standards of premises) the standard applied in determining if a crime exists is the same in a sporting incident as in any other field, although whether a prosecution occurs may depend on the prosecutor's view of the requirements of public policy. In the context of civil law a person's assumed consent to the risk of injury and exposure to normally unacceptable risks is *not* implied if there is a breach of the 'duty of care' which others must show and the test of whether there has been a breach is based on what is 'reasonably foreseeable'; that standard is objective and would be set against normal practice and current knowledge so is constantly changing as society and available knowledge changes.

DUTIES OF COMPETITORS
Duties toward other competitors

Competitors are duty bound to compete within the rules and not to resort to foul or reckless play. Adherence to this code both reduces the risk of injury and increases enjoyment of the game. The extent of competitor's consent, then, is only to action or injuries arising from the ordinary run of play within the rules, or from an associated accident. This does not include being injured as a result of foul play, which in theory amounts to a criminal or civil wrong, although the 'foul' would have to be one involving deliberate injury or completely reckless behaviour by one player towards the other, for the perpetrator to incur the risk of criminal prosecution, or to breach his 'duty of care' and be liable to a civil action for compensation if injuries result. Examples already exist.[3] Both rugby and football players in the United Kingdom have been criminally charged, and sued for damages following punches or other foul play. In the USA, ice-hockey players who have used their sticks or fists to attack others have similarly been found guilty of criminal assault. Golfers must have sensible regard for others, and indeed themselves—in a recent case, one Mr Feeney, with the single mindedness of the golfer who has hit a duff shot from one fairway on to another, crossed on to the adjacent fairway to look for and recover his ball and indeed play it, and while doing so he was struck by a ball driven by the more optimistically named Mr Lyle (but so far as is known not a relative of Sandy); the court, you might think quite sensibly held that Mr Feeney, who had not been visible, had no right of action against Mr Lyle, and it went on to say that, even if Mr Feeney had been visible, he would have been 25% to blame for any injury anyway, for having failed to check on the actions of golfers on the tee of the fairway before straying on to it.[4]

When considering prosecution of actions that might technically be criminal assaults, prosecutors will take account of the fact that the activity was a sporting activity and of the nature of the game and of its rules. Allowance might well be made for 'heat of the moment' impulsiveness, retaliation and self-defence. The 'scenario' is just as likely to make a prosecution more appropriate than less appropriate.[5] These are policy decisions, however, the question being whether it is in the public interest to prosecute; in marginal cases with no serious injury and little public profile, the decision might well be not to prosecute—but that has nothing to do with whether technically a crime has been committed. If a prosecution is taken these 'allowances' would have little relevance to a finding of guilt or otherwise, but they would come back into the reckoning after a finding of guilt in relation to sentence, and again in this regard, depending on the 'scenario' and indeed the view of the particular judge, this could make matters better for the accused, or worse. In the Johnson case (see note 2), the sentence was 6 months' imprisonment for biting an ear, which for a first offender in the context of a street brawl, would probably be seen as severe. On the other hand, a case was recently reported from the Sheriff Court in Kirkcudbright (equivalent more or less to the English County Court) where the judge found the accused guilty of a crime arising in the course of a football match but stated his view that these things should not result in court action and should be settled in the context of the game, and he admonished the accused.[6]

In the context of civil law suits, while the law from time to time may appear to change, it is more likely simply that the standards that apply to the test of 'foreseeability' constantly change. What might have been foreseeable in the light of knowledge of any particular speciality 20 years ago, may be totally different in the light of present day knowledge. This concept is very important. Every significant sporting activity now seems to have a very well organized controlling body and most of these spend considerable time and money on looking at every aspect of the chosen sport and in particular regulating the conduct of athletes and adequacy of equipment and increasing medical knowledge of the effects on the athlete of participation in particular sports. Unfortunately for the enthusiastic but badly informed organizer or instructor, or indeed medical adviser, his own particular knowledge would be largely irrelevant in any claim in the civil courts; what is relevant is the knowledge and information that is available and which he could have had. For the medical practitioner there is no such thing now as the 'nominal' or 'honorary' appointment. To a lesser extent the knowledge of these advances will be imputed to the competitor also.

A distinction has also to be drawn between the standards of proof required under the criminal and civil law respectively. In criminal law the standard is high, requiring proof of guilt of an alleged crime 'beyond reasonable doubt', with the benefit of any doubt in favour of the accused, whereas in civil law there is the less exacting standard of 'the balance of probabilities'.

The State is primarily responsible for criminal prosecutions. Under civil law, the costs of raising an action might well still deter an aggrieved party from raising a speculative action. But let the sportsman beware who deliberately assaults an unemployed, penniless opponent, who will therefore qualify for legal aid for a civil suit! While we are still a long way behind the USA, those in the medical profession will be only too aware of the new 'growth industry' in law, namely suits for civil damages.

THE LAW OF SELF-DEFENCE

The law of self-defence could rarely be directly applicable to a sporting incident and it proceeds upon different principles from the theory of 'consent'. Its basic principles provide guidelines with regard to the question of consent to injury in sport and also highlight the significance of this test of 'reasonableness'.

If a person is attacked or assaulted he may defend himself by force, but it must be roughly equivalent to the force employed against him. It must not be excessive, having regard to the danger (actual or honestly and reasonably believed to exist) to him and the nature of the attack. If excessive force is used in defence, it may in itself become an assault, even if the person against whom it is directed was the original aggressor. Of course, the 'heat of the moment' would be taken into account. Intent is also important. The defender may be deemed to have had the intention only of defending himself against the force which was applied to him or which he thought was being applied. Thus acquittals have resulted even when excessive defensive force has apparently been used. In one case, a person was attacked by an unarmed man at night. He defended himself using a knife and stabbed his attacker. In court he successfully claimed self-defence by saying that he believed he was being attacked with a knife and had therefore used what he thought was equivalent force.[7]

Violent actions performed in self-defence, in short, must be equivalent to the force used by the attacker and must stop when the attacker has been beaten or, has run off or, as might happen on a football or rugby pitch, has just stopped attacking. To strike an unconscious attacker repeatedly, no matter how vicious his attempted assault, may be regarded as a fresh assault.

Courts take mitigating circumstances into account. However, if a person had special combat-sport training and knowledge, less leeway might be allowed in assessing whether the amount of force used in self-defence was reasonable or excessive in the circumstances.

CATEGORIES OF INJURY

1. *Injury from an intended assault*. Here there is intent to produce injury and the attack is deliberate, e.g. a deliberate kick or punch directed at one player by another at football. Unless in self-defence this is a criminal assault, and the fact that it occurs in the course of a sporting activity is really irrelevant to the

question of whether a crime has been committed, or whether there is a case for civil wrong.

Evidence led will generally be eye witness evidence, or in the context of public sporting events, filmed evidence, but it could be the case that medical evidence about the injury itself from a forensic practitioner could assist a court.

2. *Injury from a negligent act.* In this category, there has been disregard for the safety of others and the action or inaction in question has resulted in injury to someone else, e.g. a rugby player recklessly driving into the ruck or raking with his boots. This sort of activity does not usually come within the sphere of criminal law. It is more relevant in the context of civil liability, and may give rise to an action for compensation for the injury.[8]

In criminal law an attacker is deemed to accept his victim as he is, weaknesses and all ('eggshell skull' theory). It is not a defence to claim the punch in question would not have injured a normal person. The risk of unexpected weaknesses in his victim lies with the assaulter. In civil law the condition of the victim is simply another strand of the foreseeability test.

Duties towards spectators

A competitor owes duties (moral or commercial) to his spectators to play within the rules and not to play in a manner which will mar their enjoyment or cause injury to them. However, injuries do happen, particularly in, for example, golf competitions and motor sport. Unless a ball was deliberately driven into the crowd or a car was deliberately driven off the track it is unlikely that a competitor would be held liable for any injuries which might ensue (but he and his employer could be if negligence is established[9]). Not so in Italy, however. When Lorenzo Bandini was involved in a collision with Jim Clark and then careered off the track, killing himself and four spectators, Clark was held to be legally liable and was unable to return to Italy for the rest of his life.

In any case, while a *participant* might not be responsible for injuries caused to spectators, the organizers could find themselves facing a civil suit, if the precautions taken by them fell short of acceptable standards.

Duties towards organizers

These are basically the same as the duties towards spectators. The game must be played properly and within the rules, so that the organizers' credit is not marred.

Conflicts between duties arise in the case of dirty play. Some

American ice-hockey players act violently on the rink. This attracts spectators and thus fulfils the requirements of the organizer. Both are satisfied but, in order to maintain the satisfaction, the violence (therefore spectator entertainment and organizers' cash revenue) must be repeated or increased. It is in these areas of increasing violence that legal intervention has occurred.

DUTIES OF SPECTATORS

Although most events are run with spectator enjoyment in mind, good behaviour on the part of the spectator, for his own and the competitors' safety, is expected. Football hooliganism, or pelting competitors or the referee with missiles, is unacceptable to all concerned and will constitute assault or some public order offence. Spectators owe duties to the organizers to follow rules laid down for their safety and the safety of participants, such as keeping clear of the track at a motor race or standing out of the firing line at a golf match. Spectators would be most unlikely to succeed in a civil claim against the organizers or participants if they had deliberately or stupidly ignored properly publicized and supervised safety precautions.

DUTIES OF ORGANIZERS

Organizers must ensure that an event is run within the rules, with all reasonable safety precautions being taken. In this respect, in particular, only competent and trained referees should be used.

When a major event takes place there may be considerable financial pressure on an organizer. This may cause him to overlook adequate safeguards in the interest of profit. As an example, the provision of cushioned floorings or qualified medical cover in some martial arts competitions has been ignored, with resultant unnecessary injuries or complications.

The organizers' duties toward spectators include efficient running of the event, suitable safe venues and, where appropriate, adequate marshalling. The Ibrox disaster in Glasgow, which caused 60 deaths in 1971, led to major changes in safety standards at football grounds throughout Britain. Inadequate marshalling at a golf match resulted in a spectator being struck on the head and an award for $265 000 being made against the organizers. A similar award has been given in a British court. Therefore, marshalls at events must be suitably trained and detailed rules on spectator control must be issued.[10]

The organizers' failure in some respect may give rise to what the court subsequently decides was a reasonably foreseeable injury to participants or spectators, and therefore actionable in law. Furthermore, the test is not subjective, but objective, so that the actual knowledge or awareness of the organizers is not relevant—what matters is what the reasonably competent organizer *of the specific activity involved* should have foreseen, as judged by the standard of the 'reasonable man'. Viewed with benefit of hindsight, the causal link between an act or omission and an injury which has in fact occurred can seem horribly 'foreseeable'.

The improved research into facilities and safety equipment, and indeed into the medical effects of participating in particular sports in the first place, can only be welcomed, so far as they make sports safer for all. However, unfortunately, as has been alluded to, the effect of all of this increased knowledge is that the standard of what is reasonable is lifted. Well meaning helpers in particular sports may find themselves at the wrong end of a court action if they are simply unaware of current medical and equipment requirements or of codes of practice set by governing bodies. Drugs in sport have now taken on a far higher profile than previously and any medical man involved in a sport would at the very least be expected to know the mechanism for seeking expert clearance for the use of what otherwise may be a medically acceptable drug. You can well imagine that if a finalist at Wimbledon was subsequently disqualified because he had been prescribed a particular drug for his hay fever by a practitioner knowing that he was a Wimbledon finalist, and that drug contained substances that caused the disqualification, the subsequent compensation claim would be irrefutable and vast. The Taylor Report following the Hillsborough disaster has led to the implementation of even more sweeping changes to try to prevent such an occurrence happening again; but just as importantly to ensure that precautions are taken to enable organizers to cope if such a disaster does occur. It probably now is the case that, be it for coping with the unexpected or for coping simply with risks that may be perceived to exist within a particular sport, organizers should have made arrangements to have suitably trained medical assistants readily available; 'suitably trained' may mean that a general medical practitioner is not good enough and that there should be specialist medical assistance available. For instance in Lord Taylor's recommendations following the Hillsborough disaster, he recommended not just that there should be medical practitioners in attendance, but that there should be medical practitioners specifically trained in first aid, which is something that many medical practitioners might not see as a specialist subject!

THE REQUIREMENTS OF PUBLIC ORDER

Some people consider that, at the moment, there is a general breakdown in society of the concept of the rule of law and a consequent increase in civil disorder or disobedience. They would see the principal manifestation of this in sport as being in football. The prime concern is to curb spectator violence and vandalism and the courts are taking a wide view of what constitutes a criminal offence. In Scotland the crime of 'breach of the peace' already covers a huge range of activities, but in a recent case, on appeal, conduct which the lower courts specifically considered 'inevitable' was nonetheless found to be a crime by the Appeal Court.[11] Two football teams, Morton and Celtic, were playing. Sadly, the two sets of supporters had to be separated by a 3 m wide gangway. A supporter was seen by two police officers to give a V-sign towards the opposition supporters and was heard to shout 'F . . . . . . w . . . . .s' or (as the case report rather tantalizingly records) 'words to that effect'. (Similarly, when approached by two police officers and warned, he replied 'I am doing f. . . all' 'or words to that effect'!) He was charged with committing a breach of the peace, which in Scotland is a 'breach of public order and decorum, to the alarm and annoyance of the public'. Usually in such cases 'the public' takes the tangible form of two policemen, who surprisingly enough seem particularly sensitive gentlemen continually alarmed and annoyed by bad language! In fact, actual alarm or annoyance is not now required to prove the offence, simply a reasonable belief that some mischief may result to the public peace. The judge in the lower court acquitted the accused, saying 'inevitably at a football match the crowd are singing and shouting and swearing, and making a great deal of noise. It is inevitable that spectators in one section will make rude gestures and hurl coarse insults at spectators in the other section.' The appeal judges clearly took a less resigned view of things and, in convicting the accused, decided that, inevitable though such conduct may be, acceptable to society it was not, but this probably just means it has become unacceptable to a society struggling with football hooliganism!

In the first edition of this book the remark was made that the effect on public order might increasingly become an important consideration in assessing the conduct not only of the spectators but also of players and organizers involved in any spectator sport, and it was noted that the Appeal Court's words would apply with equal force to provocative actions indulged in by participants and organizers, namely: 'It is the duty of the police to forestall the eruption of violence whenever possible. In the course of that duty

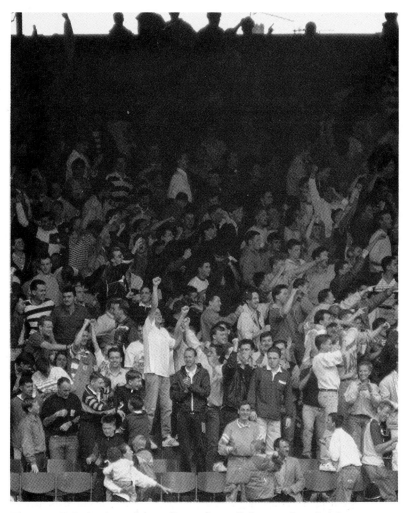

Fig. 1.7 'It is the duty of the police to forestall the eruption of violence whenever possible'—when disorder develops amongst spectators disaster can result (cf Hillsborough)

they have the power to terminate provocative conduct...by arrest, if that is necessary, before it leads to violence' Fig. 1.7. From that statement it would appear that the 'violence' need not necessarily be between those directly involved, so that the conduct of a participant or organizer could be considered to constitute a breach of the peace, if it might provoke a disturbance either on the field of play or, more pertinently, among the spectators.

Since the first edition of this book, the activities of Terry

Butcher, the then captain of Rangers, and Chris Woods, that team's goalkeeper, have rendered those remarks prophetic! Both players were found guilty of a breach of the peace for fairly violent actions which were against other players but which were over in an instant. The charge was not one of assault, but of breach of the peace and it is quite clear from the comments of the judge at the first instance, the Sheriff, and also from the comments of the Appeal Court Judges, that they were very much looking at this whole incident in the context of a football match between Rangers and Celtic specifically, which at the best of times creates intense rivalry and a degree of animosity, and what concerned the court was that the activities on the pitch might reasonably be expected to lead to spectators being alarmed or upset, or probably more specifically, resorting to violent behaviour of their own. Interestingly enough, in relation to Butcher, who was the captain of the team, the Sheriff at the first instance stated 'that these actings were unjustified by the rules of the game, his duties as captain, the heat of the contest in the course of a vigorous contact sport, or any other factors'.[12]

While these considerations apply particularly to the field of criminal law, as the law of negligence in civil law continues to develop it is certainly not impossible that a good case could be raised against, for example, a footballer by a person injured in some sort of crowd disturbance shown to have been sparked off by the conduct of the player on the field. This last hypothesis is purely conjecture at the moment, but it would be in line with the way the courts seem to be moving.

Summary

You have to look very long and hard, and probably in vain, to find legal principles and cases which are peculiar and unique to the field of sport so far as the law is concerned. The same, it is submitted, applies in relation to sports medicine and the law. Simply because previously (and still, to an extent) in the context of criminal law certain types of activity might have had a sort of 'immunity' from prosecution, it might have appeared as if the law was different from the general rule of law in these sporting contexts. Similarly in relation to civil law, because of this essential test of foreseeability as it relates to participants, and more particularly to organizers, it might previously have been thought that the law was somehow more lax and 'forgiving' in a sporting context, whereas truly if that ever was the case these results come from the way the tests were applied, the knowledge at the time, and even the attitude of judges.[13] The only safe course now, and indeed the only sensible course ever, is to accept that there is no difference in the eyes of the law. What is a crime out of the sporting arena is a crime within it. In any civil matter to which the standard of foreseeability is applied, it is going to be looked at quite objectively in the light of the mass of information and knowledge that can be available (even if it is not known to the particular defendant) and the fact that it is in the context of sporting activities, is largely irrelevant. Particularly with the recent emphasis and literature in relation to medical involvement in sporting activities, this brings, on the one hand, a new challenge for the medical practitioner, but on the other hand yet another pitfall in the field of medical negligence, and requires the medical practitioner who is involved with any sport, especially just at club level, to bring to that activity all of the skills and knowledge, not only that may be at his own individual disposal, but also those that are at the disposal of the profession generally.

In the United States of America many successful suits have been conducted against sportsmen and now in the UK legal actions for assault in rugby and football and resulting from poor organization in karate have been successful. When such cases are considered, the law takes into account the intentions of those involved, and slight excesses may be excused as being committed in the heat of the moment. 'Did he intend to commit injury?' 'Was he really going for the ball?' However, whether the action giving rise to the injury comes under the civil or the criminal law, it is no defence to say that only a slight injury was intended or should have resulted.

The footballer goes on the field to play football and to do his utmost (within the rules) so that his team may win. He does not go out so that an opponent may deliberately or recklessly foul him, breaking his leg. The perpetrator in this instance has failed in his duty to play within the rules and is therefore liable in law either criminally or civilly for the consequences of his actions.

And when the medical practitioner runs up to assist with his broken leg, being the official doctor of the club, the injured footballer has a right to expect that that doctor has not just put down his third pint of beer, has all the equipment available at his disposal to cope with this type of injury, and will know of any peculiarities that injuries obtained in this particular type of activity may bring. Spectators attend a golf or motor-racing event in the belief that all reasonable precautions for their safety have been taken, and they thereafter consent by implication to the residual risk of injury, provided it arises from some event which a reasonably competent organizer of such an event could not have foreseen. If a mishap does occur, particularly one that is well within the bounds of foreseeability, inherent in the risks of the sport, he will expect ready back-up support, including proper medical attention and equipment.

CONTROL OF CHEATING

The governing bodies of many sports are currently extremely anxious because of increasing violence in play. Rugby Union authorities have altered the rules of the game for safety reasons and have banned certain players from returning to the field. In the USA, where some spectator sports thrive on the element of violence involved, there are now an increasing number of cases brought for compensation by victims. Certain alternatives therefore present themselves regarding the cleaning-up of sports.

1. SELF-GOVERNMENT

Each governing body must take it upon itself to ensure adequate safety precautions and rules for its own particular sport. Where inherent dangers exist within a sport it is possible to alter the rules to reduce the risk. This precaution is reinforced by the immediate control exercised by the referee, umpires or marshals. Their decision must thereafter be backed up firmly by the respective governing body.

2. LEGISLATION

Governments tend to have neither the time nor the inclination to amend rules continually or to ensure their enforcement, so self-government is preferred as a method of ensuring that risks are kept to a minimum. Where self-government is seen to be inadequate, a government might have no other choice but to ban the sport or to take over its control itself.

3. BANNING

To ban a sport completely is probably an unacceptable method of controlling violence in sport. Banning may result in the activity being carried on illegally without any of the protection for competitors or provided by proper supervision or medical back-up. Thus, although the numbers participating will indeed fall, the chances of injury will in fact increase.

Guidelines for governing bodies

1. Particular attention should be paid to the creation, maintenance and regular updating of a full and definitive code of rules.
2. Referees and officials should be trained and properly qualified. Basic injury management should be part of the training.

3. All members should be registered. Some form of screening should exist so that 'bad eggs' can be excluded from participating in that particular sport.
4. Adequate facilities for coaching and premises for training should be available so that standards may be both maintained and increased. Such facilities should only be open in the correct circumstances and to the correct people.
5. Proper medical back-up should be available to cover all aspects of the particular sport.

It should be the aim of all responsible competitors and organizers to make sport safer. This will inevitably involve a change in the attitudes of the different parties concerned.

Spectators will require to realize that injury and violence are not desirable elements in sport and are on the contrary unnecessary and unacceptable. This would then relieve the competitor of pressure to commit fouls, especially if he himself is aware that strict refereeing control will ensure his future exclusion from the sport if he does so.

Prompt and well-organized medical supervision must be available in risk sports to increase the safety margin further when injuries do occur.

REFERENCE

Sports Council 1990 People in Sport fact sheet. The Sports Council, London.

NOTES

1. *White* v. *Blackmore* 1972 2QB651
2. *R* v. *Johnson* (1986) 8CAR (S) 343
3. See generally Halsbury's Laws of England volume 34 (1980); the laws of Scotland (*Stair Memorial Encyclopedia*) volume 19 (and the cases cited there); Grayson F 1990 Sports Medicine and the Law: *Medicine, Sport and the Law* (Ed) S. D. W. Payne. Blackwell Scientific, Oxford
4. *James Feeney* v. *Ian Lyle* 1991 S.L.T. 156
5. See *Butcher* v. *Jessop. Post hoc*; see note 12
6. *P.F.* v. *R. Kerr*, Kirkcudbright Sheriff Court 28 March 1991
7. *Owens* v. *HMA* 1946 JC119
8. *Condon* v. *Bassi* 1985 to ALL E.R. 453 C.A (£4900 awarded to football player whose leg was broken in a late tackle)
9. *Harrison* v. *Vincent* 1982 R.T.R. 8, C.A. An interest of this case is that liability arose from the failure of the organizers of a motor cycle event to follow an *international code of practice* by not keeping the first 100 metres of a slip road on a hairpin bend free from obstruction in that a recovery vehicle was parked protruding some 2 feet into it. The rider of a motor cycle with a side car found his brakes failed on a bend and the cycle left the track and the passenger was injured when he hit the recovery vehicle. The brakes failed because of an improperly fitted brake caliper. The passenger was able to sue (a) the rider of the cycle and his employers on the basis that they had been negligent in failing to inspect or install the

brake caliper properly, and (b) the organizers for their failure to keep the slip road free of obstruction. The Court held that, with regard to the brake failure, since this was a matter that would be attended to before the race in the relative calm of the workshop and not in the flurry and excitement of the sport, the normal standard of care applied although they further expressed the view that a modified standard might be applicable to acts done in the course of violent sport where only reckless disregard for safety or an actual intention to injure might constitute a breach of the duty of care. In relation to the organizers, the court said that they could not avail themselves of the defence of '*volenti non fit injuria*' because they could not show the passenger was aware of the presence of the recovery vehicle on the slip road—the organizers had a duty of care to take account of contingences which a 'carefree competitor' might ignore.

10. *Horne and Marlow* v. *RAC Motor Sports Association* Daily Telegraph 19 June 1989. (The RAC were held responsible for Stewards who were acting conscientiously enough but had failed to move spectators away from a dangerous part of a rally course).
11. *Wilson* v. *Brown* 1982 SLT (361)
12. *Butcher* v. *Jessop* 1989 SLT 593
    Footnote: Many Scottish Sheriffs are not at all out of touch with the world they live in but have a wonderfully dead pan way of understating the facts in written reports which may make them sound somewhat unworldly. For those who know an 'Old Firm' game at first hand, it may be worth quoting the Sheriff's notes, forming part of the Appeal that went to the High Court—these notes are for the benefit of the High Court Appeal Judges:
    Rangers and Celtic are regarded by the greater part of the Scottish Football public as representing respectively the Protestant and Catholic sects of the Christian religion. There is intense rivalry between the supporters of each team which includes an element of sectarian animosity. Games between them are usually marked by considerable excitement and tension on the part of the spectators with displays of animosity between the rival segregated fans. Even before the teams emerge there is usually a great deal of shouting back and forth between rival groups of spectators. Events preceding this match followed the pattern indicated. The fans were singing, shouting and gesticulating and a few of them were making various obscene gestures with one or two fingers across the pitch—directed presumably at the opposing fans. In addition, the majority of them seemed to be accompanying their shouts and songs by pointing in unison with their index finger in a gesture, the meaning of which was not at all clear. Etcetera! Etcetera!
13. 'Her Majesty's Judges are not weaklings. They like a manly sport as well as the next fellow … British Judges have traditionally not only played the game in court, but on the sporting field as well with the result they have evolved a law of sport that is fair, gentlemanly—and tough. In fact the quintessence of Englishness: old time style'.—Fenton Bresler *You and the Law* (Punch Publications 1975) page 58.

2. Sport and exercise in the prevention and treatment of disease

INTRODUCTION

Regular exercise is beneficial to health. This has been the policy statement endorsed by successive governments and the Sports Council. As well as creating a feeling of healthy self-awareness and improved lifestyle, a reduction in harmful habits like smoking or drinking excessive amounts of alcohol could be expected in those who exercise. Such habit changes alone would prevent premature death in many. However, there is now more positive evidence that exercise has a direct influence in maintaining health in all age groups.

Physical inactivity, at any age, reduces the individual's capacity for physical exertion. Those who are chronically inactive tolerate exercise badly and become increasingly more easily fatigued. Aside from physical incapacity people who have periods of prolonged inactivity develop physiological changes—the skeletal muscles become weaker and there is reduced bone density. When such people do undertake physical activity their anaerobic capacity is extremely limited and their energy sources are exhausted within minutes. This incapacity has been graphically demonstrated in volunteer treadmill studies when walking uphill at about 3 mph involved severe exertion for average unfit men over 35 years of age (Welsh Heart Programme Directorate 1987). This incapacity increases with age. Inactive people become progressively dependent on anaerobic conversion of glucose to lactate to generate ATP and correspondingly are more prone to fatigue upon exercising. This process can be reversed by regular aerobic activity.

At any age physical activity has dramatic effects on body function. These result in an increased cardiac stroke volume and a slowing of the pulse rate. This is called the 'training effect'. Both the vascular bed and the mitochondrial enzyme content of muscle also increase. Such trained muscle is more biochemically efficient and can utilize more lipids and less glycogen (glycogen sparing effect). This is a possible reason for the reduction in high density lipoproteins (HDL) associated with exercise. The muscle adapts by increased strength and size and by being able to extract more oxygen from the blood—changes which reduce fatigue and discomfort because less lactic acid is generated.

These effects can be demonstrated after 8–10 weeks of regular rhythmic exercise like brisk walking, cycling, running or swimming.

The clinical implications of these lifestyle changes may be more closely examined in relation to cardiovascular, metabolic, respiratory disorders and disability. Exercise is also valuable in the assessment of disease, in maintaining psychological wellbeing, in childhood and in old age.

EXERCISE IN THE ASSESSMENT OF DISEASE

In clinical practice, exercise tolerance is a valuable standard by which the effects of therapeutic agents and physical rehabilitation can be assessed. It is frequently used to assess the response to therapy in post-exertional bronchoconstriction (Phillips et al 1981). More recently, an accurate prediction of the presence and extent of coronary artery disease in patients with angina pectoris has been demonstrated (Elamin et al 1982). In this exercise test, performed on a bicycle ergometer at 60r/min against a series of incremental loads, changes in the rate of progression of ST segment depression relative to heart rate increase (ST/HR slope) was shown to be an accurate index of myocardial ischaemia, correlating well with angiographic findings. This test may therefore obviate the necessity for coronary angiography in all except those patients in whom surgery would be contemplated.

Postexertional hypotension is also an important physical sign in patients on adrenergic neurone blocking drugs, and careful measurement of erect blood pressure before and after exercise is of value in assessing patients with suspected hypovolaemia or neurodepressant drug effects (Hoffbrand 1982).

In lower limb ischaemia, exercise testing is used as part of the standard investigation of peripheral vascular disease (Laing & Greenhalgh 1980). The severity of claudication, the walking distance to onset of pain, response to stopping cigarettes and further exercises are all important in deciding whether further investigations such as arteriography are necessary.

In elderly patients, and those recovering from stroke or rheumatic disease, even the ability to lift a kettle or cup and to perform simple tasks may be the yardstick, all else being equal, between social independence and long-term care. Improved motor ability, albeit limited, also indicates a successful response to rehabilitation therapy.

CARDIOVASCULAR DISEASE

Prevention

Exercise may have a positive role in the prevention of cardio-vascular disease. Changes in blood lipids, especially an increase in HDL cholesterol from the endothelial surfaces of blood vessels and the exercise associated reduction in arterial blood pressure may prevent the development of atheroma. Furthermore, glucose tolerance is improved and fibrinolysis increased, both of which contribute to the prevention of peripheral vascular disease (Holloszy et al 1986). These hypotheses have been supported epidemiologically in groups of healthy men and women who were overweight (Wood et al 1988, Hardman et al 1989). In both studies it was observed that a combination of diet and regular exercise, in the form of jogging up to 20 km per week or brisk walking three times per week but covering about the same distance, led to weight loss and changes in the blood lipid profile with increase in the HDL fraction reflecting increased lipoprotein lipose activity and more efficient lipid transport. There were no observed changes in the LDL cholesterol level.

Exercise and hypertension

Regular exercise has been observed to produce a significant fall in blood pressure in those who are mildly hypertensive. Boyer and Kasch (1970) noted a fall of 13/12 mmHg in a group of exercised hypertensive men compared to a 0/6 mmHg fall in normotensive controls. Fitzgerald (1981) further suggested that the fall noted was maintained for 4–6 hours afterwards.

These anecdotal observations have been substantiated by Wilcox et al (1982). In a controlled study of men with uncomplicated essential hypertension (mean standing blood pressure 165/109 mmHg) treadmill exercise was performed until heart rates of 120 beats/minute were obtained and maintained for 5–10 minutes separated by 3 minutes' rest. During exercise the blood pressure rose slightly (175 mmHg systolic) but dropped by approximately 25% afterwards. The fall was maintained for up to 10 hours. These results imply that a 'good walk' twice a day might be a reasonable treatment for mild hypertension. This response among mild to moderate hypertensives (148/99 mmHg baseline) has also been observed from brisk exercise (70% maximum) taken for 45 minutes three times per week. When exercise of this nature was taken on a daily basis the reduction in blood pressure was greater (Nelson et al 1986).

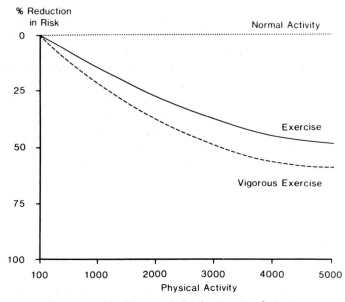

Fig. 2.1 Reduction in risk of myocardial infarction in relation to energy expended per week (kcal). Exercise = submaximal regular exercise; vigorous exercise = regular high-energy output with frequent bursts of peak exertion

Exercise and coronary heart disease

Since Morris et al (1953) published their work on London transport workers and noted a significantly lower incidence of both coronary heart disease and fatal myocardial infarction in bus conductors compared to bus drivers, many others have reached similar conclusions relating to vigorous exercise (Fig. 2.1). Morris et al (1973, 1980) extended their work in civil servants. Of the 18 000 studies they noted that active leisure time pursuits in males were associated with half the incidence of coronary heart disease of their non-active male colleagues. The effects were independent of other risk factors such as obesity, body habits, smoking and hypertension. In other parts of the world similar conclusions have been reached (Zukel et al 1959, Brunner et al 1974, Dawber 1980, Salonen et al 1982).

The confirmed benefits are unfortunately short-lived. Fitness in youth and young adulthood does not protect against coronary heart disease in later life. In fact, American College athletes who stopped exercising after graduation were at greater risk from coronary artery disease than their non-trained colleagues (Paffenburger & Hyde 1983). It has also been suggested that a minimum amount of physical activity may be required to produce a protective effect: an energy expenditure of around 2000 kcal per week, equivalent to about five hours' brisk walking or three and a half hours jogging (Paffenburger et al 1986). This observation has been further supported by work in middle-aged office workers (Morris et al 1990) where the protective effect of exercise was observed only in those taking vigorous aerobic exercise at least twice a week. Recreational activities (e.g. gardening, sawing etc.) appeared to confer no protection unless performed vigorously and very regularly. These findings imply that if exercise is to maintain its beneficial effects it must become habitual and be performed at specific levels.

Post infarction rehabilitation

Most patients who suffer an uncomplicated myocardial infarction are discharged from hospital within a few days. They are encouraged to mobilize early and may also benefit from a post-infarction exercise programme. There is some evidence that this may prevent reinfarction and accelerate the return to work (May et al 1982). The same observations apply to patients who have had coronary artery bypass surgery (CABG).

Exercise and peripheral vascular disease

Peripheral vascular disease is the commonest reason for lower-limb amputation in Britain. Of 5540 amputees who attended artificial limb and appliance centres in England and Wales in 1978, 3514 had amputations because of peripheral vascular disease. The 1977 report from the Royal College of Physicians *Smoking and Health* stated that over 95% of patients with arterial disease of the legs were reported to be smokers and that those who continued to smoke were much more likely to develop gangrene of the leg and suffer subsequent amputation than those who stopped. The number of amputations rises each year. Other symptoms of peripheral vascular disease such as crippling claudication can be reversed to some extent by giving up tobacco and performing regular exercise in the form of walking. Most patients can double their walking distance within 2–3 months of beginning exercise. The mortality rate amongst such patients is also considerably lower than those who have bypass surgery (Lundgren et al 1989).

The mechanism by which the improvement is achieved is uncertain but the long-term results over 4–6 years were good. The most striking change is an increase in oxidative enzymes in the trained muscles similar to that seen in physically-trained normal individuals as an adaptation to hypoxia. Blood flow is not mark-edly increased and the effects of such therapy are reversed by bypass surgery.

EXERCISE AND METABOLIC DISEASE
Diabetes Mellitus

Physical training increases insulin sensitivity and has been shown to have a beneficial effect on the control of the blood glucose level in maturity onset diabetes (Type III) (Trovati et al 1984). In juvenile onset diabetes the effect of exercise is less clear but anec-dotal observations imply that less insulin may be required to maintain control.

The main risks are exercise-induced hypoglycaemia or hyper-glycaemia and ketosis in diabetic patients. Patients who wish to exercise should therefore be warned not to do so when their in-sulin injection is about to have its greatest effect and also about the risk of post-exercise hypoglycaemia. Appropriate carbohydrate intake before exercise will reduce such risks and considerable individual experimentation will be required. Nevertheless, many diabetics have successful sporting careers and some have become top athletes.

Obesity

Body weight control is best effected by a combination of diet and exercise. Newsholme (1983) has suggested that regular training increases the sensitivity of substrate cycles, responsible for meta-bolic regulation, to circulating adrenaline and noradrenaline thereby increasing energy expenditure and influencing bodyweight. However, in attempting to control obesity by diet and exercise it has been observed that the capacity for exercise tends to fall off spontaneously. Nevertheless, weight loss is increased in the long term when regular aerobic exercise is added to a weight reducing diet. These observations have been confirmed in obese adult females who undertook brisk walking 5 days per week for up to 50 minutes per day and in obese children and adolescents who undertook a regime of dietary restriction and bicycle riding. In all cases greater weight loss was achieved than in control groups (Hill et al 1989, Reybrouck et al 1990).

EXERCISE IN THE PREVENTION AND MANAGEMENT OF OSTEOPOROSIS

It has been shown that weightlifters, cross country runners and ballet dancers all have a higher than average bone mass. With ageing, particularly in women, the risk of osteoporosis and fracture, especially of the femoral neck, is increased. Regular exercise will increase the bone mineral content (BMC) in both men and women. In one group of women over 80 who undertook a 30-minute per day exercise schedule three times a week an increase in BMC of 4.4% as against a loss of 2% in non-exercised controls was observed after 36 months (Nagent 1983). There is a strong case for both pre- and post-menopausal women undertaking regular exercise, which ideally should be antigravitational, to prevent osteoporosis. Mechanical stress is important, in both men and women, in maintaining bone mass (paradoxically obesity provides this in non-exercising individuals!) and moderate exercise appears to stimulate osteogenesis (Stevenson et al 1989).

EXERCISE IN THE MANAGEMENT OF OBSTRUCTIVE AIRWAYS DISEASE

In both asthmatic and bronchitic patients exercise regimes have been shown to improve performance due to a combination of increased tolerance of physical activity and improved lung function (Ries & Moser 1986).

Exercise-induced asthma can affect up to 90% of children with asthma as well as a proportion of non-asthmatics. A minority of elite performers also suffer from the condition which may be related to a thermal effect on mast cells particularly associated with airway cooling. With careful training, especially swimming, and the use of prophylactic inhalers before exercise, improved physical performance with less exercise induced obstruction will occur (Bundgaard 1985). Even in patients with severe chronic obstructive airways disease exercise combined with appropriate drug therapy (ephedrine containing compounds and corticosteroids are not permitted in sport) and not smoking, marked improvements in physical performance have been observed (Grimby 1983).

EXERCISE AFTER SCHOOL

Many people stop taking part in regular exercise after they leave school, university, the Forces, etc. At these institutions exercise is organized and often compulsory. Other factors, such as beginning to earn a living, getting married or the arrival of a baby, take up time and lead to a decrease in organized exercise. As age progresses the habit persists. In elderly people society accepts stiffness, weakness, and slowness as part of the ageing process. We tend to allow our elders to lose their independence by discouraging their physical activity. It may be quicker for us to do their

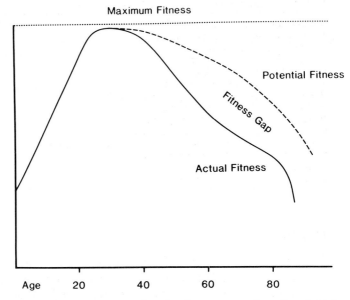

Fig. 2.2   The fitness gap (Reproduced with permission from Gray J A M 1982 British Medical Journal 285: 545–547)

and our own shopping than to do it together. The elderly are not only old but generally tend to be very unfit.

This decrease in exercise as age progresses or after major life events leads to the concept of the 'fitness gap' (Fig. 2.2). All four physical aspects of fitness—strength, stamina, suppleness and skill—can be improved at any age. These are coupled to psychological benefits, increased physical performance and better quality of life.

EXERCISE AND PSYCHOLOGICAL WELLBEING

People who exercise regularly appear to suffer less from depression or tension than those who do not. In fact, mildly anxious or depressed people may note a marked change in mood after an exercise regimen which is now increasingly being incorporated into psychotherapy (Martinson 1990). The effect seems to mediate through beta-endorphin, beta-lipoprotein activity or increased central production of monoamines (Chauloff 1989) some or all of which may contribute to the phenomenon of 'Runner's High'.

Table 2.1 Impact of exercise on health (McLatchie 1990)

- Control of mild hypertension
- Reduction of body mass due to:
  —appetite suppression
  —healthy dietary practice
- Alteration in lipid profile
- Favourable effects on pregnancy
- Prevention and alleviation of low back pain
- Reduction in cigarette smoking
- Reduction in alcohol consumption
- Reduction in anxiety; elevation in mood
- Improved self-image; reduction in antisocial behaviour
- Reduction of promiscuous behaviour
- Improved corporate image
- Improved work attendance and production

CONCLUSION

There are many beneficial effects of exercise on health (Table 2.1). Perhaps the most significant of these is the change in self-image and subsequent lifestyle which is induced by regular activity especially in groups. This has been effectively demonstrated in studies of cigarette smoking in people who take regular exercise. For example, in a study of young boxers all from social classes 4 and 5, only 1.7% smoked cigarettes compared to 42% of their peers (McLatchie 1986). The smoking habits of professional football players (less than 5% smoke cigarettes) also appear to be related to divisional status and imply that social class and cultural mores can be broken (Hutchinson et al 1986). Furthermore such groups could effectively be used in anti-smoking campaigns because of the enormous influence they can exert on their fans. Reducing the incidence of cigarette smoking would radically alter the pattern of disease in the Western World.

The benefits of exercise have also been demonstrated by work-site fitness programmes which, in Japan and the USA, lead to increased quality and quantity of production, the recruitment of premium employees and an improved corporate image (Shepherd 1988).

REFERENCES

Berger M 1983 Exercise in the prevention and management of diabetes mellitus. Exercise Health Medicine (Abstracts)

Boyer J L, Kasch F W 1970 Exercise therapy in hypertensive men. Journal of the American Medical Association 211: 1668–1671

Brunner D, Manelis G, Modan M, Levin S 1974 Physical activity at work and the incidence of myocardial infarction, angina pectoris and death due to ischemic heart disease: an epidemiological study in Israeli collective settlements (*kibbutzim*). Journal of Chronic Disease 27: 217–233

Bundgaard A 1985 Exercise in the asthmatic. Sports Medicine 2: 254–266

Chauloff A 1989 Physical exercise and brain monoamines: a review. Acta Physiologica Scandinavica 137: 1–13.

Dawber T R 1980 The Framingham study. The epidemiology of atherosclerotic disease. Harvard University Press, Cambridge, Mass. ch 10, pp 157–171

Ekroth R, Dahllof A G, Gundewall B, Holm J, Schersten T 1978 Physical training of patients with intermittent claudication: indications, methods and results. Surgery 84: 640

Elamin M S, Boyle R, Kardash M M, Smith D R, Stoker J B, Whitaker W, Mary D A S G, Linden R J 1982 Accurate detection of coronary heart disease by new exercise test. British Heart Journal 48: 311–320

Fitzgerald W 1981 Labile hypertension and jogging: new diagnostic tool or spurious discovery? British Medical Journal 282: 542–544

Grimby G 1983 Exercise and physical training in the rehabilitation of patients with respiratory impairment. Exercise Health Medicine (Abstracts)

Hardman A E, Hudson A, Jones P R M, Norgan N G 1989 Brisk walking and plasma high density lipo protein (HDL) cholesterol in previously sedentary women. British Medical Journal 299: 1204–1205

Hill J O, Schlundt D G, Strocco T, Sharp T, Pope Cirdle J 1989 Evaluation of an alternating calorie diet with and without exercise in the treatment of obesity. American Journal of Clinical Nutrition 50: 248–254

Hoffbrand B I 1982 Post exertional hypotension: a valuable physical sign. British Medical Journal 285: 1242

Holloszy J O, Schultz J, Kusnierkiewicz J, Hagberg J M, Ehsani A A 1986 Effects of exercise on glucose tolerance and insulin resistance. Acta Medica Scandinavica (Suppl) 711: 55–65

Hutchinson D R, Mountain N J, McLatchie G R 1986 Smoking habits in professional football. British Journal of Sports Medicine 20: 113–114

Kramsch D M, Aspen A, Abramowitz B, Kreimandahl T, Hood W B 1981 Reduction of coronary atherosclerosis by moderate conditioning exercise in monkeys on an atherogenic diet. New England Journal of Medicine 305: 1493

Laing S P, Greenhalgh R M 1980 Standard exercise test to assess peripheral arterial disease. British Medical Journal i: 13–15

Lundgren F, Dahllof A G, Lundholm K, Schersten T, Volkmann R 1989 Intermittent claudication—surgical reconstruction or physical training? A prospective randomised trial of treatment efficiency Annals of Surgery 209: 346–395

McLatchie G R 1986 The 'hard-man' image of the non smoker. XXIII FIMS World Congress of Sports Medicine, Brisbane, Australia

McLatchie G R 1990 A team approach central to management. In: Soft tissue injury—A Team Approach. Medical Action Communications, Surrey, UK

Martinson E W 1990 Physical fitness, anxiety and depression. British Journal of Hospital Medicine 43: 194–199

May G S, Eberlien K A, Furberg C D, Passamani E R, Demets D L 1982 Secondary prevention after myocardial infarction: a review of long term trials. Progress in Cardiovascular Diseases 24: 331–352

Morgan W P 1980 The psychological effects of exercise. Research Quarterly for Exercise and Sport 51: 50

Morris J N, Heady J A, Raffle P A B, Roberts C G, Parks J W 1953 Coronary heart disease and physical activity of work. Lancet ii: 1053–1057

Morris J N, Chowe S P W, Adam C, Sirey C, Epstein L, Sheehan D J 1973 Vigorous exercise in leisure time and the incidence of coronary heart disease. Lancet ii: 333–339

Morris J N, Everitt M G, Pollard R, Chowe S P W, Semmence A M 1980 Vigorous exercise in leisure time: protection against coronary heart disease. Lancet ii: 1207–1210

Nagent de Deuxchaisnes C 1983 Exercise in the prevention and management of osteoporosis. Exercise Health Medicine (Abstracts)

Nelson L, Ester M D, Jennings G L, Korner P 1986 Effect of changing levels of physical activity on blood pressure and haemodynamics in essential hypertension. Lancet ii: 473–479

Newsholme E A 1983 Exercise in the prevention and treatment of obesity. Exercise Health Medicine (Abstracts)

Paffenburger R S Jr, Hyde R T 1983 Epidemiology of exercise and coronary heart disease. Exercise Health Medicine (Abstracts)

Paffenburger R S, Hyde R T, Wing A L, Hsich C C 1986 Physical activity: all causes mortality and longevity of college alumni. New England Journal of Medicine 314: 605–613

Phillips M J, Ollier S, Tremlath S W, Bootis S W, Davies R J 1981 The effect of sustained release aminophylline on exercise induced asthma. British Journal of Diseases of the Chest 75: 181–189

Reybrouck T, Vinckx J, Van den Berghe G, Vanderschueren-Lodeweyckx M 1990 Exercise therapy and hypocaloric diet in the treatment of obese children and adolescents. Acta Paediatrica Scandinavica 79: 84–89

Ries A L, Moser K M 1986 Comparison of isocapmic hyperventilation and walking exercise training at home in pulmonary rehabilitation. Chest 90: 285–289

Salonen J T, Puska P, Tuomilehto J 1982 Physical activity and risk of myocardial infarction, cerebral stroke and death: a longitudinal study in Eastern Finland. American Journal of Epidemiology 115: 526–537

Shepherd R J 1988 Exercise and lifestyle change. British Journal of Sports Medicine 23: 11–22

Stevenson J C, Lees B, Davenport M, Cust M P, Granger K F 1989 Determinants of bone density in normal women: risk factors for future osteoporosis. British Medical Journal 298: 924–928

Trovati M, Carta Q, Cavalot F, Vitali S, Banardi C, Lucchina P, Fiocchi F, Emanuelli G, Lenti G 1984 Influence of physical training on blood glucose control, glucose tolerance, insulin secretion and insulin action in non-insulin dependent diabetic patients. Diabetics Care 7: 416–420

Welsh Heart Programme Directorate 1987 Exercise for health: health related fitness in Wales. Heartbeat Report 23

Wilcox R G, Bennett T, Brown A M, MacDonald I A 1982 Is exercise good for high blood pressure? British Medical Journal 285: 767–769

Wood P D, Stefamick M L, Dreon D M 1988 Changes in plasma lipids and lipoproteins in overweight men during weight loss through dieting as compared with exercise. New England Journal of Medicine 319: 1173–1179

Zukel W J, Lewis R H, Enterling P E, Painter R C, Ralston L S, Fawcett R M, Meredith A P, Peterson B 1959 A short term community study of the epidemiology of coronary heart disease: a preliminary report on the North Dakota study. American Journal of Public Health 49: 1630–1639

3. Organization and teaching of sports medicine

INTRODUCTION

Sports medicine has been defined as a discipline which includes theoretical and practical branches of the relevant basic sciences and medicine which investigate, document and measure the influence of lifestyle, exercise, training and sport—or lack of these—on both healthy and physically or psychologically ill or handicapped people in order to produce useful results for the prevention of disease or injury, treatment, rehabilitation and improvement in the education, health and overall performance of the individual and society at large (Royal Scottish Medical Colleges 1991).

In the years since the first edition (1986) there has been increasing interest in the concept and speciality of sports medicine not only as a branch of primary care and preventive medicine but also as an intensely practical 'on the field' speciality which involves the use of core skills, advanced life support systems and the transport of the seriously injured from the sporting venue (rugby field, mountainside) to centres of secondary care.

In developing sports medicine close liaison with multidisciplinary groups like sports science, coaching, physiology of training, body movement, psychology, biomechanics and bioengineering will be necessary. Parallels can be drawn with other branches of medicine where, for instance in orthopaedic surgery, prosthetic joints were developed from the collaborative efforts of different disciplines and strong associations are currently being developed between clinical sports medicine and the sports and exercise sciences.

The development of academic departments of sports medicine has yet to follow. However, many general practitioners are developing a special interest in the subject and the provision of sports medicine clinics throughout the UK has steadily increased over the last few years.

WHO DOES SPORTS MEDICINE?

For every patient with a sports-related injury or problem seen by a doctor a further nine will probably have had initial treatment from their coach or trainer, parents or teachers. Their advice, although well intentioned, may originate from an empirical base and could result in exacerbation of an acute injury, e.g. 'running through the pain' or lead to a chronic problem: 'My knee keeps giving way'. In certain situations, for instance, return to the field of play may be positively contraindicated. Therefore, those who officiate at sporting events should make an attempt to acquire a basic knowledge of the risks and gains of sport. This would involve factors like learning to recognize dangerous situations, when an injury has occurred, what to do safely and when to call for professional help. These aims could be achieved by an association, clinically and academically active, which endorses a public health education programme, based on the practical experience of injury management and prevention. The information could be passed to sports participants, coaches, school teachers and referees possibly through the official bodies which promote first aid.

The paramedic system in the USA is a further example of what can be achieved by concentrating on the development of specific life-saving skills. The educational material should, in addition, cover details of rehabilitation (what exercises and activities are safe after injury and when) and return to training. When injuries are successfully prevented or managed, standards are improved without spoiling the enjoyment of the pastime (McLatchie & Morris 1977).

TRAINING IN SPORTS MEDICINE

Although there is no formal structure for training in sports medicine within the National Health Service, interested clinicians should acquire a sound knowledge of accident and emergency medicine. It is in this branch of hospital practice that most sports injuries will be seen. In addition, knowledge of orthopaedics, exercise physiology and principles of physical training should be acquired. Probably the most important factor, however, is involvement with a sports team as its medical officer. This immediately confers responsibility for the care of athletes on the doctor and provides the stimulus to acquire knowledge on problems such as acclimatization, fitness testing, drug abuse and international travel. Physiological problems experienced by sportsmen or women can also be approached at first hand.

There are now several training courses open to doctors leading to diplomas or higher degrees (MSc, PhD). Possibly the most significant of these is the Diploma in Sports Medicine of the Royal Medical Colleges of Scotland. In an historic move in 1990 the three Royal Colleges agreed that standards should be set for doctors practising sports medicine so that the public could recognize

LIBRARY
COLBY-SAWYER COLLEGE
NEW LONDON, NH 03257

suitably qualified practitioners. The regulations and syllabus are as follows (RCP (Ed), RCS (Ed), RCPS (Glas) 1990) and there are three diets of the examination each year.

1. Candidates for the Diploma in Sports Medicine must possess a qualification registrable with the General Medical Council. Candidates from the European Community who are not registered with the GMC may also be admitted to the Examination by approval of the Board provided they have complied with all other requirements of the Regulations.
2. Candidates for the Diploma in Sports Medicine must have been engaged in the study of their profession for not less than two years after obtaining full registration.
3. Candidates are required to provide evidence of active participation in sports medicine. The examinations for the Diploma in Sports Medicine will normally be held three times each year unless otherwise stated. The dates of the examinations and fees payable for admission are available from the Royal College of Physicians of Edinburgh, the Royal College of Surgeons of Edinburgh and the Royal College of Physicians and Surgeons of Glasgow. The closing date for entry will be 6 weeks before the date of the examination. The dates of examinations and the fees payable for admission to the examination for the Diploma of Sports Medicine are set out in the examinations calendar which is available from the Royal College of Physicians of Edinburgh, the Royal College of Surgeons of Edinburgh and the Royal College of Physicians and Surgeons of Glasgow.
4. The Board may refuse to admit to an examination or proceed with the examination of any candidate who infringes any of the regulations or is considered by the examiners to be guilty of behaviour prejudicial to the proper management and conduct of the examination.
5. The examination will be as follows:
   (a) A multiple choice paper of 2 hours' duration;
   (b) A theoretical paper (short answer questions) of 1 hour;
   (c) A practical examination in three parts each of 20 minutes' duration as follows:
      (i)   Test of core skills (including cardiopulmonary resuscitation)
      (ii) Clinical examination (especially of the musculoskeletal system)
      (iii) Scenario tests to assess response and first aid;
   (d) An oral examination of 20 minutes' duration to cover the syllabus.
6. A candidate who passes the examination shall receive the Dip-

LIBRARY
COLBY-SAWYER COLLEGE
NEW LONDON, NH 03257

loma in Sports Medicine of the Royal College of Physicians of Edinburgh, the Royal College of Surgeons of Edinburgh and the Royal College of Physicians and Surgeons of Glasgow and shall receive a diploma bearing the seals of the said Royal Colleges.

SYLLABUS

This syllabus is intended to act as a guide to candidates proposing to present themselves for examination for the Diploma in Sports Medicine.

1. The relevant applied anatomy and biomechanics of the limb bones, joints, muscles, tendons and nerves; also the relevant anatomy of the spine and spinal cord, the skull and brain, the thoracic cage and its contents, the abdomen and pelvis and the cardiovascular system.
2. The physiology of exercise in relation to the muscles, the heart and circulation, the lungs, the blood and the endocrine glands; the effect of exercise on bone and joints; thermo-regulation.
3. Nutrition and diet including fluid and electrolyte balance.
4. The psychological aspects of sports medicine including re-lationships with other athletes, the coach and the doctor.
5. The effect of environmental conditions, including heat, cold, hyperbaric pressure, altitude and travel.
6. The female athlete: gender assessment, gynaecological aspects and osteoporosis.
7. Child and adolescent athlete: the relevant anatomy of the musculoskeletal system and growth; abnormal growth pat-terns; effects of exercise.
8. The application of the knowledge of anatomy and physiology in training methods; the assessment of all modalities of fitness.
9. The effect of exercise in particular groups: the elderly; the physically handicapped; those with chronic medical con-ditions, asthma and other respiratory disorders, diabetes mel-litus, renal disease and transplantation, cardiovascular disease; mental handicap and psychiatric illness.
10. Sports injuries:
    —Epidemiology and causes in relation to different sports.
    —Over-use injuries and injuries from trauma, their diagnosis, first aid, investigation, treatment and rehabilitation.
    —Head, neck and eye injuries—eye safety.
    —The prevention of injuries; sports equipment.
    —The role of physiotherapy and the physiotherapist to include a knowledge of techniques and strapping.

11. Cardiopulmonary resuscitation.
12. Infections in sport: conditions directly related to partici-
    pation including herpes, hepatitis and AIDS; infections en-
    countered at home and abroad unrelated to participation in
    sport.
13. The role of the team doctor at home and on tour, including
    audit.
14. The use, abuse and control of drugs in sport; blood doping.
15. The organization and administration of medical cover at
    sporting events.
16. The medical, legal and ethical aspects of sport.

The Society of Apothecaries of London instituted a Diploma in
Sports Medicine in 1988 which is open to registered medical practitioners who have worked in the field of sports medicine or who
have had other definite experience and attended a recognized
course of instruction. There is one examination held in June each
year. Requirements include the submission of a dissertation, a
critical analysis of at least six case reports of patients who have
been under the care of the candidate and the examination itself
which consists of a multiple-choice question paper, a written
paper, a clinical and oral section.

The London Sports Medicine Institute (LSMI) ran a course for
general practitioners in sports medicine which was complementary to the Apothecaries' Diploma and led after one year to an examination for a certificate in sports medicine.

There is a one-year university course in sports medicine which
is based at London University. It is full-time and expensive so both
leave of absence and sponsorship have to be sought. There is a
research fellowship available from Smith and Nephew for this
course of study.

The University of Nottingham invites applications for a two-
year part-time course leading to an MSc in sports medicine. This
involves one day per week in Nottingham with visits to other
centres. Bursaries are available and PGEA recognition is approved
for ten sessions of each of the two years. Further details are available from the Department of General Practice, Queen's Medical
Centre, Nottingham NG7 2UH.

The University of Bath is instituting a Diploma course in sports
medicine due to start in the academic session of 1992/3. This is
open to suitably qualified medical practitioners.

In the North East of England the University of Sunderland in
liaison with Hartlepool Health Authority is in the process of establishing a series of courses leading to degrees (MSc and PhD) in
sports medicine for doctors and degrees and diplomas (BSc, Dip.

Sports Med.) for paramedical personnel (nurses, physiotherapists, coaches) as well as specific sports science degrees (MSc, PhD) for those already holding a BSc or equivalent in exercise or sports science. These are planned over the academic sessions 1992–1995.

Sports science courses

Loughborough University runs several courses which lead to degrees in sports science (BSc, MSc). One such course is an MSc in physical education and sports science. Further details of the courses and cost can be obtained from Professor Clyde Williams, Department of Physical Education and Sports Science, University of Technology, Loughborough, Leics LE1 3YU.

Henry Moore's University at Liverpool has a full-time BSc (Hons) course in sports science run since 1975 designed to give a multidisciplinary scientific education applied to sport. There are also short courses commencing in October of each year and running for one evening each week (3 hours) for 10 weeks. The emphasis is on practicalities and the courses are run in collaboration with the Department of Orthopaedic and Accident Surgery, University of Liverpool. The short courses lead to a Certificate of Professional Development. There is also a one-year full-time course leading to a Diploma in Science and Football. This includes the physiology of training; match play; nutrition; fitness testing and evaluation; injury prevention; psychology of soccer; motivation; skill analysis; talent identification; player management; club resources; computerized match analysis and patterns of play. Elements of the course are conducted in collaboration with professional clubs. Applicants are invited from people with a practical background in association football. Further details of all the courses are available from Professor T Reilly, Centre for Sport and Exercise Sciences, School of Health Sciences, Henry Moore's University at Liverpool, Bryan Street, Liverpool L3 3AF.

Three universities run both medical degrees and sports science courses: St Andrews, Birmingham and Glasgow.

St Andrews has a longstanding first-year course and plans to extend this to a three-year degree entitled 'Sports and Exercise Sciences'. Unfortunately due to revisions of the sports science curriculum the course is no longer attendable by medical students.

At Birmingham there is a three-year degree (Hons) in 'Sport and Exercise Science'. This is, however, in the Science Faculty and medical intercalations are currently only permitted within the Medical Faculty. Medical students could, however, contemplate an exercise physiology project, done in the Department of Sport and Exercise Sciences but as part of a physiology degree. Further details of both these universities' courses can be obtained from Dr Martin Farrelly at St Andrews University and Professor Merwyn Davies, School of Sport and Exercise Sciences, University of Birmingham, PO Box 363, Birmingham B15 2TT.

Glasgow University remains the only medical faculty in which undergraduate students can receive formal training in sports science/sports medicine. Options available include:

1. A summer project within the medical curriculum
2. A one-year intercalation for an ordinary BSc
3. A two-year intercalation for honours.

Currently 4–5 medical students per year opt for 3. The course contains more physiology, medical and paramedical content than other typical sports science/kinesiology degrees in the UK and may contain less mainstream sports science especially in relation to the elite performer but with its practical medical content it is a degree particularly appropriate for the intercalating medical student. Further details of the degree (Physiology and Sports Science) are available from Dr Neil Spurway, Department of Physiology, University of Glasgow, Glasgow G12 8QQ.

STANDARDS OF PRACTICE—ETHICS

The World Medical Association has drafted ethical guidelines for doctors involved in sport. These are:

1. The doctor has a responsibility to recognize the special physical and mental demands placed upon sportsmen.
2. Children present a special group and first consideration must be given to their growth and stage of development.
3. Where professional sportsmen are involved due regard should be taken of occupational medicine directives. Potentially harmful methods of training and improving performance should be opposed. These include:
   (a) Procedures which modify blood constituents or biochemistry by artificial means;
   (b) The use of drugs to modify performance;
   (c) Procedures which mask pain when participation would be inadvisable;
   (d) Measures which artificially change features appropriate to age and sex;
   (e) Training or competing when it is not safe to do so, e.g. through viral illness.
4. The athlete, now a patient, should be informed of the implication of the injury or condition and its long-term effects and should be guarded against any pressure which might encour-

age the use of dangerous methods. Where children are involved, the long-term effect of training procedures or methods must be spelled out to parents and coaches.

5. The doctor involved in sport must always give his objective opinion and leave no doubt as to his conclusions.
6. In competition, it is the doctor's duty to decide whether the player can remain on the field or return to the game. He must not allow his decisions to be overruled and priority must always be given to the best interests of the patient and not to the outcome of the competition. If the doctor has to be absent for any reason, individuals to whom he has delegated responsibility must adhere strictly to the instructions he has given them.
7. The doctor's authority must be upheld by the governing body of sport and by the referee during the game. Such decisions should not be prejudiced to favour the interest of any third party whatsoever.
8. The patient's general practitioner must be fully informed of facts relevant to treatment.
9. Professional confidentiality should be observed as far as is possible. It must be realized, however, that many clinical decisions may have to be made in the presence of thousands of spectators. Where a decision cannot be made in such circumstances, the athlete must be removed from the field for private examination in the club changing room or first aid room.
10. A doctor involved in sport should not be party to any contract which obliges him to reserve particular forms of therapy exclusively for any single patient or group of patients.
11. Team doctors visiting foreign countries should ideally enjoy the right to carry out their specific functions when accompanying a team to another country. This concession may not be given in some countries and may not be covered by insurance in the USA.
12. When safety regulations are being drawn up, the team doctor should be present (World Medical Association 1981).

SPORTS COUNCIL INITIATIVES

In 1983 the Scottish Sports Council established a consultative body comprising sport scientists, sport physicians, psychologists and coaches. Its responsibilities are to act as an advisory body to the Sports Council on medical problems and training matters, to act as a catalyst in sport education for participants and members of the lay public involved in sport, to generate research interest in sports medicine and science, to liaise with sports medicine and science organizations already in existence and to assist them to establish such courses or research as may be relevant. In particular localities, it aims to assist with the establishment of sports medicine clinics. Its publication, entitled *Sport Update on Medicine and Sciences SUMS* is produced three times a year. This is a four-page pamphlet, distributed to all the governing bodies in sport in Scotland and available from the Sports Council to other interested parties. It covers methods of training and basic sports injury clinics, fitness assessment centres and the official organizations already established in sport at national and local level.

In the last few years a network of Sports Medicine Centres has been set up throughout Scotland as a result. The main objectives have been to diagnose, treat and rehabilitate those participating in sport who have been injured and to educate and give advice where needed (Knill-Jones 1990).

The Sports Council (England) established the first National Sports Medicine Institute based in London in 1992. In the North-East of England a consultative body in sports science and sports medicine has been established with the aim of improving sports science and sports medicine provision in the region (Northern Regional Sports Council).

THE TEAM DOCTOR

Doctors have become increasingly involved in sport over recent years—an association which can now no longer be casual. Ethical standards have been set and a completely professional approach is expected.

The team doctor's is an activity-based interest. While it is not essential to have played the sport covered oneself, it is vital to get to know the game and its rules, as well as the players, officials and coaches. There should be an initial meeting to discuss the organization of the sport concerned and identify and recognize respective duties.

Disqualifying conditions

The doctor should determine the health status of the players from the outset. There are certain disqualifying conditions which apply particularly to contact and combat sports. These are:

1. Loss of one of a certain pair of organs, e.g. kidney or eye.
2. Three knockouts in one year. This disqualifies the player from participating in combat or contact sports for the rest of that year. Further participation should take place only after specialist examination.

3. Prolonged coma, a neurosurgical procedure (for the treatment of serious head injuries) or serious neurological illness.
4. Persistent hypertension (at rest 160/100).
5. Anatomical abnormalities, e.g. a long neck which may predispose to cervical injury in rugby football, especially in the scrum.

TEMPORARY DISQUALIFYING CONDITIONS

1. Chronic infections.
2. Acute infections.
3. Osteochondritis or other orthopaedic defects.
4. Hernia, cryptorchidism and other conditions requiring minor surgical procedures. Cardiovascular or renal disease needs to be evaluated individually.

Diabetic and epileptic patients have successfully taken part in combat sports but should also be individually assessed. Impaired vision may not be so important as a restricted visual field but advice should be sought. Those with recurrent dislocations should seriously consider giving up their particular contact or combat sport, especially if the shoulder joint is involved.

Medical evaluation

At the beginning of each new season, the team members should be examined or assessed for fitness to compete, thus providing a baseline from which changes can be recorded. The aims of the examination should include:

1. The health status of candidates before participation in competition.
2. Advice on the management and prognosis of current problems or injuries.
3. The identification of at-risk players.

Attendance at matches and competitions

It is not always possible to attend all practices and games. Nevertheless, the team doctor should be aware of the training methods used and the type of equipment. Advice regarding the timing and type of meals before games and training is important.

When injuries occur, they may be serious enough to require professional treatment before the athlete is moved. This is particularly so with head and neck injuries, and the doctor should be available at the touchline or ringside to deal with these. The referee should be informed as to whether or not a player can return to

WEST HARTLEPOOL RUGBY FOOTBALL CLUB
Brierton Lane, Hartlepool

HEAD INJURY WARNING

Name ....

The above named player has sustained a head injury on

....

1.　He should be seen by an Accident and Emergency Department as soon as possible.

2.　He should not play rugby for 3 weeks but he can, however, attend training sessions (no contact).

3.　If he develops vomiting, weakness of a limb, any abnormal movement or excess drowsiness or confusion he must be seen by a hospital immediately.

4.　He must not drink alcohol for 24 hours.

Fig. 3.1　Head injury card

competition, and the injured player, officials or his or her relatives should be made aware of the implications of the particular injury sustained.

Communication with players and officials

Even if the doctor is able to attend all the games his or her advice may be either forgotten or ignored by the injured player and team officials. To prevent this problem occurring we introduced a card system. After speaking to the injured player a card is given to him or her (or coach or team official in cases of head injury) advising the player or officials of the nature and management of the injury, so that the medical advice given is recalled. This system became standard in 1986 at West Hartlepool Rugby Football Club. Both

---

WEST HARTLEPOOL RUGBY FOOTBALL CLUB
Brierton Lane, Hartlepool

Soft Tissue Injury Card (STI)

Name: ....

You have sustained a soft tissue injury. Over the next 24 hours you should:

1. Cool the injury area by intermittent ice application to the protected skin, i.e. ice pack for 10 minute intervals for 1 hour (5 minutes between applications).

2. Take soluble aspirin or disprin 2 tablets 3 times per day for the next 3 - 5 days.

3. Bandage the affected limb (after cooling).

4. Begin gentle movements 24 hours after injury. Walking is enough at first.

5. On days 3, 4 and 5 begin gentle active exercise provided there is no pain.

6. Do static stretching to regain muscle length.

IF PAIN AND SWELLING PERSIST CONSULT YOUR DOCTOR AS SOON AS POSSIBLE.

Fig. 3.2   Soft tissue injury card

home and visiting players benefit, and many clubs have adopted the idea (Figs 3.1, 3.2).

ESTABLISHING A SPORTS INJURY CLINIC

The main responsibility of a sports injury clinic is to diagnose, treat and rehabilitate athletes to their full potential in the shortest possible time after injury, without increasing the risk of recurrence. Overall fitness should be maintained if possible and advice should be given on both injury avoidance and basic initial care and treatment.

All injuries—acute or chronic—should be treated. Many do not differ significantly from those seen in general practice, but there will also be a proportion of sports-specific 'overuse' injuries. Patients will be encouraged to attend because of the provision of easier access to staff with a specialized interest and because they then have a greater expectation of recovery after injury.

Guidelines

1. The clinic should be under medical supervision.
2. The medical supervisor should advise the local Medical Committee of his proposal to establish a clinic and seek its co-operative approval of the clinic's aims. Staffing, patient referral, documentation and communication with the patient's own doctor must be clearly established and agreed upon.
3. Confidentiality must be observed and no medical advertising should be permitted.
4. Access to the clinic should be through a receptionist.
5. All medical and paramedical staff should be members of the appropriate professional bodies.
6. Standardized documentation for medical and physiotherapy records should be so structured so as to facilitate clinical audit.
7. The medical and paramedical staff should ensure good communication with the patient's own doctor and, where agreed with the athlete, the coach.
8. Drug prescribing policies should be clearly defined and should involve liaison with the patient's family doctor.
   a. The use of free samples should be strictly controlled and documented.
   b. Drug prescribing should be prompt and only essential drugs should be given.
9. Access to investigative facilities should be defined. Laboratories and X-ray departments should be used efficiently, but local arrangements may dictate that investigations are arranged through the patient's own general practitioner or the accident and emergency department of the local hospital.
10. Financial arrangements must be clearly defined. The fees charged should be readily available for inspection and expenses identified, e.g. staff, equipment, accommodation, insurance, etc.
11. The clinic should identify whether it is profit- or non-profitmaking.
12. The medical and paramedical staff should advise their defence associations of their involvement in a sports injury clinic.

REFERENCES

Knill-Jones R 1990 Survey of activity in Scottish Sports Medicine Centres. Sports Coaching, Sports Medicine and Sports Sciences. Performance Bulletin 1

McLatchie G R, Morris E W 1977 Prevention of karate injury—a progress report. British Journal of Sports Medicine 11: 78–82

Royal Scottish Medical Colleges Board in Sports Medicine 1991 Statement from joint Board Meeting. Edinburgh and Glasgow

Vinger P F, Hoerner E F (eds) 1981 Sports injuries—the unthwarted epidemic. PSG Publishing, Littlejohn, Mass

World Medical Association 1981 Ethics in sports medicine. Journal of the World Medical Association

4. Women in sport

INTRODUCTION

In parallel with changes in sports participation at all levels, there has been a dramatic increase in the number of female athletes in the last two decades. Girls now start intensive training, particularly in swimming and gymnastics, at an early age. Nine- and ten-year-olds also train and compete in athletics, with the result that overuse injuries, which were once rare in this age group, are being reported more frequently.

Performance times for women have also improved in the last decade, especially in long-distance events. Greta Weitz, who won the World Championship women's marathon in Helsinki in 1983, is in the upper fifth percentage of male marathon runners. Her best time would have won the men's marathon race in the 1948 Olympic Games and she would have been second in 1956. In swimming events too, women have moved closer to men, although in track and field events, the 800 metres, the high jump and long jump records are still poor by comparison with male performances (Fox & Mathews 1981).

PUBERTAL CHANGES

Before puberty there is relatively little difference between the average weight and height of either sex. Girls of 8 to 13 tend to be heavier and taller than their male counterparts due to their earlier prepubertal growth spurt, which occurs in girls before the menarche (De Vries 1980).

After puberty, although the average male is taller and heavier than the average female, male and female athletes from the same sport tend to have similar body compositions. Gymnasts tend to be smaller and lighter than average whereas basketball players and shot-putters tend to be much taller.

Body fat content before puberty is similar in both sexes. After puberty, the average female has 25% body fat compared to 15% for the average male (De Vries 1980), but there is a wide variation in the percentage body fat among trained female athletes (McArdle et al 1981), which is sport-related. Athletes who participate in endurance events and train at high intensity for long periods have relatively low amounts of fat, and this has been associated with menstrual disturbance (Frish et al 1973). Levels as low as 6% have been reported. Females with high percentages are at a distinct disadvantage in athletic events which involve speed, strength and power.

RESPONSE TO TRAINING

Weight training is now an important integral part of the training schedules of most athletes who compete at top level. Both males and females demonstrate increased strength in response to a weight training programme. Increases of up to 44% have occurred in women with very little increase in muscle bulk (Browne & Wilmore 1974). The increase in muscle bulk which occurs in males as a result of training is due to their higher level of plasma testosterone. Women who weight-train, take anabolic steroids or have high natural levels of testosterone will tend to develop increased muscular hypertrophy.

The maximum oxygen uptake (VO_2max) is similar in both sexes before puberty but thereafter it tends to fall in women to 70–75% of the VO_2max of males (Åstrand et al 1973). After puberty, trained females have higher values than untrained males and females and there are no changes in the maximum oxygen uptake as a result of the menstrual cycle. Women have smaller hearts than men but demonstrate a similar response to aerobic training by increasing their left ventricular dimensions (Cahill et al 1979).

Unfit women are less able to tolerate exercise in hot environments than trained women and tend to lose heat by radiation. Fit women tend to lose it by sweating and are able to maintain their body temperature with a lower sweat rate (Morimoto et al 1967). The ability of trained athletes to maintain their stroke volume and cardiac output helps them to tolerate both heat and dehydration. In hot humid climates, working at the same relative exercise intensity, women have greater heat tolerance than men. This is probably due to their larger body-surface-area:weight ratio, which facilitates heat loss through radiation and convection. Kizer (1981) found that in scuba diving women lose heat more rapidly in water, where heat conduction is 25 times faster than air. However, because of their high percentage of body fat, women may feel hotter than men in wet suits before they get into the water.

NUTRITION

In general terms women have a lower basis metabolic rate than men, which varies during the menstrual cycle. The nutritional requirements for women are highest during pregnancy and lactation, while the nutritional demands of the male are greatest during adolescence. Dietary problems occur frequently in female athletes particularly in the so-called feminine sports (Brooks-Gunn et al 1987).

There is an increased incidence of musculoskeletal problems in amenorrheic athletes. Those who are hypooestrogenic have a reduced bone mineral density in trabecular bone, i.e. the body of the vertebrae and the neck of the femur (Cann et al 1984, Drinkwater et al 1984, Nelson et al 1986). Osteoporosis in young female athletes is sports specific; there is a much greater incidence in marathon runners and it is associated with age of onset of training, the intensity and volume of training, diet and stress— vegetarians are most at risk (Riggs 1981). The mean bone mineral density is comparable in some cases to a 60 year old woman. If untreated they are guaranteed stress fractures at the menopause.

The calorific and nutritional requirements for women athletes tend to be inadequately supplied by their normal diet. Many limit their food intake at times because of popular vogues to slim. Up to 40% of women aged between 20 and 50 years have signs of iron deficiency, and the mean haemoglobin concentration is lower in female endurance athletes than in non-athletes (Pate 1983). Endurance athletes may therefore require more iron because of their increased demand. Myoglobin is increased in muscle fibres as a result of endurance training. This is accompanied by the breakdown of red cells. Iron is also required by cytochrome oxidase, which plays a part in the transfer of oxygen in muscle tissue. Appropriate cushioning in running shoes reduces the breakdown of red cells in long-distance runners. Regular serum iron, ferritin and haemoglobin estimates should be carried out in female athletes.

Vitamin C taken with a meal increases the absorption of non-haeme iron (Rossander et al 1979), while tea reduces the absorption of non-haeme iron by 60% and some oral contraceptives interfere with the metabolism of folates and vitamin B_{12}.

SEXING

A normal female has 46 chromosomes, 44 autosomal and two X sex chromosomes. A variety of chromosomal abnormalities may occur: XO or XXX and occasionally there may be a mixture or mosaic of chromosomes which have developed from two or more stem lines. If a Y chromosome is part of the mosaic, the athlete would be disqualified from competing as a female. Routine sex tests are carried out at major international competitions and at all Olympic Games.

MENARCHE

The time of menarche varies in different countries. The average age now is between 12 and 15. Many factors influence its onset. These include nutrition, body type, family size and skeletal maturity. Ballet dancers, gymnasts and athletes who start training early have a late menarche. In fact for each year of training before expected menarche, the actual menarche is delayed by an average of 5 months. On the other hand, no significant difference in the age of menarche was found in a study of two groups of ballet dancers, one who did heavy training before and one group who started after the menarche. Girls who mature late are often taller, with less weight per centimetre of height. They are more likely to do well in athletics than those who mature early and develop other interests (Malina et al 1978).

Several theories have been postulated to explain delayed menarche. That there must be at least 17% body fat for menarche to occur has not been confirmed and, even though menarche and breast development may be delayed in some groups, the age of onset of pubic and axillary hair is not affected. This leads to the suggestion that high-intensity exercise may impair gonadotrophin-mediated ovarian maturation. High-intensity exercise is associated with raised levels of plasma prolactin which may interfere with normal hypothalamic–pituitary function by suppressing the action of follicle-stimulating hormone (FSH) (Mathews & Fox 1976).

THE MENSTRUAL CYCLE AND ATHLETIC PERFORMANCE

The effect of the menstrual cycle on performance is highly individual and is as variable as menstruation itself. Gold medals have been won by women in all phases and there are no medical contraindications to participating in sport—including scuba diving—provided the athlete is comfortable.

Premenstrual tension

Women with marked premenstrual tension will have problems in sports where fine judgement is required. Weight gains of several pounds may also occur. Women with severe premenstrual tension are more accident-prone (Dalton 1960). Regular strenuous exercise may either improve or have no effect on premenstrual tension but does have a beneficial effect on dysmenorrhoea (Ryan 1976).

MENSTRUAL IRREGULARITIES

Before 1970 few investigations reported abnormal menstrual cycles in athletes, but since then the intensity and duration of training has increased. There is a high incidence of irregular cycles, oligomenorrhoea and secondary amenorrhoea, particularly in long-distance runners (Baker et al 1981). The exact mechanism is still being investigated.

Menstrual disturbances have also been reported in a wide variety of other athletes, including those participating in rowing, swimming and ballet. The athletes with the most intense training schedules and those who have been running for the longest time have the highest incidence of oligomenorrhoea and amenorrhoea, but changes have been reported in runners who only do between 5 and 30 miles a week. Exercise-related menstrual changes are commoner in younger nulliparous athletes with a late menarche, and there is a higher incidence of prior menstrual irregularities and amenorrhoea in long-distance runners (Schwartz et al 1981). They weigh less, have a lower percentage of body fat and run faster. Diet also plays a part in inducing menstrual irregularities and there is a higher incidence of amenorrhoea in vegetarians.

Many regular menstruating athletes have a shortened luteal phase and low progesterone. Oestrogen deficiency in young athletes can cause demineralization of bone. Casper et al (1984) suggest that the chronic increased metabolic clearance of gonadal steroids in endurance-trained athletes results in decreased circulating oestrogen and progesterone levels which in turn affect the hypothalamic pituitary axis leading to luteal phase defects. Steroid hormones are metabolized to a considerable extent in adipose tissue; therefore changes in body fat may alter endocrine functions.

Changes in prolactin due to exercise have also been documented (Boyden et al 1981) and high levels of prolactin can affect the hypothalamic pituitary ovarian axis. Hyperprolactinaemia is a well-known cause of amenorrhoea and infertility in non-athletic women. Athletes with menstrual problems should be screened for hyperprolactinaemia and pituitary tumours.

Stress also plays a part in secondary amenorrhoea. After 2 months summer training camp, three-quarters of the female West Point Cadets were amenorrhoeic. After 18 months only 8% were amenorrhoeic (Anderson 1979). Menstruation frequently returns when the stress of intense training and competition is reduced.

Oligomenorrhoea and amenorrhoea may cause problems for athletes if they require an X-ray, because of the 10-day rule.

In pregnancy there are many benefits due to exercise (Warren

1991). Regular exercise in pregnancy should not increase the heart rate above 140 beats per minute and strenuous exercise should not exceed 15 minutes, particularly in warm humid conditions (Am. Coll. Obs. Gyn. 1985) when the increase in body temperature and the diversion of blood from the foetus to the exercising muscle may have an adverse effect (Clapp & Dickstein 1983). Regular exercise during pregnancy can increase VO_2 max (Clapp 1989). Ideal exercise for pregnant women are swimming, cycling and aerobic walking. Exercise after delivery should be sports specific (Shangold 1982). After vaginal delivery exercise may be started after 1 week (cf. Liz McColgan) but any sport that requires rotation of the spine or stress on the sacroiliac joints should be avoided until at least 6 weeks later to prevent the possibility of prolapse. In general exercise in pregnancy leads to a shorter labour and increased pre and post natal self esteem.

INJURIES

Women were once considered to be more at risk from injuries than men, but recent surveys have shown they both sustain the same types of injury. The incidence of injury is related to the level of fitness and conditioning and to the sport itself (Rosegrant 1982, Haycock & Gillette 1976). The most common injuries are to ankles and knees, the least common to the heart (Haycock & Gillette 1976). Because of the wider pelvis in the female, there is a greater tendency to genu valgum. The normal pull of the quadriceps tends to pull the patella laterally. As a result, chondromalacia patellae is a relatively common problem.

An injury peculiar to females occurs in water skiing during the take-off period. Failure to rise from the sitting position produces forceful retrograde douching which can cause haematoma of the vulva or tearing of the vaginal wall. Wearing a wet suit will prevent this.

Poor posture associated with weak abdominal muscles predisposes to back problems in some sports. The increasing incidence of low back pain in female gymnasts is giving rise to concern. There is a higher incidence of Scheurmann's and pars interarticularis fractures in gymnasts compared with runners (Jackson et al 1981). Female gymnasts with hyperlordosis, decreased mobility of their shoulder joints, short hip flexors and weak abdominal muscles are more at risk of developing low back pain and should be carefully supervised.

All gymnasts and athletes should be examined when they enter a sport. Those with structural abnormalities should be advised against participation in particular risk sports. Minor abnormalities such as inflexibility, muscle imbalance, leg length discrepancies, poor abdominal muscles and poor posture should be actively corrected.

REFERENCES

American College of Obstetrics and Gynecology 1985 Exercise during pregnancy and the postnatal period in ACOG home exercise programs. Washington DC ACOG

Anderson J L 1979 Sports and Fitness Programmes at US Military Academy. Physician and Sports Medicine 7: 72–80.

Åstrand I, Åstrand P O, Hallbaeck T, Kelbohm H 1973 Reduction in maximal oxygen uptake with age. Journal of Applied Psychology 35: 649–654

Baker E, Mathew R, Kirk R, Williamson H O 1981 Fertility and Sterility 36 2: 183–187

Boyden T W, Oamenter B S, Gross D, Stanforth P, Rolkis M D, Wilmore J 1981 Prolactin responses, menstrual cycles and body composition of women runners. Presented at the Endocrine Society Meeting, June, Cincinnati, Ohio

Brooks-Gunn J, Warren M P, Hamilton L H 1987 The relationship of eating disorders to amenorrhoea in ballet dancers. Medical Science Sports and Exercise 19 1: 41

Browne H C, Wilmore J 1974 Effects of maximum resistance training on strength and body composition of women athletes. Medicine and Science in Sports and Exercise 6: 174

Cahill N S, O'Brien M, Rodahl A, Allen J F, Knight D, Dolphin C 1979 Pilot study of left ventricular dimensions and wall stress before and after submaximal exercise. British Journal of Sports Medicine 13: 122–129.

Cann C E, Martin M C, Genant H K, Jaffe R B 1984 Decreased spine mineral content in amenorrheic women. Journal of the American Medical Association 251: 66

Casper R F, Wilkinson D, Cotter E 1984 The effect of increased cardiac output on luteal phase gonadal steroids: a hypothesis for runners amenorrhoea. Fertility and Sterility 41 3: 364–368

Clapp J F 1989 Oxygen consumption during treadmill exercise before, during and after pregnancy. American Journal of Obstetrics and Gynecology 161: 1458

Clapp J F, Dicksteins C 1983 Maternal exercise performance and pregnancy outcome. 13th annual meeting of the Society for Gynecologic Investigation: 104

Dalton K 1960 Menstruation and accidents. British Medical Journal 5210: 1425–1426

De Vries H A 1980 Physiology of exercise for physical education and athletes. 3rd edn. William Browne, Dubuque, Iowa

Drinkwater B L, Nilson K, Chestnut C H 1984 Bone mineral content of amenorrheic and eumenorrheic women runners. New England Journal of Medicine 311: 277

Fox E L, Mathews D K 1981 Physiological basis of physical education and athletics. WB Saunders, Philadelphia: 346–394

Frish R E, Revelle R, Cook S 1973 Components of the critical weight at menarche and at initiation of the adolescent spurt, estimated total water, lead body mass and fat. Human Biology 45: 469

Haycock C E, Gillette J 1976 Susceptibility of women athletes to injury. Journal of the American Medical Association 236: 163–164

Jackson D W, Wiltse I L, Dingemen R D, Hayes M 1981 Stress reactions involving the pars interarticularis in young athletes. American Journal of Sports Medicine 9: 304–312

Kizer K 1981 Women and diving. Physician in Sportsmedicine 9: 85–92

Malina R M, Spirduso W W, Tate C, Baylor W M 1978 Age of menarche and selected menstrual characteristics in athletes at different competition levels. Medicine and Science in Sports and Exercise 10: 218–222

Mathews D K, Fox E L 1976 The physiological basis of physical education and athletics. W B Saunders, Philadelphia: 446–487

McArdle W D, Katch F I, Katch V L 1981 Energy, nutrition and human performance. In: Exercise Physiology, Lea and Febiger, Philadelphia; 288

Morimoto T, Slabochova A, Naman R K, Sargant F 1967 Sex difference in physiological reaction to thermal stress. Journal of Applied Physiology 22: 526–532

Nelson M E, Fischer E C, Catsos P D 1986 Diet and bone status in amenorrheic runners. American Journal of Clinical Nutrition 43: 910–916

Pate R R 1983 Sports anaemia—a review of the current research literature. Physician in Sportsmedicine 11: 115–131

Riggs B L, Wahner H W, Dunn W L, Mazess R B, Offord K P, Melton L J 1981 Differential changes in bone mineral density of the appendicular and axial skeleton with ageing. Relationship to spinal osteoporosis. Journal of Clinical Investigations 67: 328–335

Rosegrant S 1982 Conditioning reduces injuries. Women's rugby. Physician in Sportsmedicine 10: 142–146

Rossander L, Hallberg L, Bjorn-Rosmussen E 1979 Absorption of iron from breakfast meals. American Journal of Clinical Nutrition 32: 2484–2489

Ryan A J 1976 Sports during pregnancy and other questions. Physician in Sportsmedicine 4: 82

Schwartz B, Cumming D C, Riorden E, Selye M, Yen S, Rebar R W 1981 Exercise associated amenorrheoa: a distinct entity? American Journal of Obstetrics and Gynecology 141: 662–670

Shangold N M, Levine H S 1982 The effect of marathon training upon menstrual function. American Journal of Obstetrics and Gynecology 143: 862

5. Principles of training

There is a current drive to promote Sport for All—for all ages and abilities—but to do this we must help people to pick up skills throughout their life. (Radford 1990)

SELECTION OF SPORT

If people are to develop a sporting habit they should ideally be introduced to sport early and also stay involved. The concept of exercise adherence should be developed with goals being set and success experiences engineered to provide encouragement (Table 5.1). How people select a sport depends on both extrinsic and intrinsic factors with age being a major influence (Table 5.2). Most children, for instance, are introduced to a sport like swimming by a family member whereas complex sports like team games are introduced by a PE instructor or teacher. As the child gets older intrinsic factors such as interest and motivation become more important but physiological factors like body size exert increasing influence in sport selection. By mid-life intrinsic factors predominate. In old age extrinsic factors like availability and finances have greater influence.

Table 5.1 Support for an individual to keep going in sport (Reproduced by kind permission of Medical Action Communications)

Self:
- intrinsic motivation
- self-help

The Coach

Medical support:
- injury prevention
- injury treatment
- drugs—what to avoid
         —what is safe
- dental care
- dietary advice

Family and friends
- moral support and encouragement

Institutions
- club
- leagues
- school
- district council, etc.

Table 5.2 Factors influencing introduction to sport
(Reproduced by kind permission of Medical Action Communications)

Intrinsic Factors
- Physchological
  —interest
  —motivation
  —self-belief
  —knowledge
- Physical/physiological
  —gender
  —body size
  —muscle ultrastructure
  —body composition, etc.
- Medical
  —health status

Extrinsic status
- People
- Resources
- Local facilities
- Time
- Tradition and culture

The age factor is very important. The earlier a person is introduced to a sport the better his/her performance is likely to be. Those introduced early to swimming believed they could swim further than people introduced later (Fig. 5.1). There is also sup-

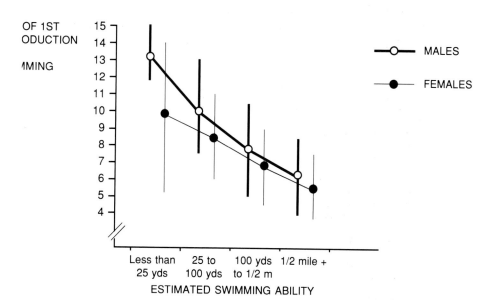

Fig. 5.1 Self-estimated swimming ability and age of first introduction (*n* = 496) (Reproduced by kind permission of Medical Action Communications)

port for the theory that early introduction to sport induces self-confidence and increases self-esteem in the young child and that this confidence in his/her ability is expressed in other skills learned throughout life.

Sport is, therefore, a special opportunity which has powerful social implications. As a means to an end it can produce educational, social, fitness and health benefits but as an end in itself it can lead to performance and excellence (Radford 1990).

Long before the advent of the academic discipline of Sports Science and Training Theory, athletes and their coaches/trainers had developed a pragmatic approach to their problems. Scientific methods have, more recently, been used to evaluate the old methods and to suggest new ones, and today the modern coach/trainer has a rich mixture of traditional and modern methods from which to select.

The purpose of training for sport is to improve athletic performance in order to succeed in competition. To achieve this, attention has to be paid to the skill, mental attitude and tactical sense of athletes, as well as to their physical conditioning, but in this chapter the physical aspects alone will be considered. It must be remembered, however, that the skilled coach will include certain training activities for many reasons. Some activities do not improve performance directly, but may rehearse certain aspects of competition, reduce the chance of injury or improve consistency.

An athlete's training is, therefore, a patchwork quilt, including a number of different activities, and these will change as the athlete's needs change from one part of the year to another, or from one part of his/her career to another. They will also vary from athlete to athlete, but most of all will vary from one sport to another, for one of the first principles of training for sport is that training benefits are *specific* to the training activities that produce them.

SPECIFICITY OF TRAINING

Except in sports that are dominated by skill or tactics, athletes cannot hope to improve simply by participating in their sport; they must engage in a training programme which develops the qualities required for their sport.

In recent years much effort has gone into analysing the physical demands of a wide variety of sports, and assessing how different training programmes help athletes meet these demands. This has revealed important elements of specificity in the development of strength, speed, skill and endurance. For example, the adenosine triphosphate (ATP) required for the contraction of muscles can be delivered by three different metabolic pathways: the phosphagen portion of anaerobic metabolism, heavily relied on during brief but intensive activities of a few seconds; the longer anaerobic system resulting in the production of lactic acid, which is relied on when intensive work is sustained up to a limit of about 50 seconds; and the aerobic system, which will continue to meet the muscles' moderate demand for ATP for several minutes or even hours but of course cannot provide the fuel for contraction at the rate demanded by very intensive activities.

In deciding which activities to include in an athlete's training, the coach/trainer must, therefore, be aware of the metabolic systems that deliver the fuel for muscular contraction, and the length and intensity of work that calls each into action.

THE TRAINING LOAD

Selecting the correct training programme is, therefore, much more than using the appropriate activity; if the correct metabolic systems are to be trained the activities must be performed at the necessary intensity and for the necessary length of time to produce the desired training effect.

It is often convenient to think of an athlete's training as a *load*, which must be sufficient to produce the desired adaptation response in the specific system that is needed. If the training load is insufficient, no training effect takes place, and so the training load must be increased. This can be done by increasing the training

—frequency
—duration, or
—intensity.

Overload

Not all exercise is training, for if the exercise load is not sufficient, no training effect ensues. Even at the very outset, therefore, training must impose a work stress greater than that experienced in everyday life and later, as the athlete adapts to his/her training, the load must be increased sufficiently to provoke further adaptation. Training must, therefore, be *progressive*, for a constant load will in time not be sufficient to ensure a continuing training effect.

PHASES OF TRAINING

When dealing with a beginner, it is usual to start by developing tolerance for the training process, so training *frequency* is increased first, with the duration of each training session, and its intensity, deliberately held in check. The next phase is then usually to increase the *duration* of training, with an increase in *intensity* coming later. 'Intensity' is of course a relative term which describes at what distance from maximum effort an athlete is performing. In many ways it is the intensity of an athlete's training that is the crucial variable. In most sports, athletes must eventually learn to perform with increasing intensity for progressively longer periods while recovering in ever shorter periods of time.

Once initial tolerance to training has taken place, a more rapid training response is produced if the athlete trains more intensively, but there is often a price to pay. As training intensifies it becomes more likely to cause a breakdown or produce injury, and long periods of intensive training involve such a high energy output that athletes must be given the necessary time to recover. Even highly experienced athletes, therefore, cannot sustain high-intensity training work indefinitely, and so coaches produce cycles of work of varying intensity, volume and emphasis so that their athletes have the least chance of injury or breakdown and the best chance of producing their best performance at the time required.

Training is so specific that it is difficult to generalize about all training for all sports, but it is frequently true that athletes need to train more than one energy system. Many sports are not 'continuous' in the sense that a 100 metres sprint on the running track or a marathon road race are: many, such as soccer, tennis and basketball, involve intermittent effort where the athletes must be capable of periods of brief, high-intensity work, periods of lower-intensity work, and even some periods of relative rest, spread sometimes over as much as an hour and a half. The cycle of physical training in these circumstances will often be:

Phase 1: Aerobic endurance training
Phase 2: Anaerobic endurance training
Phase 3: Anaerobic—speed training
Phase 4: Competition

These phases would not usually be discrete, but would taper one into another, and other elements involving mastery of technique and tactics would be included at all phases.

All sports have their own requirements and therefore their own pattern of training cycles and phases. Training for squash is unlike training to run 200 metres, and training for weight lifters is unlike training for a front row forward in rugby. In all sports the skill of the coach lies in no small part in knowing how to blend together all the elements of training to obtain the desired progressive effect.

Recovery, rest and detraining

Rest and recovery is an important part of all training, and athletes who train too intensively, too long or too frequently, in the mistaken belief that this will produce a more rapid training effect and so help them steal a march on their rivals, find instead that it leads to chronic fatigue and a tendency to break down. Herein lies a dilemma for the athlete and coach, for once training is stopped all the adaptations achieved begin to reverse. It is this fear that leads so many athletes to return to training too soon after illness or injury. The skilful coach, therefore, must study rest and recovery as much as he/she studies training loads, for they are related subjects.

Developing strength

To develop strength the athlete must use muscular forces against some form of resistance. Strength training used to go by the name of 'weight training' but is now often described as 'resistance training'. The nature of the resistance dictates to a great extent the type of strength that is developed.

FREE WEIGHTS (I.E. BARBELLS, DUMBBELLS, ETC.)

These are still very popular and have survived all the training fads and fashions. A variety of exercises can be prescribed to strengthen any muscle group, and gradation and progression of loading is easy to achieve. One drawback is that most training with free weights is anti-gravity and so in the vertical plane only, and it is not always easy to convert the strength gained in this way into improvement in specific sports skills. The classic system developed in the 1940s was based on the concept of the repetition maximum (RM). A 10 RM was a load that the athlete could lift ten times only before fatigue prevented any further lift; a 5 RM was a load that could be lifted only five times, and a 1 RM was a weight that could be lifted only once.

A traditional programme is for the athlete to perform three sets of each exercise:

Set 1: 10 repetitions with ½ 10 RM load
Set 2: 10 repetitions with ¾ 10 RM load
Set 3: 10 repetitions with 10 RM load

Training should take place three times per week and strength improvements should be measurable in 5 or 6 weeks.

Experienced lifters still find the three-set system beneficial, but 5 RM to 7 RM weights are increasingly popular, and five sessions a week are commonly prescribed. Systems with stacked weights have replaced free weights in many places. These stacked systems have certain advantages: they are safer to use and with the use of wires and pulleys permit work at a greater variety of angles and directions which can better mimic the requirements of individual sports.

ISOMETRICS

This is no longer a favoured training method (although it is still the most popular among researchers). The main drawback is that static contractions are not a common feature in most sports. Strength gains achieved through isometric training tend to be limited to the limb position and angle used in the training.

When isometrics is used, strength gains are apparent after 5 weeks, if training has taken place at least three times per week and each contraction is held for approximately 6 seconds and repeated up to 10 times.

ISOKINETICS AND VARIABLE RESISTANCE SYSTEMS

There are several commercially available systems that produce a resistance by employing hydraulics, compressed air, fly-wheels, cams, etc. These are designed to produce resistances either of a pre-set velocity or to match the ability of athletes to apply forces throughout the whole range of a movement.

The great attraction of these systems is their specificity and the way they can load a muscle group continuously throughout a movement. Drawbacks are that the strength gained at one velocity of training may not always be transferable to another velocity, and that many sports skills require *acceleration* through the movement and not a constant velocity. Many machines are required to meet the whole range of an athlete's needs.

BODY WEIGHT

Body weight can be used as a resistance to work against, either directly, as in jumping and bounding, or indirectly as in hill running.

By working against their body weight athletes can develop an explosive strength easily channelled into their own sports. Pliometrics, or the system of depth-jumping from and to various heights and at various speeds, or distances, encourages the rapid recruitment of forces to train not only elastic strength and power but also the CNS, in the recruitment of high-threshold motor units and the synchronous firing of motor units.

SKILL-SPECIFIC RESISTANCE

Many sports skills can be performed against a resistance which allows the most skill-specific form of resistance training possible.

Rubber tubing has been used to resist golf swings, tennis serves and hurdlers' trailing legs. Athletes have run, swum and rowed towing partners or some retarding object. Swimmers train wearing drag suits to increase the water resistance. These all have the advantage of developing strength within the context of the athlete's pattern of skill. Care must be taken, however, not to disrupt or interfere with the skill, and the use of ankle weights by runners may so interfere with their normal motor patterns that any strength gains that do occur are offset by other losses.

Anaerobic speed training

'Speed' is a problem term in training and the coach/trainer must be careful to distinguish, for example, between speed based on skill and strength, as in discus throwing, speed based on aerobic efficiency, such as the final 200 metres of a middle distance race, and the anticipatory and perceptual speed of a slip fielder in cricket.

For the speed/power athletes such as sprinters, training will include skill and resistance work but aerobic fitness must also be developed. Above all, these athletes must develop the ability to work at high intensity, so the phosphagen system needs to be developed.

Phosphagen stores in the muscles are rapidly depleted, but also rapidly restored. In speed/power events athletes usually perform repetitions followed by rest. Sprinters commonly perform sprints of 7–10 seconds in duration, with a slow walk-back recovery of 2–3 minutes. If this cycle is completed intensively this ensures the depletion of the phosphagen stores and gives time for their virtual full recovery. Sprints of this kind provide the training stimulus to improve the storage, delivery and recovery of the high-energy phosphates necessary for their sport. A trained sprinter can perform a very large number of repetitions in this way before he/she shows any sign of progressive fatigue.

Aerobic endurance training

To improve aerobic capacity continuous work of both low and high intensity is required, and during some periods of training interval training will often be used.

Heart rate is the index most commonly used to determine how fast the training rate should be. The vogue for running very long distances slowly is now over, except early in training; it may also occasionally be as a rehearsal for a long race or to develop exercise tolerance. It is now known that aerobic adaptation takes place more rapidly when training is more intensive. Continuous aerobic work forms the core of modern endurance training, which is now commonly performed at 85–90% of maximum heart rate, with daily sessions. It takes only a few weeks to produce measurable improvement in VO_2max if the athlete is at the start of his training. Further improvement, such as the acquired ability to work at a higher percentage of VO_2max takes very much longer.

Interval training is also used either for variety or during the pre-training or early season. The advantage of interval work is that highly intensive work at race pace or even above can be experienced and the recovery periods can be manipulated to produce the desired effect.

Despite modern training innovations, interval training is still an ideal way to bring aerobic and anaerobic training together, and can be adapted to any sport on land or water.

Training for well-being and health

Non-athletes of all ages have turned to exercise in recent years to keep fit and feel well. They are, of course, as trainable as athletes. Advice for such people varies enormously. Although most are agreed that aerobic work should comprise the core of their programme, there is increasing evidence to suggest that a balanced programme which also includes flexibility, relaxation and strength work gives the most benefit.

The aerobic work should be regularly undertaken, perhaps on alternative days, and the work period should last 30 minutes or so. Any exercise that elevates the heart rate and keeps it elevated to at least 60% of the range between resting heart rate and maximum heart rate is acceptable.

It is usual to estimate maximum heart rate by using the simple formula

Maximum heart rate = 220—age in years

Resting heart rate can be taken, with practice, each morning immediately on waking.

It is unwise to be too precise or dogmatic about workloads, duration, intensity and frequency of training for non-athletes. Maximum heart rate can vary quite markedly from one person of the same age to another: body weight, exercise history, etc. will all be important factors to consider; nevertheless, gentle, regular aerobic exercise combined with other exercises for flexibility, relaxation and strength can and should form part of most people's lives.

For the overweight, or those who have not been engaged in regular exercise for several years, thought should be given to non-weight-bearing forms of exercises such as swimming or cycling.

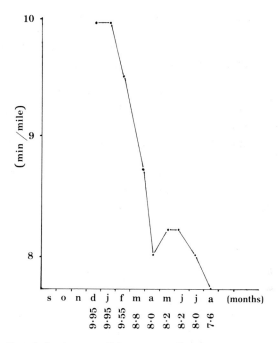

Fig. 5.2   Pace (minutes per mile) over a 6-mile test run

This will reduce the risk of injury to the knees, feet and ankles, which may otherwise object at first to the new demands being placed upon them.

Figures 5.2–5.5 show how one non-athlete who took up jogging at Glasgow University responded over his first 12 months of training. He was in his mid-thirties and at the beginning, in September, was incapable of sustained continuous running over 400 m. By April (7 months after the start) his total mileage had risen to 150 per month. There was no running test for the first 3 months, but thereafter, when tested on the same 6-mile course his fastest pace each month improved from almost 10 minutes per mile to about 7½ minutes per mile (Fig. 5.2).

Figure 5.3 shows very similar trends for his resting heart rate. After an initial rise when he began his exercise programme, the subject's heart rate dropped steadily. There is an interesting parallel rise in Figures 5.2 and 5.3 showing an increase in resting heart rate and a decrease in running speed in May and June. This reflects a 4- or 5-week period of partial rest: an excellent example of the reversibility of training.

Throughout this period the subject was also given four

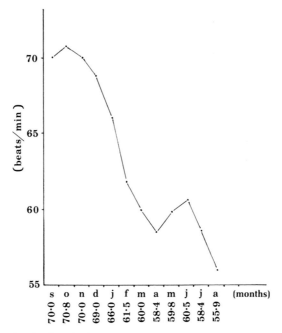

Fig. 5.3   Resting heart rate

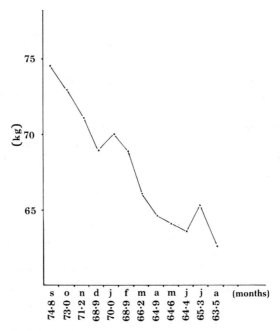

Fig. 5.4   Body weight

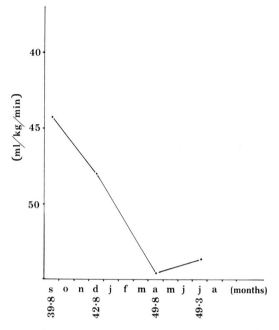

Fig. 5.5 Estimated VO$_2$max

sub-maximal tests on a bicycle ergometer to estimate his maximum VO$_2$, and these show an increase of almost 25% in his aerobic efficiency (Fig. 5.5).

The improvements in cardiorespiratory and aerobic efficiency reflected in Figures 5.3 and 5.5 brought with them not only an improvement in running performance (Fig. 5.2), but also a substantial reduction in body weight (Fig. 5.4), even though this was not the stated objective of the training. Perhaps the greatest penalty for following a programme such as this is a financial one: the cost of a new wardrobe of clothes!

REFERENCES

Åstrand P O, Rodahl K 1977 Textbook of work physiology, 2nd edn. McGraw-Hill, New York

Dick F W 1980 Sports training principles. Lepus Books, London

Fox E L 1979 Sports physiology. W B Saunders, Philadelphia

Harre D (ed) 1982 Principles of sports training. Sportverlag, Berlin

Nicholas J A, Hershman E B (eds) Clinics in sports medicine 3. W B Saunders, Philadelphia

Pollock M J, Wilmore J H, Fox S M 1978 Health and fitness through physical activity. John Wiley, New York

Radford P 1990 Sport for all. In Injury in sport—a team approach. Medical Action Communications, Surrey: 7–8

Shephard R J 1982 Physiology and biochemistry of exercise. Praeger, New York

Tancred B, Tancred G 1984 Weight training for sport. Hodder & Stoughton, London

Watson A W S 1983 Physical fitness and athletic performance. Longman, Harlow

Wilmore J H 1982 Training for sport and activity, 2nd edn. Allyn & Bacon, Boston

6. Laboratory assessment of performance

The assessment of performance is a skill which is continually being carried out during a sporting event. The most common and valuable tool to a coach is the ability to observe and make subjective assessments of performance. However, whether the result of the performance was the outcome of skill, fitness or mental attitudes can be difficult to discern. The problem with subjective assessment is that its accuracy is subject to the knowledge and the experience of the assessor. Even with the most experienced observer there are many times when inaccurate judgements have been made because one of the many factors, governing performance, has been compensated for by an inadequacy in another. Objective assessments are more valuable for they give some dimension to the result, e.g. time, distance, score. Unfortunately, unless some subjective assessments are made, objective assessments may give little indication of how that dimension was accomplished. The means by which a coach can assess the present state of a performer's capacity would be to administer certain tests which would provide objective measurements relating to total performance. In order to do this, the specific component of performance would have to be objectively measured independently of the others, thus providing a more accurate insight to its value.

The intention of this chapter is to concentrate on physiological fitness and how it can be objectively assessed within the laboratory. While making the reader aware that this is an important factor of performance, it does not wish to detract from the importance of the other factors such as skill and mental attitude and will show, at a later stage, how both of these important factors can affect the validity of results in a test. Likewise, field testing is a useful means of acquiring the results of fitness parameters for it is often simple to administer and requires inexpensive equipment. Unfortunately, it has many drawbacks in producing reliable results. The laboratory setting eliminates some of these deficiencies and although it may have its own related problems, it does provide a suitable environment in which testing procedures can be standardized and provide greater accuracy for more meaningful results.

Before any method of assessing fitness can be carried out, certain important considerations must be accounted for, these include:

1. Pre-test procedures
2. The purpose and intention of the test
3. The suitability of the test and the equipment used
4. The statistical criteria for the test
5. The use of the test results.

PRE-TEST PROCEDURES

The test must be preceded by an ethical screening questionnaire (BASS 1988, Lange-Anderson et al 1971). This document should contain general information such as name, date of birth, age, occupation and sport (event or position), it should ascertain certain features relating to the subject's lifestyle and hereditary factors concerning cardiovascular disease and the related risks of smoking, drugs and alcohol. It is important that it be known to the tester any reason why the subject is presently being treated for injury or taking any form of medication. Before continuing with the next stage the questionnaire must be approved by the tester and signed by the subject to its accuracy.

The next procedure is to take certain measurements of the subject relating to spot health checks. These include height, weight, body fat, blood pressure, lung function and haemoglobin tests. The upper limits for systolic and diastolic blood pressures which have been approved by the local ethical committee for testing of athletes must be adhered to and tests which would be of a potential danger to a subject with hypertension must not be carried out. If possible, prior visits to the laboratory before the actual tests are to be administered provide an opportunity for habituation to the facility and the equipment, a chance to establish a friendly relationship between the performer and the test administrators and a time for reinforcing the procedures of the tests.

Safety of the subject must be of paramount importance, equipment must be checked and calibrated, blood sampling must follow a strict code of practice and where tests are to be carried out to maximal limits of exhaustion a medical practitioner must be present or resuscitation equipment made available, with someone having the knowledge of how to use it. An efficient laboratory will have facilities for first aid, medical support and knowledgeable laboratory technicians.

PURPOSE AND INTENTION OF THE TEST

Total fitness is comprised of certain components:

1. Strength
2. Speed
3. Flexibility
4. Endurance

Strength and speed are products of power.

i.e. Power = strength × speed (watts)
         = force × velocity

It would seem simple enough to state that the intention of a test was to measure 'fitness'. However, when it is known that fitness is made up of several components, one test alone cannot fulfil the requirements. It is usual that if one wishes to establish an assessment of total fitness, that a physiological profile is built up which consists of a battery of tests, (AAHPER 1965) each one reflecting the measurement of a fitness component. In many cases this is unnecessary for one or two tests may reflect the demands of the performance and the effects of exercise and training. The intention of any test becomes more apparent when the physiological demands of the performance are known and the magnitude to which each component of fitness is required. Therefore, the purpose and intention of any fitness test is to choose one which relates to the physiological profile of the performer and reflects the physiological demands of the performance.

THE TESTS AND EQUIPMENT

Prior to a fitness component test the true definition and an understanding of the component must be established. This will enable the tester to choose the most appropriate test and equipment.

Strength

Strength is the maximum force which a muscle can exert in a single contraction. However, muscles can contract either isometrically, isotonically or isokinetically and tests for these types of muscle contraction can be performed using strength dynamometers, free weights and isokinetic strength testing machinery respectively. The method by which this gross strength can be ascertained is to perform one single, maximal contraction. Strength testing is essential in sports and events which demand great amounts of strength e.g. shot-putting. It is necessary also in certain muscle groups which are constantly in use.

Speed

This can be defined as the minimal movement time of a single limb 'limb speed' or the total body 'body speed' between two fixed points. It can be recorded simply as a time (seconds) or if the distance is known can be given in units of velocity (ft/sec., m/sec.). The time for a short sprint (less than 60 m) or a karate chop are examples of speed tests and when technical equipment is used such as lasers or light sensors linked to either a multisecond timer or computer, greater precision and accuracy is guaranteed.

Flexibility (Montoye 1978)

This is the range of movement of a given joint or combination of joints. Various pieces of equipment which are used to measure this component range from simple protractors to highly sophisticated goniometers. The procedures involve recording the displacement of a bone, in a linear or angular dimension, to the adjacent bone with which it articulates. In sports where great amounts of flexibility are demanded the testing of this component is essential, e.g. gymnastics. However, tests on an injured joint compared to its counterpart can give an indication of limited movement.

Endurance

Endurance is defined as the ability to repeat muscular contractions without fatigue. Fatigue is a decline in the level of performance. The performance in this case relates to muscular contraction and as all our skeletal muscles depend upon different energy sources, which in turn depend upon the duration and intensity of the contractions, appropriate tests must reflect the predominant energy source used for these contractions.

Aerobic endurance

This is the ability of the body to supply oxygen to the working muscles and extract waste products which are transported in the bloodstream and the airways, to the atmosphere. The ultimate test for measuring the ability to perform aerobically is the Maximal Oxygen Uptake Test (VO_2max) (Sinning 1975). The test is designed to elicit the highest possible oxygen uptake a performer can achieve and can be administered using various work ergometers, the two most commonly used being the *cycle ergometer* and the *treadmill*. The protocol, which can be continuous or discontinuous, is similar irrespective of the work machine used. The

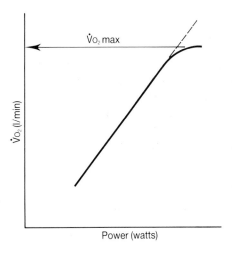

Fig. 6.1   Graph to show the point at which VO_2max has been reached. Note: If the point of deflection shown on the graph, is not achieved there are other criteria which can be considered in establishing whether VO_2max has been reached (BASS 1988). The final figure for VO_2max is usually expressed in units of millilitres of oxygen per kilogram of body weight per minute (ml/kg/min)

continuous method is the most widely used especially when testing sport performers. It consists of the subject working at a constant rate while measurements of the volume of expired air are being taken during the steady state of work. The expired air is then analysed for oxygen content and from the results the amount of oxygen used can be calculated. This procedure is repeated for further increments in work load and the test is terminated when the subject reaches a state of exhaustion and can no longer continue. If the values for oxygen uptake are plotted against their corresponding values of work or power the graph should be linear to a point where there is no further increase in oxygen uptake with further increases in work load. This point of deflection is known as the VO_2max (Fig. 6.1).

The equipment used for gas analysis and collection can range from a sophisticated on-line, fully computerized system or the more reliable and accurate on-line collection bag system. The latter involves collecting the expired air at each increment of work with a large plastic bag or rubber balloon. An extract from each bag is then analysed for oxygen content using either a modern electronic gas analyser or the more accurate, yet time consuming, chemical analyser.

Estimates for the value of VO_2max are often made by measuring heart rate (HR) at the same point as oxygen uptake (VO_2). If several measurements are made at submaximal levels the value of HR can be plotted on a graph against its corresponding value of VO_2. From the linear relationship which these two measurements form, the estimated value for VO_2max can be extrapolated using the criterion of maximum HR = 220 – Age (Fig. 6.2).

When gas analysis equipment is not available an estimated value of VO_2max can be made by recording the HR at the appropriate level of work and plotting this figure on an Åstrand Nomogram (Åstrand & Rodahl 1986).

Another test which does not give a direct value for VO_2max but which is widely used and related to the aerobic efficiency of the performer is the Physical Work Capacity Test (PWC). This can be taken at any level of HR but the most common is the PWC_{170} test which relates to the physical work capacity extrapolated at a heart rate of 170 beats/min (Wahlund 1948). This is a value which is considered for the majority of people to be a high but well tolerated working level. However, for sport performers an extrapolation would be more applicable if taken at maximum HR = 220 – Age.

Lactate endurance

This is the ability of the muscle to rely on anaerobic metabolism at any given point of submaximal intensity of exercise. The end product of this anaerobic metabolism is lactic acid and if not

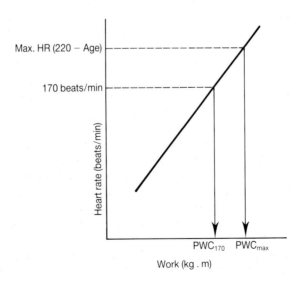

Fig. 6.2   Graph to show the physical work capacity at 170 beats/min and maximum HR

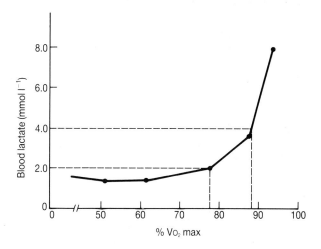

Fig. 6.3   Graph to show sudden increase in blood lactate

removed then muscle fatigue will inevitably occur. The test which ascertains the work level at which there is a dramatic increase in blood lactate is known as 'The onset of blood lactate accumulation test' (OBLA). This term is preferred to the old term of anaerobic threshold (Brooks & Fahey 1984). The test can be administered in conjunction with the VO_2max test. Blood sampling (finger prick of 50 microlitres) commences at a work load corresponding to 60% of the maximum and a further three collections made up to approximately 90% of maximum work load. When the figures for blood lactate are plotted against the corresponding values of % VO_2max it can be seen that at the blood lactate levels of 2mmol.1^{-1} and 4mmol.1^{-1} these are the limits between which there is a sudden and steep rise in blood lactate concentration (Fig. 6.3).

   This sudden rise in blood lactate level indicates a rapid rate of muscle glycogenolysis. This can result in glycogen depletion and consequent muscle fatigue. A rise in blood lactate levels indicates that the lactate entry into the blood is higher than can be removed and kept at reasonable levels. A failure to cope with lactate production during a performance will cause the pH of the blood to fall thus causing an additional fatigue factor during aerobic endurance activity.

   Therefore, it is important to realise, that when testing an endurance athlete the VO_2max test is not the sole criterion for assessing the aerobic capabilities of the performer (Skinner & McLellan 1980). Ultimately the VO_2max test gives an indication of the per-

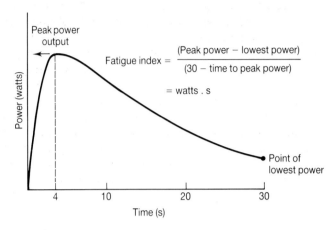

Fig. 6.4   Cycle-ergometer power curve

former's potential but does not indicate the level at which the performer can operate without higher levels of fatigue setting in.

Anaerobic endurance

This is the ability to maintain high levels of work intensity. In order to recover from such bouts of activity, ultimately will depend on the performer's tolerance to high levels of lactate produced locally within the muscle. The test most widely used to ascertain this ability is the 'Wingate Anaerobic Test' (Bar-Or 1987). This test consists of pedalling a front-loaded cycle ergometer which has a special timing device attached to the flywheel. This device measures fractions of a revolution of the flywheel and is linked to a computer. On command, the subject pedals the cycle at maximum speed and with a fixed load previously worked out according to body weight (Dotan & Bar-Or 1983). The number of revolutions is fed into the computer which, on termination of the test, prints out the results in a graph form of power (calculated by the fixed load and distance travelled in intervals of time) against the time interval (up to a maximum time of 30 seconds) (Fig. 6.4).

Instantaneous power

This is the ability of the body to explode into immediate action and relies exclusively upon the high energy phosphates stored within the muscles. Short bouts of high speed performance are synonymous with instantaneous power generation and the tests which are used to indicate this ability are of 10 seconds or less in duration. A simple test is the standing vertical jump which requires very little expensive equipment other than a vertical board marked in centimetre height intervals. The purpose of the jump board is to measure the standing vertical jump from standing reach, to jump and reach. The height obtained combined with the weight of the performer can indicate the explosive power output. A more sophisticated piece of equipment used to measure this component is the force platform. This registers the maximum downward force exerted by the subject at take-off. A sprint cycle test of a 10-second duration administered in an identical way to the 30-second *anaerobic endurance* test will provide the maximum peak power output.

STATISTICAL CRITERIA

Having decided upon the test and the equipment to be used, the next stage is to make certain that the test procedures follow certain statistical criteria:

- Validity
- Reliability
- Objectivity

Validity

This is a fundamental requirement of all testing procedures and asks whether the test measures what it is intended to measure. It indicates the relevance of the test and should take into consideration the principle of *specificity* (Sharkey 1988) of measurement, i.e. that the test corresponds as closely as possible with the purpose and mode of the exercise or training which it is intending to assess. Testing can be quite meaningless if the procedures employed are not specific to the sport in which the performer competes or the pattern and speed of movement of the various used muscle groups are not reconstructed within the test. A good example of non-specificity would be for a sprint cyclist to be tested on a treadmill for an aerobic assessment. Whether or not the principle of specificity can be adhered to will ultimately depend upon the type of equipment available within the laboratory and the different sport participants wanting to be assessed. Swimmers for example are very difficult to assess specifically, because they should be measured within the water and swimming at their own particular stroke. This would involve the use of a swimming flume—a very expensive piece of equipment.

A great deal of innovative design has gone into the specificity of laboratory testing equipment. This has helped to stimulate the various sports such as rowing, canoeing, skiing and skating. The obvious location for testing would be the environment in which the performance takes place and without restricted equipment such as tubing and mouthpieces. A system of telemetry overcomes this problem but the environmental changes which cannot be controlled make life very difficult for accurate results to be obtained.

As mentioned in the first part of this chapter a skill performance does not depend on fitness alone, for skill and mental attitudes play a significant role. As all physical tests measuring performance demands a certain level of skill the movement patterns of the performer must be reflected in the test. Running on a treadmill necessitates a different skill to running on the track and a test on a cycle ergometer is alien to a cyclist who is accustomed to a racing machine. Similarly, if a performer is not motivated enough to do well in a test this will reflect the results. It is important that the tester is aware of the precise reasons why test results have not achieved their expected limits.

Reliability

This implies that variables are accounted for and that the tests do measure what they are supposed to measure. The next criterion is, can the tests follow the same procedures under the same conditions and produce similar results? If this is so, they can be said to be *reliable*. In order to accept the reliability of a test a certain level of correlation must exist between the two sets of test scores.

Laboratory assessments score high on this criterion because there is a greater control over the environmental variables.

Objectivity

One of the problems which exists with the testing of sport performance is that one laboratory may have different equipment, procedures and trained personnel from another. This may affect the results of a subject who decides to be tested at two different venues. However, if the two sets of results are shown, as in reliability, to be highly correlated then the *objectivity* criterion is satisfied. The Sports Council in conjunction with the National Coaching Foundation have made a considerable effort to eliminate some of the objectivity problems. They asked members from the physiological section of the British Association of Sports Scientists (BASS) to develop test procedures and to recommend how testing centres may be staffed, equipped and managed. As a result of this exercise BASS produced an excellent document which states the guidelines to assist laboratories in ensuring that adequate precision and reliability of measurement is achieved and ensures consistency of procedures between different testing centres is available. They recommend that centres that may wish to implement the testing of human performance apply for creditation, thus ensuring that this criterion is satisfied on a national network. Only when a reliable network of national testing centres is established will there be a national data bank of reliable information available. This information will provide sport scientists and coaches a set of norms on which to compare the results of their tests.

THE USE OF TEST RESULTS

Providing the tests, the procedures and the criteria for testing have all been satisfied, one of the most important questions remains to be asked, 'What will the results of the test be used for?' The results of a fitness test, as sound as the intentions may have been, are quite meaningless if they are presented to the coach as a set of statistical data. The following criteria can be used as guidelines for the use of test results.

1. If reliable national norms are available and the test satisfy the criterion of objectivity, then the results can be compared to similar performers in the same sport, age and gender categories.
2. If the tests are reliable and repeated at regular intervals then the results can be compared to the performer's own, previous test results. This is particularly useful in assessing the benefits of training programmes and performance before and after injury.
3. If national norms are not considered to be reliable, or the laboratory uses different procedures, then the results can be compared to other performers under identical conditions in the same laboratory.

Whichever one of these criteria is chosen for the use of the results, the final outcome must provide the sport scientist, the coach, the performer, the medical practitioner and the physiotherapist with vital information from which they can evaluate the essential aspects of their important work in preparation for sport performance. A combination of the information acquired before and after the tests provides an educational base from which all concerned can co-operate to gain a greater understanding of the enhancement of sporting performance.

REFERENCES

AAHPER 1965 Youth fitness test manual (revised edition), NEA Publication, Washington DC

Åstrand P O, Rodahl K 1986 Textbook of work physiology 3rd edn McGraw Hill, New York

Bar-Or O 1987 The Wingate anaerobic test: an update of methodology, reliability and validity. Sports Medicine IV, 381–394

BASS 1988 Position statement on the physiological assessment of the elite competitor, second edn. White Line Press, Leeds

Brooks G A, Fahey T D 1984 Fundamentals of human performance. Macmillan, New York

Dirix A et al (eds) 1988 The Olympic book of sports medicine vol. 1, 121–150. Blackwell Scientific Publications, Oxford

Dotan R, Bar-Or O 1983 Load optimisation of the Wingate anaerobic test. European Journal of Applied Physiology 51: 409–417

Lange-Anderson K et al 1971 Fundamentals of exercise testing, World Health Organization, Geneva

Montoye H J 1978 An introduction to measurement in physical education. Allyn and Bacon, Newton, Mass

Sharkey B J 1988 Specificity of testing taken from advances in sports medicine and fitness. Vol. 1: 25–43, Year Book Medical Publisher, Chicago

Sinning W E 1975 Experiments and demonstrations in exercise physiology. W. B. Saunders, New York

Skinner J S, McLellan T H 1980 The transition from aerobic to anaerobic metabolism. Research Quarterly in Exercise and Sport 51: 234–248

Wahlund H 1948 Determination of physical working capacity. Acta Medica Scandinavica 132 (supplt.) 1

7. Diet in sport

It is being increasingly recognized that the basic nutritional needs of athletes do not differ significantly from those of non-athletes except in calorific requirements. Nevertheless, diet in sport has traditionally been subject to fads and nutritional quackery. The gullible athlete may then be lured into unnecessary expenditure in search of his competitive goals. Although most dietary indiscretions are harmless, certain among them, especially use of the supervitamins, may lead to deterioration in health.

GENERAL REQUIREMENTS

Approximately 90% of people in the United Kingdom have access to sufficient food abundantly to satisfy their nutritional needs. However, it has been demonstrated that some athletes living on their own do not take a well-balanced diet (Wagner 1976). Therefore if an athlete underperforms in comparison to his previous achievements, inadequate dietary intake should be excluded first in the search for an explanation.

Protein

Most European and American people obtain about 10–12% of their dietary energy (in a 2000–4000 kcal/d intake) from protein. This is equal to 50–120 g of protein daily. Protein losses occur by excretion in the urine, and this is not increased significantly during exercise. Protein is also lost in the faeces in a mean of 12 mg of nitrogen/kg of body-weight. Again, exercise does not seem to influence this loss in any way. Losses also occur during sweating, and thus during heavy activity this kind of nitrogen loss will increase. However, even exhausting exercise performed for 4 hours each day would produce a loss of only 1.2 g of nitrogen. This would require only 7.5 g of protein to replace and, since most physically active people take in at least 50 mg of protein daily, this is easily achieved (Norgan et al 1974). In brief, protein depletion is not a hazard, even in strength athletes.

Fat

Approximately 30% of dietary intake should derive from fats. Of these, vegetable fats should predominate.

Fat can only be used up in athletic activity if oxygen is present for its combustion and for the oxidation of free fatty acids. If, on the other hand, anaerobic metabolism takes place, carbohydrate is used as a fuel: it is broken down to lactic acid, which may inhibit the mobilization of free fatty acids. So the utilization of fats in strenuous activity will depend on the maximal oxygen uptake of the individual. Fit athletes are therefore more capable of using fat as an energy source than unfit people.

Carbohydrates

Fifty to sixty per cent of food intake should consist of carbohydrates. Although they yield only half as many calories per gram as fat, more calories per litre of oxygen are released by carbohydrates than fat. They are also necessary for glycogen storage in both muscle and liver.

During short periods of maximal exercise carbohydrate is probably the only energy source, but in prolonged, severe exercise a gradual decrease in muscle and liver glycogen will occur (Fig. 7.1). When exhaustion occurs the glycogen stores may be

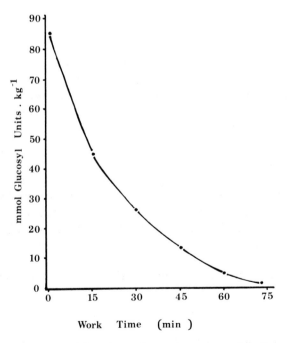

Fig. 7.1   Muscle glycogen content during 75 minutes of cycling at 85% maximal oxygen uptake

depleted (Hermanson et al 1967) but prolonged exercise can still be performed at less than 60–70% of maximal oxygen uptake, provided that the supply of free fatty acids (FFA) is adequate. It has also been noted that during such prolonged exercise glycogen stores are depleted to a greater degree in the slow twitch (type I) fibres which suggests that they are implicated in a major way in such activity (Costill et al 1973).

HEPATIC OUTPUT OF GLUCOSE DURING EXERCISE

Muscle lacks the enzyme glucose-6-phosphatase, which converts glucose-6-phosphate to glucose. Muscle glycogen cannot therefore be involved directly in blood glucose regulation, and this is done by the liver, the glycogen of which can be converted to glucose. Thus, during exercise, the output of glucose increases with the intensity and length of the exercise. Glucose elaborated from the liver may supply up to 40% of the energy of working muscle (Ahlborg et al 1974). Glucose output from glycogenolysis varies from 25–90% during exercise depending on whether the person takes a low- or high-carbohydrate diet.

Lactate is the most important source of gluconeogenesis and may account for as much as 50% of the hepatic glucose output at moderate work loads.

VITAMINS AND MINERALS

Since athletes undertake more strenuous activity than others it has been argued that their vitamin requirements may be significantly increased and also that deficiencies may occur if supplements are not taken. However, no properly controlled study in the world literature supports this contention.

Vitamin A

Vitamin A is present in animal fats and its precursor is found in carrots and green vegetables. Deficiency is associated with decreased immunity to infection and, in the young, eye complaints or stunted growth. These features are uncommon in the Western World and more attention has been given to overdose which can be fatal.

Athletes taking a reasonable diet are unlikely to suffer a lack of vitamin A.

Vitamin D

Sources include animal fats, cod and halibut oil. Vitamin D can be synthesized in the skin by the action of ultra-violet light on its precursor. This is important in people who have a low dietary intake of vitamin D. The limited sunshine in the West of Scotland was said to be responsible for the reappearance of rickets among Indian children. Adequate dietary intake is the ideal. However, supplements may have to be given to vegetarians.

Vitamin E

It has been observed in certain species of animal that lack of vitamin E causes dystrophic changes to occur in muscle. Under stress, it is postulated, an athlete could potentially suffer deficiency and subsequent decreased performance. Initial studies by Prokop (1960) suggested that administration of vitamin E did improve performance. However, in 1957 Thomas failed to demonstrate any benefit, and more recently Sharman et al (1976) found no increased performance in swimmers on large doses compared to a placebo group. It is therefore a reasonable conclusion that vitamin E has no ergogenic properties, at least under the conditions of these studies.

Vitamin C

Ascorbic acid (vitamin C) is inexpensive, but it is most unlikely that deficiency will occur with the normal British diet. There is no evidence that supplements improve athletic performance (Gey et al 1970), despite the enormous quantities that must be flushed away daily in toilets all over the world. Vitamin C is involved in adrenal metabolism.

Vitamin B

Thiamine, riboflavin and niacin are the best known of this complex. All are involved in carbohydrate metabolism and they are the only vitamins which may have significance for muscular activity and performance in people who are not suffering from malnutrition (Durnin 1982). Supplements have not been shown to improve performance but deficiency will adversely affect training. Daily intakes should be 0.44 mg of riboflavin, 0.35 mg of thiamine and 6.6 mg of niacin per 1000 kcal (DHSS 1969).

VITAMIN B_{15}

Pangamic acid (vitamin B_{15}) is occasionally represented to athletes as the missing ingredient for excellence. One of the so-called 'supervitamins', its use can, however, be associated with toxicity. It is a combination of dichloroacetate and dimethylglycine hydrochloride (DMG). When this latter substance reacts with saliva, dimethylnitrosamine, a potent carcinogen is formed. The use of supervitamins without evidence of efficacy from controlled clinical trials must be vigorously discouraged. This is our responsibility and can only be achieved through coach and athlete education (Smith 1982).

Minerals

Of the minerals, iron is worthy of comment, mainly because of its role in the formation of the haemoglobin molecule but also because there is a sharp contrast in requirements between the sexes. There are very few diets in which inadequate intake of iron would exist in exercising males whereas women may not even have an adequate intake from an ordinary mixed diet. For a healthy woman the average daily requirement is 12–15 mg. Many female athletes, therefore, undertake exercise with ranging degrees of anaemia. Regular blood checks should be carried out and supplementation medically prescribed. Anaemia should not be regarded as a nutritional problem which is to be self-managed. If it is not corrected with supplementation under supervision further investigation is obviously required.

FLUID AND MINERAL REPLACEMENTS DURING TRAINING

In endurance sports such as marathon running, cycling or tennis fluid loss through sweating can become quite significant. For instance up to 8% of body weight may be lost during a marathon despite fluid ingestion (13–14% of body water). Dehydration is poorly tolerated with exercise. Both heart rate and body temperature climb and heat exhaustion results.

During sweating more water than ions is removed from the body fluids (Costill & Miller 1980) so that there is an increased concentration of remaining electrolytes. This stresses the point that fluid replacement (with water) is more important than increased ion/ electrolyte intake.

The temperature of the ingested fluid is important both in relation to its absorption and cooling effects. Good evidence exists (Costill & Miller 1980) that small quantities of cold water in volumes of 150–180 ml taken three to four times per hour are more effective than warm fluids. Large volumes do empty more rapidly from the stomach but gastric bagging and breathing discomfort may be experienced. There is no evidence that cold fluids produce cramping, and distress is more related to the volume intake than the temperature.

Small amounts of fluid, preferably water or hypotonic solutions of glucose or electrolytes, minimize the risks of dehydration in heavy exercise if taken regularly and have dramatic effects on plasma volume when compared to similar exercise conditions without fluids. In cool weather conditions where dehydration is not a major problem the athlete should ingest larger quantities of solutions containing carbohydrate, but less frequently. The slow gastric release of carbohydrate may then provide a steady energy source for the active tissues.

During repetitive exhaustive exercise over days or weeks the risk of chronic dehydration is also reduced by the same fluid regimens. Renal conservation of sodium and potassium occur to a degree and provided that there is a dietary intake of approximately 80 mmol/d of potassium, chronic electrolyte depletion and dehydration are not major problems.

DIETARY MANIPULATION
Anabolic steroids

The strength athlete above all is tempted to improve his performance by the use of anabolic steroids. Despite intense interest there are a very few authoritative reports on the short-term effects of these and even less on their long-term effects. The reasons for this shortage are ethical—it is inappropriate to carry out long-term studies on human volunteers.

The use of steroids is increasing and there is evidence of drugs being self-administered in large doses. In one study doses of > 400 mg of methandienone daily were noted (Fitzgerald & McLatchie 1980). Anecdotally, the athlete on steroids is less susceptible to fatigue (Freed et al 1975) and injury. However, Sharp (1979) had suggested that tendon injuries may occur more commonly during steroid administration because of a disproportionate increase in muscle strength in relation to tendon strength.

There are well-documented complications of steroid ingestion. In the prepubertal male, accelerated epiphyseal development and diminished height have been reported (Marginal comment 1973), as had gynaecomastia (Laron 1962). Acne is one of the most unacceptable complications to the user of steroids (Marginal comment 1973). After puberty adult sexual function may be altered because of the suppression of pituitary luteinizing hormone. Animal experiments confirm this. There is resultant diminution in the production of testosterone and in spermatogenesis. Theoretically, normal testicular maturation can also be disrupted (Bovis & Stevenson 1970). Alteration in liver function tests has been observed in all age groups during administration. Cholestatic jaundice, abnormal thyroid function tests and changes in plasma proteins have all been observed. These changes revert after cessation of administration.

In weightlifters the most common reasons for stopping the drugs were acne, headache, nausea or dizziness.

The orally active steroids are hepatotoxic if chronically ingested and they have been associated with primary liver cancers (Wynn 1975). Hyperinsulinism has also been noted. This has been identified as a significant factor in the development of atherosclerosis, especially of the coronary arteries. Abnormal glucose tolerance curves may also occur, leading to diabetes mellitus (Wynn 1975).

In Britain use of steroids is illegal and detection techniques are becoming more accurate. Radio immunoassay is a standard method. However, as athletes use more testosterone-related steroid refinements even this method can fail. Who can accuse a man of cheating just because he has too much testosterone in his body?

There is another side to the coin. From Eastern European countries we receive anecdotal reports of the medical monitoring of athletes on steroids. After their careers are over they are weaned safely off them. No official reports have been published, but if the athletes remain in good health and given that large numbers of athletes in all countries will continue to abuse steroids this would appear to be one method of preserving their health. Doctors may have ethical objections to the use of steroids but still have a responsibility to their patients. Perhaps if we cannot eradicate steroids throughout the world (and this could only be done by effective international liaison and life bans on all offenders) we should, as doctors, at least monitor those of our patients who use them.

Glycogen loading

Glycogen loading is a dietary technique developed to enable endurance athletes (especially marathon runners) to build up stores of muscle glycogen. Work output and subsequent recovery are increased but it is not clear how frequently the dietary regime can be repeated with good results. There is also some suggestion that for older athletes the technique can be dangerous because of the risk of inducing water retention.

TECHNIQUE

The aim is to deplete existing muscle glycogen stores by moderately heavy exercise. Then a high protein diet is taken for a short period. Thereafter for the 2–3 days before the race the diet

Table 7.1 Muscle glycogen as influenced by diet (Sharman 1981)

	Glycogen content g/100 g muscle	Average walk time (min)
After a normal mixed diet	1.75	126
After protein fat diet	0.63	59
After almost wholly carbohydrate diet	3.3	189

Table 7.2 High-protein–fat diet (Sharman 1981)

Breakfast:	Lean bacon Eggs 1 slice starch-reduced bread, diabetic marmalade Tea/coffee, synthetic sweetener, milk
Lunch:	Lamb chop/steak Brussels sprouts, runner beans Yoghurt/cheese Tea/coffee/milk
Supper:	Grilled cod Cauliflower/tomato Cheese, one slice starch-reduced bread Tea/coffee/milk

Table 7.3 High carbohydrate diet (Sharman 1981)

Breakfast:	Porridge/cornflakes, milk, sugar Toast, marmalade Tea/coffee, milk, sugar
Lunch:	Sausages, chipped potatoes, baked beans in tomato sauce Gateau Tea/coffee, milk, sugar
Supper:	Soup Roast beef, Yorkshire pudding, potatoes, peas Canned peaches, custard Tea/coffee, milk, sugar

consists almost exclusively of carbohydrate. Typical diets are illustrated in Tables 7.1–7.3.

ADVANTAGES

1. Increased muscle and liver glycogen stores
2. Lower fluid requirements during a marathon
3. Shorter recovery time

DISADVANTAGES

1. Slight increase in body weight (? due to water retention: glycogen retains water)

2. Increased water retention could be dangerous for the older or post-coronary marathon runner
3. The advantageous effects may not be reproducible on repeated loading
4. Heavy meals of carbohydrate may be dangerous for middle-aged athletes

Although a slight increase in body weight occurs this does not seem troublesome and is partially offset by the weight loss while on the protein diet (Heeley et al 1975). The dangers of heavy meals in middle-aged runners have been emphasized by a case report of one runner who ate almost two whole loaves at one sitting and developed chest pain (Mirkin & Spring 1973). Such excesses should obviously be avoided.

One final point is that while glycogen loading may assist marathon runners it is probably only of value to runners who exercise at 75–80% of their maximal oxygen uptake. Most people in popular marathons do not train or run at anything near this level. They do not therefore make any great gains from excessive carbohydrate loading. Such people should be encouraged simply to maintain a mixed diet with increased carbohydrate to meet their training requirements.

Making the weight

Weight reduction is important in sport. Widely used methods include voluntary fasting or dehydration for weight-loss. Plastic and rubber suits are used during practice as are saunas, steam rooms and artificial heat devices. Diuretics and cathartics are commonly used. Even voluntary spitting is resorted to, in an attempt to lose extra ounces. All these methods promote water loss.

When fluid and food restriction is practised, water, fat and protein are all lost. Such dehydration is accompanied by major side-effects:

1. Reduction in muscular strength
2. Decreased work performance
3. Increased heart rate when attempting to perform the same degree of work
4. Dehydration associated with decreased glycogen storage in the liver.

All of these changes impede normal growth in the young athlete and will produce profound weakness in the adult.

The ideal weight should be determined by skinfold measurements and the recommended weight for the individual's height and build should be aimed at, taking into account the sport involved. The desired weight should be identified early in the training season and the athlete should reduce to this over at least 4 weeks. This is best done by modest dietary reduction accompanied by a modest increase in training.

For weight-gain the aim is to increase muscle mass through increased intake and increased training, usually with weights. Increased food intake can be achieved by adding two or three extra snacks per day and the diet should be low in fat but high in carbohydrate.

Caffeine as a stimulant

Coffee or tea drinking (containing up to 200 mg and 80 mg of caffeine per cup respectively) have been used by athletes to stimulate the cardiovascular system in the hope that better performance will result. Other sources of caffeine include certain soft drinks, such as cola and Lucozade. The training effect sought is reduced heart rate and blood pressure in response to increased exercise load. However, both are increased with caffeine and sleeplessness or cardiac arrhythmias can result even from relatively light ingestion (Goldstein et al 1969, Clark & Olson 1973). While there may be some benefits they have yet to be demonstrated in a controlled study. We recommend temperance in tea and coffee drinking while strongly encouraging an effective training programme.

DRUG ABUSE IN SPORT

In the late 1960s following the amphetamine related deaths of several cyclists, the International Olympic Committee (IOC) set up a Medical Commission in charge of eradicating drug abuse in Olympic sports. Testing for drugs first took place in the Mexico Games of 1968 and steroid detection was made possible in Montreal in 1976 after the development of a reliable, radio-immunoassay technique at St Thomas' Hospital, London. This revolutionized doping control by testing urine samples for banned substances with the ultimate aim of eradicating the use of performance-enhancing drugs.

Definitions

The doping definition of the IOC Medical Commission is based on the banning of pharmacological classes of agents so that new drugs, some specifically designed for doping, may also be banned.

DOPING CLASSES

1. Stimulants
2. Narcotics
3. Anabolic steroids
4. Beta blockers
5. Diuretics
6. Peptide hormones and analogues

DOPING METHODS

1. Blood doping
2. Pharmacological, chemical and physical manipulation

CLASSES OF DRUGS SUBJECT TO CERTAIN RESTRICTIONS

1. Alcohol
2. Marijuana
3. Local anaesthetics
4. Corticosteroids

Prevalence

Official estimates of the prevalence of drug taking is usually about 2% of all samples. This is based on the failed urine test at major championships, but is generally recognized as an underestimate due to sample bias. The Dexa Institute, the Italian branch of the Gallup research institute interviewed 1015 athletes and 216 technicians (coaches, doctors, managers) on the prevalence of drug abuse. The two most popular drugs amphetamines and steroids were estimated as being used by between 10 to 20% of athletes and considered to be effective. The dangers were also appreciated by more than 80% of those interviewed. Nevertheless many athletes were willing to risk serious side-effects. Most (63%) felt that winning was the main motivating force. Supplies of illegal drugs were readily available and those abusing them had been encouraged to do so. However, 66% of the survey population supported tighter control on drug abuse. Paradoxically despite this general attitude the introduction of random drug testing in the USA has provoked controversy through the Fourth Amendment of the United States Constitution which states that 'citizens must be secure from unreasonable searches and procedures'. Legal precedent states that random urine testing is a search, but is it unreasonable? As a result several cases of legal action are already underway against sporting authorities and it has been suggested that sporting authorities may have to return to health promotion campaigns until these legal questions are answered.

SAFE PRESCRIBING FOR SPORTS PARTICIPANTS

Doctors may unwittingly be manipulated into prescribing banned substances by unscrupulous individuals or quite innocently prescribe agents for common ailments which are illegal in sport and lead to the athlete being banned. Full information of the banned list is available from the Sports Council, Walkden House, 3–10 Melton Street, London NW1 2EB, telephone 071–383 5667/5411.

The International Olympic Committee (IOC) on the advice of the Medical Commission has drawn up a list of banned substances all of which have been abused at some time.

Banned substances

Drugs to avoid prescribing include:

- *Systemic corticosteroids*
- *Non-selective adrenoreceptor agonists* like adrenaline, noradrenaline isoprenaline, ephedrine, pseudo-ephedrine. Medicines containing phenylpropanolamine used in relief of the common cold, will be banned in the future.
- *Selective beta 2-adreno-receptor agonists* are permissible only by inhalation or insufflation. They are banned parenterally or orally.
- *All opiates.* Some are found in antidiarrhoeal compounds and cough mixtures.
- *Local anaesthetics*—lignocaine, cocaine, etc.—unless injected on its own into a synovial space with or without corticosteroid. The date given and diagnosis must be declared before a competition.
- *Diuretics.* These have been abused in strength and combat sports to make the weight. All are banned.
- *Beta-adreno receptor antagonists.* These drugs are effective in bowling and shooting because they control tremor and slow the pulse.

Permissible agents under certain circumstances

- *Topical steroids*
- Selective beta 2-adreno-receptor agonists *by inhalation*
- *Sodium cromoglycate* (but INTAL is banned by the IOC because it also contains isoprenaline)
- *Aminophylline or theophylline formulations*
- *Loperamide* and *combinations of diphenoxylate and atropine* are permitted, also *hyoscine,* for the treatment of diarrhoea and relief of abdominal colic respectively.

- *NSAIDs* may be used freely for pain relief.
- *Anticonvulsants* may be taken provided they are declared.
- *Hypnotics* may be prescribed freely except in modern pentathletes. Further information should be sought when dealing with these athletes.

REFERENCES

Ahlborg G, Fehg P, Hagenfeldt L, Hendler R, Wahren J 1974 Substrate turnover during prolonged exercise in man. Journal of Clinical Investigation 53: 1080

Bovis A, Stevenson R H 1970 Comparative androgenic myotrophic and anti-gonadotrophic properties of some anabolic steroids. Steroids 15: 61–65

Clark A, Olson C B 1973 Effect of caffeine and isoprenaline on mammalian ventricular muscle. British Journal of Pharmacology 47: 1–7

Costill D L, Gollnick P D, Jansson E C et al 1973 Glycogen depletion pattern in human muscle fibres during distance running. Acta Physiologica Scandinavica 89: 374–383

Costill D L, Miller J M 1980 Nutrition for endurance sport. Carbohydrate and fluid balance. International Journal of Sports Medicine 1: 2–14

DHSS 1969 Recommended intakes of nutrients for the United Kingdom. Department of Health and Social Security Reports on Public Health and Medical Subjects 120. Her Majesty's Stationery Office, London

Durnin J V G A 1982 Muscle in sports medicine—nutrition and muscular performance. International Journal of Sports Medicine 1(3): 52–56

Fitzgerald B, McLatchie G R 1980 Degenerative joint disease in weightlifters—fact or fiction. British Journal of Sports Medicine 14(283): 97–101

Freed D L J, Banks A J M, Longson D, Busley D M 1975 Anabolic steroids in athletes: crossover double blind trial on weightlifters. British Medical Journal 2: 471–474

Gey G O, Cooper K H, Bottenberg R A 1970 Effect of ascorbic acid on endurance performance and athletic injury. Journal of the American Medical Association 211: 105

Goldstein A, Kaizar S, Whitby O 1969 Psychotropic effects of caffeine in man. IV. Clinical Pharmacology and Therapeutics 10: 489–492

Heeley D M, Sharman I M, Cooper D F 1975 Variations in the composition of blood and urine following the ingestion of a high protein diet. Proceedings of the Nutrition Society 34: 69A

Hermanson L, Hultman E, Saltin B 1967 Muscle glycogen and prolonged severe exercise. Acta Physiologica Scandinavica 71: 129–139

Laron Z 1962 Breast development induced by methandrostenolone (Dianabol). Journal of Clinical Endocrinology 22: 450

Marginal comment 1973 American Journal of Diseases in Childhood 125: 479

Mirkin G, Spring S 1973 Carbohydrate loading: a dangerous practice. Journal of the American Medical Association 223: 13, 1511–1512

Norgan N G, Ferro-Luzzi A, Durnin J V G A 1974 The energy and nutrient intake and the energy expenditure of 204 New Guinean adults. Philosophical Transactions of the Royal Society of London 268: 309–348

Prokop L 1960 Die Wirking von naturlichem Vitamin E auf Sauerstoffverbrauch und Sauerstoffschuld. Sportarztliche Praxis 1: 19

Sharman I M 1981 Glycogen loading: advantages but positive disadvantages. British Journal of Sports Medicine 15(1): 20–23

Sharman I M, Down M G, Norgan N G 1976 The effect of vitamin E on physiological function and athletic performance of trained swimmers. Journal of Sport Medicine and Physical Fitness 16: 215

Sharp N C C 1979 Sports injuries (lecture). Department of Physical Education, University of Birmingham

Smith N J 1982 Nutrition in the athlete. American Journal of Sports Medicine 10: 253–255

Thomas P 1957 The effects of vitamin E on some aspects of athletic efficiency. PhD Thesis, University of Southern California, Los Angeles

Wagner R 1976 Nutrition in athletics. Coach and Athlete 28, 29: 36–37

Wynn V 1975 Metabolic effects of anabolic steroids. British Journal of Sports Medicine 9, 2, 60–64

8. The value and limitations of protective equipment

The risk of injury can be reduced considerably by protective equipment. Although its efficacy and design may in certain sports, be dictated more by social values than by biomechanical characteristics, it should fulfil the following criteria:

1. It should be light, durable and comfortable
2. It should permit a full range of normal movement
3. It should be protective and remain so through a wide temperature range
4. It should be safe to wear.

HEAD PROTECTION

Sports which make use of headgear are increasing—American football, winter sports, cricket, climbing and aerial sports. The value of protective headgear in reducing the incidence of head injury in motor-cycle and autosport racing accidents has been established (Dooley & Trinca, 1978, Whitaker 1976). In steeplechasing also, primary serious head injury and cumulative brain damage have been reduced after the recommendations of Foster (1976), Allen (1976) and d'Abreu (1976). The helmet design now in use is similar to the motor-cycle crash helmet.

During boxing training sessions head protection is regularly worn and in those countries which have made headgear compulsory for boxers a decrease in the frequency of knockouts from 4% to 0.3% of all fights has been observed (Schmid et al 1968). In addition, the use of padded or sprung flooring also protects against serious head injury in combat sports (Fig. 8.1).

Helmet design

The design should take into account the risk of injury in the particular sport. In order to be effective certain design criteria must be satisfied:

1. The physical efficiency of the helmet is dependent on the type of material used and its absorptive capacity. There is an optimum which varies with temperature.

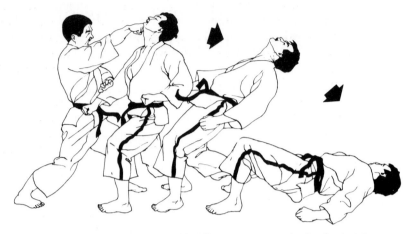

Fig. 8.1   The use of sprung or padded flooring prevents further brain injury after knockdowns, falls or throws in combat sports

2. Shell deflection is related to the rigidity of the material. A totally ungiving helmet provides the best deflection but would be too heavy to wear. It also increases the risk of neck injury by increasing flexion or extension of the neck during acceleration/deceleration of the head.
3. Energy absorption space permits a lighter structure. Two variations of this concept are a foam-lined helmet shell and a suspension helmet. The latter has an advantage over the foam-lined helmet in its ability to absorb energy. However, in rapid decelerations the head may strike the inside of the shell.

Dangers of headgear

The balance to be achieved in helmet design would appear to lie between rigidity (and therefore weight) and efficiency. The dangers of heavy helmets have been highlighted in sports parachuting, where they can weigh as much as 2 kg. On landing, exaggerated cervical flexion can occur to such a degree that sternal fracture and atrial rupture results (chin–sternum–heart syndrome, Simson 1971).

In motor sports, when an integral crash helmet (full-face) is often worn, rebreathing has been described as occurring, leading to transient light-headedness or blackout. Attention should be paid to the air-conditioning of such helmets, especially when worn with flame-proof balaclavas and bibs (Greenbaum et al 1982).

In American football sternal rupture, cardiac rupture and abdominal visceral injury have followed butting tackles by helmeted players. But, contrary to popular belief, the American National Athletic Injury/Illness Reporting System (NAIRS) has not confirmed that helmets increase the risk of cervical injuries in American football (Clark & Powell 1979).

Too little protection may be given by traditional types of protective headgear. Fatal accidents are more common among horse and pony riders than in those taking part in motor or motorcycling sports and head injuries are extremely common. Although legislation now compels younger equestrians to wear proper protective headgear fashion appears more likely to persuade them to do so. Under the Young Riders Protective Headgear Bill, which became Law in 1990, children of 14 and under must wear an approved hat, suitably harnessed, when riding on the highway (Fig. 8.2).

In the Pony Club, it is compulsory for competing riders to wear either an approved jockey skull cap (BS4472) or a riding hat with a flexible peak (BS6473). Stable lads are not insured unless wearing ND4472 type caps and a change in attitude towards the use of this type of cap by the 3 million people who ride for pleasure would be welcome and probably reduce the high incidence of head injuries sustained in riding accidents.

EYE PROTECTION (See Chapter 17)

In racket sports the eyes are best protected by protective spectacles/visor or goggles, which deepen the orbital margins thus preventing the entry of missiles (Fig. 8.3). One prerequisite of the design of such protection is the preservation of good peripheral vision. In contact sports, e.g. hockey, ice-hockey, and combat sports like fencing, face–eye protectors are of most value. Such measures have reduced the number of injuries by as much as 90% and they are now universally accepted (Pashby 1977).

In water activities goggles prevent keratitis and offer better underwater vision than contact lenses because they keep air in contact with the cornea. This allows for clearer vision.

Dangers of eye protection

Firm contact lenses have produced corneal oedema in divers, and soft lenses have caused infection. Globe rupture is a risk if goggles rebound and elastic strapping has been incriminated in cases where this has happened. Wearers of goggles should be made aware of such dangers.

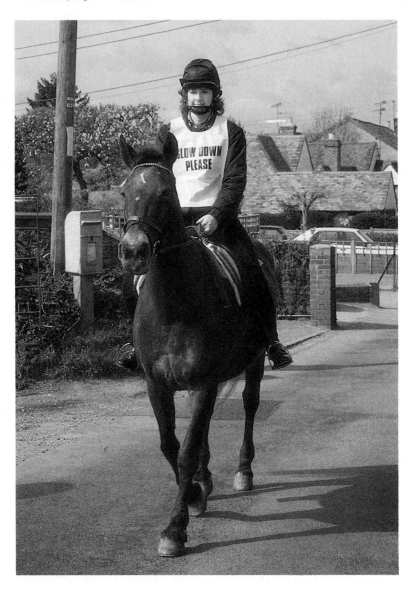

Fig. 8.2   Protective clothing for horse-riding

MOUTH PROTECTION
Gumshields

Dental injury is almost totally preventable in collision sports, including squash. The most effective shield is one designed by a

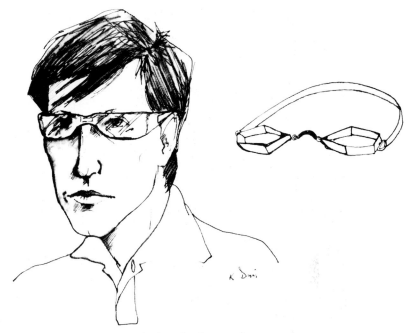

Fig. 8.3   Protective spectacles/goggles for squash

dental surgeon. In the case of children and adolescents regular fittings are recommended. This may involve extra expenditure but the long-term gains in dental preservation are well worthwhile.

DANGERS OF GUMSHIELDS

A poorly fitting shield will produce problems. This commonly results from the use of preformed or self-fitting shields. While inhalation is unlikely, discomfort and dental injury are extremely common.

PROTECTION OF THE NECK

Most neck protection in sport is from penetrating trauma, as in fencing and kendo (Fig. 8.4). It is known that the current equipment is satisfactory but freak accidents have occurred because of poorly fitting protective gear.

In collision sports neck strengthening, referee awareness and skill training are the most important factors in injury prevention. Silver (1983) reports that, due to more efficient headgear, serious cervical injury is being seen more commonly after motor accidents. Such patients would previously have succumbed to head injuries.

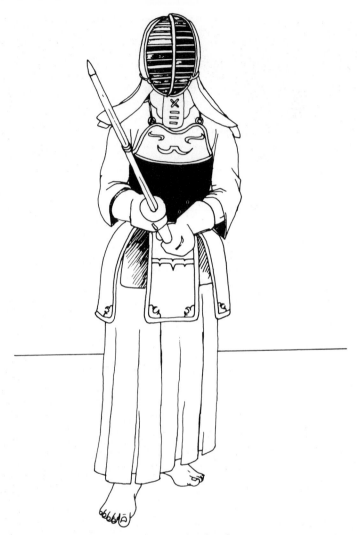

Fig. 8.4   Traditional protective gear used in kendo

ARM AND HAND PROTECTION

Padding of various types is effective in reducing bruising to the
arms. Fractures will still occur, however, if the impact is violent.
In boxing, bandages are effective in reducing the incidence of hand
injuries and gloves protect both the fighter and his opponent. The
incidence of hand and facial injuries was considerably reduced in
karate after the introduction of protective hand padding (Fig. 8.5).
The only remaining danger was that in the controlled-contact style

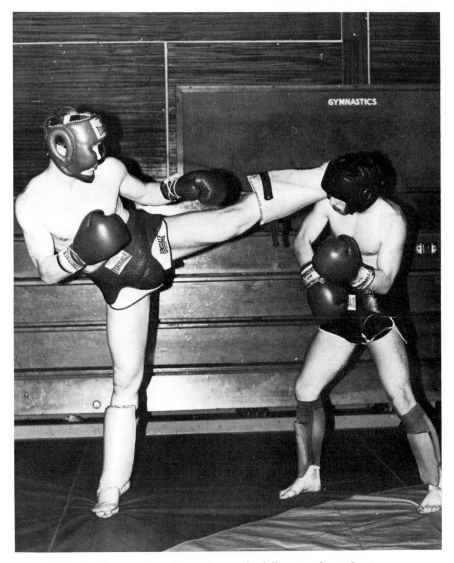

Fig. 8.5 Correct protective equipment for full contact karate/boxing

blows might be landed with unmitigated force instead of pulled just short of target (McLatchie & Morris 1977).

GROIN PROTECTION

In combat and missile sports such as cricket the competitor is protected by a groin guard. However, many players do not wear

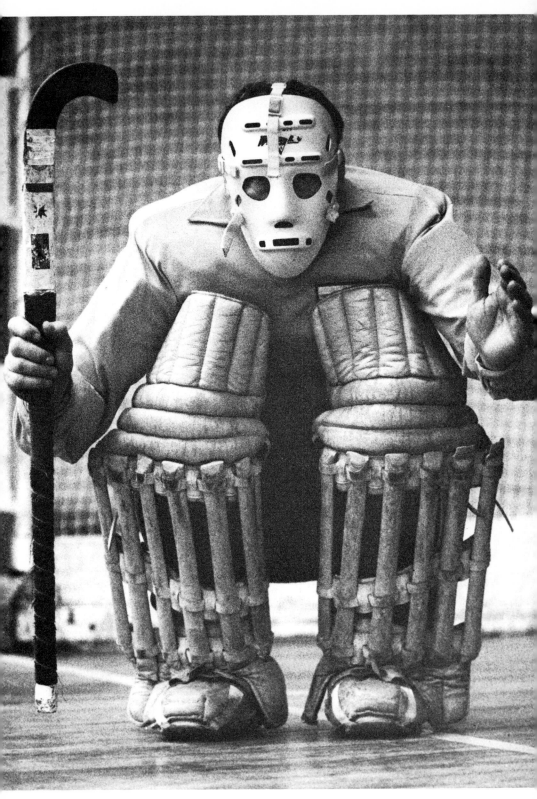

Fig. 8.6 Example of protective equipment in hockey

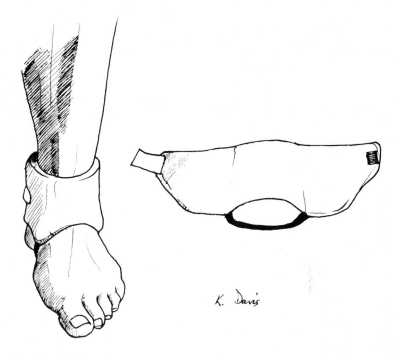

K. Davis

Fig. 8.7   Ankle pads

them. In karate not wearing such a guard results in disqualification, which is rough justice since the discovery is usually made after the injury is sustained!

The standard cricket box is adequate but can produce extensive bruising if struck firmly. It may also easily be dislodged by a rising kick. The most efficient guards are those worn by boxers, but they tend to be expensive.

THIGH AND LEG PROTECTION

Padding extending up the thigh is now standard for cricket batsmen, hockey goalkeepers (Fig. 8.6) and American footballers. It prevents haematoma of the thigh and anterior tibial compartment. In Scandinavian countries footballers are not insured unless they wear shin pads. The incidence of lower limb fractures is considerably reduced when shin pads are worn.

ANKLE AND FOOT PROTECTION

Protection of the ankle in football is a recent innovation. Modern low-cut football boots afford little protection to the ankle. The pads

used consist of heavy-duty reinforced foam with an outer covering. They are held in position by an elasticated Velcro-snap
fastening at the back (Fig. 8.7).

In outdoor sports such as skiing, hill walking and climbing,
protection of the ankle is achieved by the design of the boot. Proper
riding boots are recommended in equestrian sports. Ski bindings
also provide a protective mechanism which prevents injury. However, they have limitations of which the skier should be aware.
They will not protect the leg under all circumstances, although
their effectiveness can be increased by proper installation, maintenance and an anti-friction device (Bahniuk & Zamir 1976). Without question, however, the skill of the participant is the major
factor in preventing skiing injuries (Garrick & Requa 1977).

REFERENCES

Allen W 1976 Brain damage in jockeys (letter). Lancet 1: 1135
Bahniuk E, Zamir I 1976 Characteristics of antifriction devices used for ski
    bindings. Orthopaedic Clinics of North America 7(1): 105–115
Clark K, Powell J 1979 Football helmets and neurotrauma—an epidemiological
    overview of three seasons. Medicine, Science and Sports 11: 138
D'Abreu F 1976 Brain damage in jockeys (letter). Lancet 1: 1241
Dooley B J, Trinca G W 1978 Value of protective headgear in reducing head
    injuries. In: Heulke D F (ed) Proceedings of the American Association for
    Automotive Medicine, 22nd Conference, Illinois. A A A M 49
Foster J 1976 Brain damage in National Hunt jockeys. Lancet 1: 981
Garrick J G, Requa R 1977 The role of instruction in preventing ski injuries.
    The Physician and Sportsmedicine 5 12: 57–59
Greenbaum R, Malino A F, Davies R, Baskett R J F 1982 Rebreathing in a
    subject wearing an integral crash helmet. British Medical Journal 284:
    774–775
McLatchie G R, Morris E W 1977 Prevention of karate injuries—a progress
    report. British Journal of Sports Medicine 11: 78–82
Pashby T J 1977 Eye injuries in Canadian hockey. Phase II. Canadian Medical
    Association Journal 117: 671–678
Schmid L, Hajik E, Blonstein L 1968 Experinece with headgear in boxing.
    Journal of Sports Medicine and Physical Fitness 8: 171
Silver J 1983 Interview statement. 'Mind How You Go', BBC Television
Simson L R 1971 Chin–sternum–heart syndrome—cardiac injury associated
    with parachuting mishaps. Aerospace Medicine 42: 1214
Whitaker J 1976 Motor cycle safety: accident survey and rider injuries,
    supplementary report 239. Transport and Road Research Laboratory, Bucks

9. General medical problems in sport

INTRODUCTION

Participation by the general public in a wide range of sporting activities is increasing as a means of improving levels of fitness. Doctors must now be prepared to give advice on many aspects of participation in such sports. Three areas of advice are particularly relevant:

1. General advice to be given to anyone, particularly if aged over 35, who wishes to participate in vigorous sport.
2. Advice to those patients with pre-existing chronic disease who wish to continue their participation, or take up a sport despite their disease.
3. Specialized advice about the medical problems that may arise in sportsmen and women, of all levels of ability, as a result of their sporting activities.

GENERAL ADVICE

Anybody aged over 35 who wishes to take part in vigorous sport should have a comprehensive medical examination similar to that for a life assurance policy. This will identify potential risk factors such as excessive weight, smoking, heavy alcohol intake, or family history of ischaemic heart disease. Such an examination may also reveal pre-existing, but previously undiagnosed disease such as hypertension or diabetes. Any suspicious symptoms such as chest pain means that further investigation, including the appropriate specialist referral, is mandatory before allowing that individual to participate in any form of sport. Any identifiable risk factor should be corrected. Most deaths in sport occur in those individuals with clearly identifiable risk factors that have not been corrected (Opie 1975).

ADVICE TO PATIENTS WITH PRE-EXISTING DISEASE

The detection or pre-existence of any chronic disease such as hypertension is not an absolute contraindication to an individual's participation in sport provided that appropriate advice is obtained regarding choice of sport and the intensity of participation. Many chronic diseases grossly restrict the choice of sport.

Such diseases include most forms of chronic inflammatory arthritis and neurological disorders such as multiple sclerosis or traumatic paraplegia. Such chronic problems are best catered for by the many sporting organizations now in existence for the disabled athlete.

However many diseases do not severely disable. The most common diseases in this category include hypertension, asthma, diabetes and epilepsy.

Cardiovascular diseases

Chest pain in athletes is not always due to angina. Other causes are common and include tracheitis or musculo-skeletal pain. Similarly a systolic murmur detected on examination may well be benign. However a cardiologist's opinion may be required to exclude structural defects such as valvular diseases or coronary artery obstruction. Medical examination in these cases may include exercise testing and angiography. Hypertension is a risk factor for myocardial infarction and the risk is accentuated by prolonged severe exercise, particularly isometric exercise. Advice to sportsmen and women with hypertension is thus to refrain until their diastolic blood pressure is well controlled and to choose a sport which does not require prolonged isometric exercise. Additionally they should maintain a normal weight and a regular exercise programme and probably undergo an exercise stress test to determine the blood pressure response to exercise.

A previous history of myocardial infarction does not present a major hazard to subsequent exercise and sporting activity. Rehabilitation programmes for such patients are now widely advocated and practised and an increased wellbeing and ability to cope has been demonstrated in patients who have undergone these programmes (Gloag 1985). It is also likely that such a training programme ultimately reduces myocardial oxygen requirements for a given exercise load and thus enhances myocardial oxygen delivery in patients with coronary artery disease (Nagle et al 1983). A further possibility is that exercise elevates HDL lipoprotein levels and thus increases protection against subsequent coronary artery disease (Altekruse and Wilmore 1973).

Respiratory disease

The commonest respiratory disease affecting athletes is asthma, but there is no reason why participation in sport should be limited. The cardinal symptoms are wheezing and breathlessness which comes on five to ten minutes after exercise. Such patients are frequently symptom-free at rest. The most likely mechanism for such exercise-induced asthma is increased respiratory heat exchange associated with an increase in minute ventilation (McFadden & Ingram 1979). Inhalation of a beta–2-agonist before exercise is the treatment of choice in mild asthma although more severe cases may require suppressive treatment with regular inhalation of steroid. Exercise-induced bronchospasm is directly proportional to the intensity of exercise and the mechanism is related to expiratory heat exchange. Swimming is thus less likely to provoke attacks than running or cycling (Fitch & Morton 1971).

Diabetes

Any diabetic participating in vigorous sport should have a precise and clear idea of their diabetic control using frequent urinalysis, or more preferably capillary blood monitoring. They should be aware of their own particular signs of loss of control due to either hyper- or hypoglycaemia. Modification of their insulin requirements using small doses of insulin before exercise, or supplementary carbohydrate afterwards, may be required depending on their sport activity. Diabetes however, is not a contraindication to sport, as demonstrated by the increasing number of top class sportsmen and women who are insulin dependent diabetics. A graded programme may stabilize the diabetic's insulin requirements (Cuppers 1984) and may possibly prevent cardiovascular complications.

Epilepsy

Similar advice should be given to epileptic athletes as to epileptic car drivers. They should only participate in sport when their fits are adequately suppressed and they should refrain from dangerous or solitary sports such as mountaineering or scuba diving.

SPORT-RELATED ILLNESS

Pre-existing medical conditions may thus alter the choice of sport or stop participation. Fit athletes however, provide a very different problem for a doctor as many conditions may arise as a result of their energetic participation in sport.

Cardiovascular disease

Bradycardia is commonly found in fit athletes and is usually part of the 'athlete's heart syndrome'. This occurs when the heart muscle hypertrophies due to regular training, and comprises sinus bradycardia and moderate cardiomegaly as seen on chest

X-ray (Hutson et al 1985). Palpitations due to ventricular ectopic beats are also a common finding, but often of no significance, during the recovery phase from severe exertion. Sometimes fainting due to syncope may occur, again after severe exertion, and should be investigated to exclude cardiac anomalies such as hypertrophic cardiomyopathy (HCM).

Gastrointestinal disease

Nausea, vomiting and abdominal pain are common symptoms in trained athletes, particularly before competition. Often they are caused by nervous tension, but more commonly from food or food intake before strenuous exercise which inhibits gastric emptying (Ramsbottom and Hunt 1974). Thus approximately 4 hours should elapse between competition and the last meal. Abdominal pain may also be due to 'the stitch', probably caused by abdominal muscle spasm or stimulation of nocioceptive nerve fibres in the ligament of Trietz. Any long lasting abdominal pain requires further investigation. Gastrointestinal bleeding, resistant to investigation, has also been described in long-distance runners.

Diarrhoea is also common in athletes and it has now been established that there is a direct relationship between intensity of training, the distance run, and the degree of diarrhoea (Fogoros 1980). This is called 'runners' diarrhoea' and possible causes include intestinal ischaemia, changes in intestinal secretion and absorption, or changes in intestinal motility. Any athlete participating abroad should be aware of 'travellers' diarrhoea', a common syndrome of gastroenteritis due to native strains of *E. coli* to which the traveller's intestine is not acclimatized. It is self-limiting and best avoided by strict supervision of the diet and drinking water. Treatment is usually with an antibiotic, doxycycline, and rehydration powders such as Dioralyte, Rehidrat, etc., in combination with Imodium or Lomotil are often essential to permit resolution of the illness. Where giardiasis is the cause of diarrhoea the most effective treatment is with oral metronidazole (Flagyl).

It is also suggested that a regular prophylactic agent such as Ciproxin can effectively prevent travellers' diarrhoea if taken twice daily on a regular basis while abroad.

Renal function

Abnormalities of renal function detected on urinalysis in athletes usually result from two benign conditions, traumatic haemoglobinuria, and pseudo-nephritis, also called 'jogger's nephritis'. The former is the result of haemolysis and can be found in sports such as long-distance walking (march haemaglobinuria), but is also found in sports with repeated direct trauma such as karate

(Davison 1969). 'Jogger's nephritis' occurs after prolonged exercise and is characterized by the detection of red cells and protein in the urine (Gardner 1956). Violent exercise can result in decreased renal blood flow and lead to proteinuria. Treatment of both conditions is temporary rest.

Any form of prolonged exercise can result in loss of plasma water (up to 20%) with resultant hypovalaemia and diminished renal function. It is thus vital that all athletes are conversant with the principles of adequate fluid replacement namely:

1. Drink water in excess of thirst requirements
2. Replace salt also, but in hypotonic solution. Glucose solutions are well absorbed from the gastrointestinal tract and thus glucose solutions with salt in hypotonic amounts should be taken while undergoing endurance training.

Gynaecological problems

Amenorrhoea is more common in female athletes than the general population. There is clear association between the intensity of training and the incidence of menstrual disturbance (Erdeley 1976). Amenorrhoea tends to be more common in athletes with a low body weight and low body fat (Fishman et al 1975). Treatment is by reduction of exercise with the consequent resumption of periods usually within two to three months.

Following pregnancy, training can be resumed immediately after delivery, but competition should be avoided for at least the first month.

Infections

There is risk associated with severe physical exertion during any infection, especially where there is an associated pyrexia, even if the illness is mild and viral. Pyrexia is a manifestation of raised core temperature and increased metabolic rate. The additional strains imposed by exercise may induce cardiovascular collapse. Convalescence from any viral illness, particularly glandular fever or influenza can be prolonged by exercise. Advice to athletes should therefore be directed to achieving an adequate period of convalescence, although it is usually safe to continue exercise with the common cold.

TRAVEL ABROAD

Competition, and training for competition, now involves considerable overseas travel. The sports doctor must therefore be conversant with immunization needs and the medical problems associated with exercise in unusual environments such as high altitude or extreme heat.

Immunizations

Compulsory immunization against smallpox and cholera, i.e., that requiring an international certificate of vaccination, is no longer required as smallpox is now considered extinct and most countries accept that cholera vaccination should also no longer be mandatory. However yellow fever vaccinations are mandatory for athletes passing through the yellow fever belts in Central Africa and Central America.

Immunization against infectious disease should be considered depending upon the environment to which the athlete is travelling.

Tetanus

It is extremely important to be protected against tetanus through-out the world. A reinforcing dose 10 years after the primary course and again 10 years later maintains a satisfactory level of protection which will probably be life-long. For immunized adults, booster doses at less than 10-year intervals are not recommended since they have been shown to be unnecessary and can cause consider-able local reaction.

TETANUS PRONE WOUNDS

These are defined as:

1. Any wound or burn sustained more than 6 hours before surgical treatment
2. Any wound or burn which after some time shows one or more of the following:
   a. Evidence of devitalized tissue
   b. Puncture wound
   c. Contact with soil or manure
   d. Evidence of sepsis

In all such cases thorough surgical toilet must be undertaken irrespective of the immunization status of the patient (Immunis-ation against Infectious Diseases 1990).

Diphtheria

Diphtheria is practically unknown in the developed world but must be considered by travellers to Africa, the Middle East and the Indian subcontinent.

Typhoid vaccination

Typhoid vaccination is also recommended for those travelling to areas where typhoid is endemic.

Further information about immunization schedules can be obtained from the *Handbook of Immunisation* issued by the Department of Health (1988).

Acclimatization

The sports physician must also be prepared to give advice regarding acclimatization to extremes of environment not encountered in the athlete's home country.

HEAT

The usual problem encountered is one of heat acclimatization. Heat illness results from failure of the normal temperature regulatory mechanisms to prevent a rise in core temperature, combined with progressive loss of body fluids by sweating and is usually compounded by inadequate replacement of water and salt. There are several stages, from mild heat exhaustion associated with fatigue dizziness and syncope, to heat stroke with hallucinations, progressive loss of consciousness and convulsions. This is a medical emergency and should be suspected in any patient whose mental status changes while exercising in a hot climate. Treatment is by cooling the body by removal of clothing, and iced water bathing. Replacement of at least 1.5 litres of fluid four-hourly is required and major electrolyte disturbances are often present. The increasing emphasis on fluid replacement throughout athletic participation has greatly decreased the incidence of heat stroke although this is still one of the commonest avoidable causes of death amongst athletes. Heat acclimatization is extremely efficient to prevent heat stroke. The physiological changes are an increase in plasma volume and increased sympathetic stimulation of the sweating mechanism. These physiological effects are similar to those induced by endurance training and most athletes achieve acclimatization in hot climates very quickly within one week. In practical terms the most important point on arrival in a tropical climate is to ensure adequate fluid and salt intake, and 2 litres of fluid should be taken for every 10°C above body temperature thereafter.

ALTITUDE

The other extreme of climate that might be encountered is increase in altitude. The partial pressure of oxygen diminishes progressively in the atmosphere with increasing altitude. The haemoglobin oxygen dissociation curve compensates for this in the delivery of oxygen to the tissue up to a critical point. Below 1500 metres there is no impairment of oxygen transport but then aerobic power decreases by approximately 4% for every additional 300 metres. The minimum threshold for pulmonary oedema is approximately 2500 metres (Singh et al 1965). Acclimatization is relatively slow, requiring approximately 3 to 4 weeks at altitudes greater than 2000 metres. Higher altitudes need considerably longer stays for acclimatization to be complete. It is important to have an understanding of the syndrome of acute mountain sickness, the manifestations of which include fatigue, headache, personality changes, breathlessness, anorexia, nausea and vomiting (Sutton 1983). Exercise increases the hazards of acute mountain sickness particularly if undertaken without acclimatization at altitudes over 3000 metres.

DRUGS AND SPORT

It is an unfortunate fact that athletic competition at the highest level is now associated with drug taking. Determined athletes and coaches, often with the help of their doctor, may go to extreme lengths to succeed in competition. The sports physician must therefore be aware of the ever increasing list of banned substances imposed by the International Olympic Committee on the advice of its Medical Commission, in order to prevent sportsmen or women under his or her direct care, from infringing the rules.

Most governing bodies of sport follow the recommendations of the International Olympic Committee although exceptions are made depending upon the sport. Apart from being unfair, drug abuse can also be dangerous. In particular the use of anabolic steroids has been linked with aggressive and psychotic behaviour. The association between long-term use and cancer of the liver and prostate has also been well established.

Drugs to avoid prescribing in all forms of sport include systemic corticosteroids, non-selective adreno-receptive agonists, selective beta–2-agonists, opiates, analgesics and diuretics. Under certain circumstances, if the athlete is suffering from a chronic disease such as asthma or epilepsy, their usual medication may be taken provided a declaration is made before competition (Harries 1990).

The list of banned drugs is enormous and it is best to prescribe from a list of medicines that is safe to use. Athletes should be warned to seek advice from their doctor particularly when buying over the counter formulations which may be on the banned list. Full information and a copy of the banned list is available from the Sports Council.

REFERENCES

Altekruse E B, Wilmore J H 1973 Changes in blood chemistries following a controlled exercise programme. Journal of Occupational Medicine 15: 110–113

Cuppers J H 1984 Fitness training aids. Type II diabetes. Diabetes Dialogue 3: 31

Davison R L J 1969 'March', or exertional haemoglobulinuria. Seminars in Haematology 6: 150

DHSS 1988 Immunisation against infectious disease. In: Handbook of Immunisation HMSO, London

Erdely G J 1976 Effects of exercise on the menstrual cycle. Physician and Sports Medicine 4 3 79–80

Fishman J, Boyar R N, Hellman L 1975 Influence of body weight on oestradiol metabolism in young women. Journal of Clinical Endocrinal Metabolism 41: 989–991.

Fitch K D, Morton A R 1971 Specificity of exercise in exercise induced asthma. British Medical Journal ii 577–581

Fogoros R N 1980 Runner's trots, gastro-intestinal disturbances in runners. Journal of the American Medical Association 243: 1743–1744

Gardner K D 1956 Athletic pseudo-nephritis: alteration of urinary sediment by athletic competition. Journal of the American Medical Association 167: 803–813

Gloag D 1985 Rehabilitation of patients with cardiac conditions. British Medical Journal 290: 617–620

Harries M 1990 Prescribing for sportsmen and women. Prescribers Journal 30 6: 247–253

Hutson T P, Puffer J C, Rodney W M 1985 The athletic heart syndrome. New England Journal of Medicine 313: 24–31

McFadden E R, Ingram R H 1979 Exercise induced asthma: observations on the inducing stimulus. New England Journal of Medicine 301: 763–769

Nagle et al 1983 The effect of physical training on left ventricular failure after acute myocardial infarction. Circulation 68 supp III (abstract)

Opie L H 1975 Sudden death and sport. Lancet 1: 263–266

Ramsbottom N, Hunt N J 1974 Effect of exercise on gastric emptying. Digestion 10: 1–8

Singh et al 1965 High altitude pulmonary oedema. Lancet 1: 229–234

Sutton J R 1983 Man at altitude. Seminar in Respiratory Medicine 5

10. Infections in sport

The ever widening spectrum of sporting activities, nationally and internationally, and the increasing number of participants mean that almost every form of infection may be acquired directly or indirectly, in the pursuit of sport. Until recent years, sport-related infections were largely confined to septic cuts and abrasions, fungal dermatoses (athlete's foot) or respiratory infections (influenza, viral 'sore throat' etc), and on occasion life-threatening tetanus.

While the potential for all of these remain, some 'new' infections have emerged in recent years. 'Scrumpox' or 'herpes gladiatorum' in one form or another has always been around, but 'herpes' has nowadays taken on a new meaning for many along with the fear of acquiring viral hepatitis or the human immunodeficiency virus (HIV). This has largely been due to heightened public awareness and anxieties concerning the possible risks of acquiring HIV infection while participating in sport, and in particular combat or contact sports and others where the spillage of blood may feature.

Increased attention has also been given to the chronic debilitating effects of other virus infections such as glandular fever and Coxsackie B, which are associated with the 'chronic fatigue syndrome'. In addition there is increasing evidence to suggest that premature return to physical activity following influenza or similar 'feverish' illnesses, may have irreversible damaging effects on cardiac muscle.

Sport, whether on club tours or in competition, in recent years has increasingly taken on an international dimension involving overseas travel on a world-wide basis. In consequence more and more athletes (and officials) become exposed to foodborne and environmentally related infections such as 'travellers' diarrhoea' in its various guises or more serious conditions such as cholera, typhoid, dysentery, etc., or to malaria, the malignant form of which may result in death if improperly treated.

SPORT-ASSOCIATED INFECTIONS

The circumstances whereby athletes may acquire infection vary within sport and its related activities.

Exposure to infection may occur:

- During sporting activity *per se* e.g. scrumpox, tetanus, other wound infections (Fig. 10.1A).

- Within the changing room environment e.g. fungal infections, verrucae, respiratory infection (Fig. 10.1B).
- During travel to and from sporting events, particularly overseas e.g. 'food poisoning', 'travellers' diarrhoea', malaria (Fig. 10.1C), and
- As a consequence of leisure time activities peripheral to sport e.g. glandular fever, sexually transmitted diseases (Fig. 10.1D).

   Infection may be acquired by:

- Person-to-person spread via:

   1. Direct personal contact
   2. Airborne droplets
   3. Bloodborne transmission.

- Contact with a contaminated playing arena or changing room environment
- Insect bites
- Consuming contaminated food or water.

DURING SPORTING ACTIVITY

In the course of sporting activity, infection may be acquired directly by person-to-person spread or from a contaminated playing arena (pitch, court, pool, etc.) with contact sports, water sports and field sports posing most risks. Indirect spread may also occur as a consequence of contact with or sharing contaminated communal equipment (towels, clothing, etc.).

Scrumpox

As the name suggests this infection is most frequently associated with rugby football, and in particular among those playing in the scrum where direct person-to-person contact is greatest. During the 1970s, outbreaks due to the herpes simplex virus were reported among rugby clubs in England (Anonymous 1974, Shute et al 1979), and also occasionally affected international touring teams visiting the British Isles. More recently impetigenous scrumpox affected school rugby teams in Scotland (Sharp & Adam 1990). The presence of skin 'lesions' along with the abrasive effects of facial stubble, facilitate the spread of infection.

   The condition also occurs in other combat sports such as judo or wrestling. Outbreaks of 'herpes gladiatorum' among wrestlers have been reported on several occasions from the USA in particular. Most recently in July 1989, 60 participants (35%) attending a high school wrestling camp in Minnesota were infected with

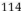

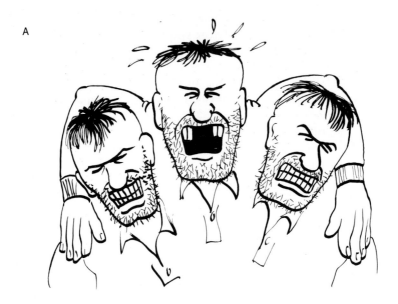

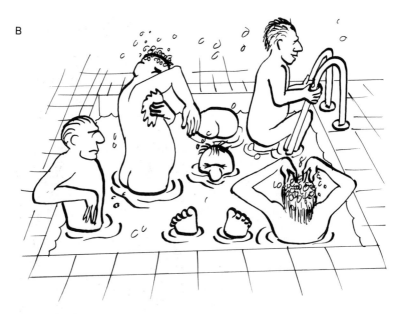

Fig. 10.1   Exposure to infection may occur: **A** During sporting activity **B** Within the changing room environment **C** During travel to and from sporting events, particularly overseas **D** As a consequence of leisure time activities peripheral to sport

C

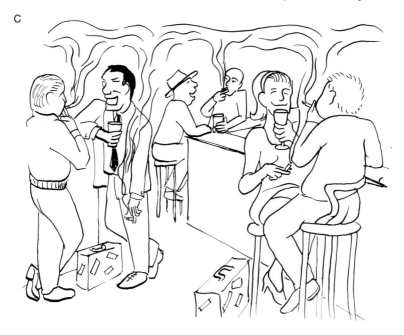

D

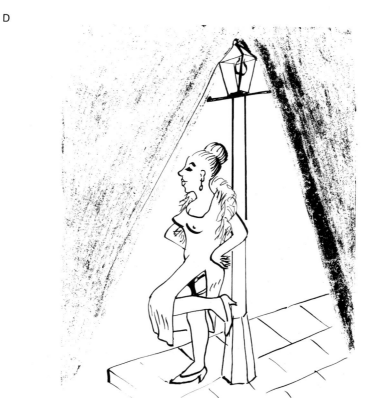

herpes simplex virus, five of whom developed herpetic conjunctivitis (Goodman et al 1990).

Scrumpox may be caused by several infectious agents, which
may be viral (herpes), bacterial (streptococcal, staphylococcal) or
fungal (tinea barbae) in origin.

HERPES

This is the most common form of 'scrumpox' and is caused by the
Herpes simplex virus type 1, the agent of herpes labialis ('cold
sore'). This should not be confused with Herpes simplex virus
type 2, the cause of genital herpes. Herpes is highly infectious
spreading directly from person-to-person or indirectly via the
sharing of infected towels, clothing or equipment, and on
occasion may result in encephalitis. Prevention depends upon
the maintenance of high standards of personal hygiene. Treatment requires the use of acyclovir, a specific anti-viral available
as a cream or tablets.

IMPETIGO

This form of scrumpox due to *Streptococcus pyogenes* or
Staphylococcus aureus, is less common. The use of topical anti-
septics may help in minimizing the spread of infection.

ERYSIPELAS

The least-common form, caused specifically by *Streptococcus
pyogenes*, is potentially the most serious. Treatment requires the
use of appropriate antibiotics such as flucloxacillin or erythro-
mycin.

TINEA BARBAE

A fungal infection which spreads similarly to other forms of
scrumpox. Treatment with fungicidal creams or tablets is usually
necessary.

An unusual consequence of scrumpox caused by a particularly virulent strain of *Streptococcus pyogenes*, affected several
forwards in a hospital rugby team in London in 1984 following a
match against a team experiencing an outbreak of impetigo. In
addition to being transmitted to front row forwards of yet
another team the following week, two girlfriends of affected
players in the hospital team were similarly affected one month
later, following which salpingitis developed in one girlfriend
and acute glomerulonephritis in one player (Ludlam & Cookson
1986).

Tetanus

Of all sport-related infections tetanus is the most serious, being potentially life-threatening. In Scotland in recent years two rugby players and one soccer player developed tetanus from cuts acquired during play, only one of whom survived.

Infection is caused by *Clostridium tetani*, an anaerobic bacillus which has the capability of:

1. Spore formation, which are omnipresent in human and animal faeces and may readily contaminate sports fields, and
2. The production of a potent neurotoxin.

Penetrating wounds with low oxygen levels and/or 'dirty' wounds where other contaminating microorganisms are also likely to be present, facilitate bacterial growth and toxin production. Treatment is invariably required in an intensive care unit providing sedation using curare-like drugs and life-support facilities. Administration of antitoxin (specific anti-tetanus immunoglobulin) is necessary to neutralize any unbound toxin present. Long-acting penicillin is usually also required to inhibit any continued bacterial growth and further toxin production.

All wounds which are deep and/or 'dirty' require early prophylactic treatment with thorough cleansing and debridement where necessary, complemented by penicillin, tetanus toxoid and/or antitoxin, depending on the *known* immunization status of the individual. Recovery from clinical disease however does not provide immunity from further infection, and such patients therefore require to be reimmunized.

Tetanus is preventable by active immunization, the basic course of which requires boosting doses at 10-year intervals and possibly every five years for those persons (e.g. rugby, soccer players) exposed to contaminated playing surfaces. Too frequent boosting doses however may result in the development of hypersensitivity reactions.

Other wound infections

Any wound or abrasion leading to a breaking of the skin surface may become infected by a range of other bacteria (e.g. *Staphylococcus, Streptococcus, Pseudomonas*), which may be present in the playing or changing room environment, on clothing or equipment, or on the skin or respiratory tract of otherwise healthy carriers. Infection may be localized or may invade other body tissues leading to lymphadenitis, cellulitis or bacteraemia, and in consequence require appropriate antibiotic treatment.

Consideration has also to be given to the possibility that infection with hepatitis B virus (HBV) or the human immunodeficiency virus (HIV) may be transmitted directly from person-to-person via open wounds (*v. infra*).

Insect bites may also pose problems to cross-country runners and orienteerers participating in environments where Lyme disease and other vector-borne infections (including malaria in parts of the world where the disease is endemic) are prevalent.

Water-related infections

Water sports can pose infection hazards to various body systems, particularly so if participating in natural or unchlorinated waters. Infections thus acquired may affect the eye (conjunctivitis), ear (otitis externa), skin (folliculitis), intestine (giardiasis, cryptosporidiosis), liver, kidneys or brain (leptospirosis) or lungs (legionellosis).

An outbreak of giardiasis in 1985 affected groups of swimmers in New Jersey, USA who had been using an inadequately chlorinated pool (Porter et al 1988). More recently a windsurfer in Scotland was similarly affected following immersion in an inland waterway into which sewage effluents discharged, while a water skier in England developed Weil's disease and died. Participation in water-sports and other water-related recreational activities have increasingly become an important risk factor in leptospirosis in the UK. Increasing recognition has also been given in recent years to infection by *Aeromonas hydrophila*, which can cause gastrointestinal illness as well as cutaneous and pulmonary infections.

In early 1988, swimmers, curlers and other persons at a leisure complex in the West of Scotland were infected by *Legionella micdadei* in an outbreak of a hitherto undescribed form of non-pneumonic legionellosis, subsequently named Lochgoilhead fever. Airborne spread of infection occurred via the ventilation system, with the source traced to a contaminated 'jacuzzi' within the swimming pool area (Goldberg et al 1989).

WITHIN THE CHANGING ROOM ENVIRONMENT

The changing room with its shower/bathing area where athletes ·are inevitably in close or adjacent contact with each other in a crowded, warm, moist atmosphere, particularly if poorly maintained, lends itself readily to the transmission of a wide range of respiratory infections (influenza, 'sore throats', colds etc.), fungal infections (tinea pedis, etc.) and/or verrucae. Other 'highly contagious' infections such as chickenpox have also been known to spread among team members as experienced by a professional soccer club in Scotland in early 1991.

Most of these infections are largely of nuisance value and are readily preventable or treatable. Influenza however poses potentially more serious problems to both the individual and to fellow-athletes, which may have both short-term and long-term effects. Influenza not only incapacitates the individual, but may also be readily transmitted to others, resulting in depleted teams affecting results or the fulfilment of fixtures. All too often affected individuals may try to 'run off' their flu in a mistaken attempt to compete or 'not to let the side down'.

More serious are the potential longer-term effects of viral infections on the heart as a consequence of continuing to train or resuming prematurely. In a study in Canada, three of 32 previously well persons were found to have had segmental ventricular effects, while 17 others showed evidence of pericardial effusions during the acute and recuperative phases of flu-like illness (Montague et al 1988). Type A virus has been isolated from the cardiac muscle of patients who died following influenza illnesses, including one previously healthy young woman in Finland (Engblom et al 1983). The effects of influenza virus on the metabolism of cardiac muscle has been shown experimentally in mice (Ilback et al 1984a). In a parallel study the effects of exercise on the clinical course of infection were also demonstrated (Ilback et al 1984b). Other viruses, in particular Coxsackie virus, are also known for their capability of infecting the heart.

DURING TRAVEL

Over 28 million people from Britain travelled overseas in 1988 (J. H. Cossar, personal communication). With the expansion of air travel, more and more countries worldwide are being visited, in many of which infections formerly commonplace in Europe are still prevalent.

The most common problems experienced by overseas travellers are bowel infections (eg. travellers' diarrhoea, salmonellosis, dysentery, cholera, typhoid and paratyphoid fevers), malaria and viral hepatitis A. With the exception of malaria, all may be acquired from the consumption of contaminated food or water, including ice.

It should not be forgotten however that 'food poisoning' can be as much a problem in Britain and other developed countries, with hotels, restaurants, social functions, etc. often featuring as the locus of outbreaks. During the summer of 1990 in the UK, several outbreaks of salmonellosis were associated with food served at various soccer, bowling, cricket and golf events.

Travellers' diarrhoea

This is usually a self-limiting condition of varying aetiology affecting newly arrived travellers from Western Europe and North America to Third World countries. Changes in food, climate and hygiene standards probably contribute to many such episodes. Nevertheless, many such infections are due to exposure to a wide range of microorganisms to which the local population has developed gut immunity.

Respiratory infections

Respiratory illnesses are common among travellers exposed to infection in crowded aircraft, terminal buildings or hotels where droplet spread readily occurs, compounded by the dehydrating effects of the low humidity encountered in aircraft.

Malaria

There are four different forms of malaria, caused by *Plasmodium vivax, P. falciparum, P. ovale* and/or *P. malariae* respectively, with incubation periods varying from 2 weeks up to 9–12 months. Malignant malaria (*P. falciparum*) is particularly dangerous and potentially fatal if diagnosed late or incorrectly treated.

Despite intensive efforts towards eradication, malaria has increased again in recent years in many countries in Africa, Asia and South and Central America. In parallel with increasing resistance to insecticides by the mosquito vector, some strains of *P. falciparum* in areas of South-East Asia, South America and Africa have developed resistance to chloroquine and other drugs, presenting additional problems in prophylaxis and treatment (*v. infra*).

Other infections

A wide range of other infections may potentially be acquired by travellers. Only smallpox has been eradicated on a global basis. Tuberculosis is still prevalent in many countries, while few are free from rabies. Lassa fever and other viral haemorrhagic fevers have affected travellers to West Africa. Typhus is present in the Far East, including Northern Australia where scrub typhus is endemic. Bubonic plague is prevalent in areas of central and South-East Asia, Southern Africa and America including some

Western states of the USA. Brucellosis may be acquired by eating goats' milk cheeses which are popular in most Mediterranean countries.

LEISURE TIME ACTIVITIES

Relaxing in or around a swimming or whirlpool bath, may result in exposure to a range of environmentally acquired infections, most of which (respiratory or fungal infections, verrucae, etc.) are usually of nuisance value only.

Acquiring a sexually transmitted disease as a consequence of other leisure time activities, can be a more serious problem. Gonorrhoea, trichomonas, herpes genitalis, etc. are prevalent worldwide. HBV and HIV infections however pose more far-reaching medical and social problems, and have the potential of being acquired through any one of sport-related situations, viz. during sporting activity, within the changing room environment or in association with travel and/or leisure time. The relative risks vary however from the very low while participating in sport to increasingly possible as a consequence of leisure time activities, especially during overseas travel.

VIRAL HEPATITIS B

HBV infection is acquired through contact with infected blood (or blood products) or by sexual spread from a carrier of the disease. The severity of the illness can vary considerably from mild to being rapidly fatal. The infectious state usually begins some weeks before becoming ill, remaining so throughout the acute illness. Chronic carriers, detectable by the presence in the blood of 'e' antigen, rarely have a recognizable illness yet they can remain infectious for many years.

The main emphasis in the prevention of spread within sport is in improving overall hygiene standards rather than by imposing undue restrictions on individuals known to be HBV carriers. Such persons need not categorically be excluded from participating in sport, including contact sports. Injuries, cuts or grazes that bleed are nevertheless potential sources of infection and should invariably be cleansed and securely covered. Any person who is known to be a carrier of the virus should always shower rather than share a communal bath, particularly if they have suffered any skin damage.

While the risk of spread during sporting activities is small, there have been reports of cases of hepatitis B acquired via contaminated thorn-pricks during orienteering events in Sweden in the 1960s (Berg et al 1971) or among barefoot runners.

HIV INFECTION

The routes of transmission of the human immune deficiency virus (HIV) are virtually identical to those of the hepatitis B virus. The potential risk of infection by HIV during sport, in particular contact sports, via abrasions, cuts or through communal bathing, has caused considerable anxiety to athletes and sports administrators alike. In the USA for example the Nevada Athletic Commission introduced mandatory HIV antibody testing of boxers fighting within that state, while in New Jersey ringside seconds are required to wear plastic gloves (Gunby 1988).

The main dangers of acquiring HIV infection are those arising from the direct, and possibly even frequent, exposure to the blood, semen or vaginal discharges of infected persons. Nevertheless, if a cut or abrasion occurs during sporting activity, bleeding should be controlled and the wound cleansed and securely covered, where possible with a waterproof 'island' type dressing, as a matter of priority. Nose bleeds require similar early attention. Particular attention should also be given to using a Brooke's type airway or Laerdal Pocket-Mask when applying mouth-to-mouth resuscitation where bleeding is present.

In view of the increasing concern, the World Health Organization convened a consultative meeting in Geneva in January 1989, which was attended by representatives of the International Federation of Sports Medicine, the International Federation for Wrestling and the International Rugby Football Board. A consensus statement was agreed, the basis of which stated that:

1. No evidence exists for a risk of transmission of HIV when infected persons engaging in sports, have no bleeding wounds or other skin lesions.
2. In contact sports there exists a potentially low risk of transmission where bleeding occurs.
3. There is no medical justification for testing or screening for HIV infection prior to participation in sports activities, and that
4. Persons who know they are infected should seek medical counselling prior to participation in sports in order to assess risks to their own health, as well as the theoretical risk of transmission to others.

Since then HIV seroconversion has been reported from Italy in an apparently previously healthy soccer player with no *admitted* risk factors, who collided head-to-head with an opponent, a drug-abuser who was known to be HIV positive; both players sustained severe eyebrow wounds with copious bleeding (Torre et al 1990). Less directly, a young rugby player in Paris similarly with no known risk factors, was found to have symptomatic seroconversion attributed to a course of acupuncture 3 months previously for the treatment of tendonitis (Vittecoq et al 1989).

PREVENTIVE MEASURES

Prevention of infection in sport can be multi-factorial, amongst which the maintenance of individual standards of personal and environmental hygiene are of paramount importance, which require to be maintained at as high a level as possible. Among more specific measures the communal sponge should be replaced by individual disposable wipes, while showering is always preferable to the communal bath.

Guidelines on hygiene have been produced in recent years by various sports bodies (e.g. The Sports Council of Wales, The Scottish Sports Council) and others (Loveday 1990), much of which relates to the prevention of spread of HIV infection. A more comprehensive review of 'Infection and Sport', giving guidance on the dangers and precautions for athletes, officials etc. has been prepared by the Scottish Sports Council, and published in booklet form in 1989.

Immunization

An increasing range of vaccines (or toxoids) have become available in recent years affording protection against many infections, only one of which viz. tetanus, has an everyday relevance to sport. While most athletes nowadays should have received a basic course of tetanus toxoid during childhood, booster doses are required at regular intervals in order to maintain effective immunity.

Influenza vaccines are worth considering for all athletes, particularly those participating in winter-orientated sports. Due to the periodic changes in the antigenic structure of the influenza A virus, and to a lesser extent the influenza B virus, immunity is poorly maintained and repeat doses of vaccine are required every 1–2 years or so.

For the purposes of international travel documentation to certain countries, immunization may be necessary against yellow fever (tropical Africa and South America) and possibly also cholera by a few countries, although this is no longer recommended by the World Health Organization as an effective control measure. Immunization against typhoid, polio, diph-theria, Japanese B encephalitis, etc. may be recommended for certain parts of the world and during certain seasons of the year.

Protection against viral hepatitis A in the form of immuno-globulin may be required for sero-negative persons travelling out-side Europe, North America and Australasia. Hepatitis B may also be considered advisable for certain types of athletes competing in Third World countries where the disease is endemic and there is a known high HBV carrier rate.

Anti-malaria prophylaxis

Advice on the current appropriate anti-malaria prophylaxis recommended for different areas of the world can be obtained by medical practitioners in the UK from several sources such as the PHLS Malaria Reference Laboratory, London School of Hygiene & Tropical Medicine (071–636 3924: for *urgent* enquiries 071–636 8636) or the Liverpool School of Tropical Medicine (051–708 9393).

In addition any practitioner with access to a terminal or compu-ter with a modem (such as that which links with Prestel) can regis-ter to use the weekly updated service on malaria prophylaxis and immunizations, provided by the Communicable Diseases (Scot-land) Unit, Ruchill Hospital, Glasgow (041–946 7120).

Other measures

Prophylactic medication does not by itself however provide ab-solute protection against malaria and should be complemented with other measures such as the use of protective clothing and insect-repellant creams.

There are as yet no vaccines available to protect against most infections (i.e. gastrointestinal) to which overseas travellers may be exposed. Reliance has to be placed primarily on general health precautions and high standards of personal hygiene, along with the avoidance of uncooked foods, untreated fluids, ice, etc. The prophylactic use of antibiotics is less frequently recommended nowadays, but may have a role in individual circumstances.

Sterile equipment packs containing sterile needles, syringes, drip needles, IV giving sets and plasma expanders, etc, for over-seas travel are available from Medical Advisory Services for Travellers Abroad Ltd (MASTA), London School of Hygiene and Tropical Medicine, Keppel Street, London WC1E 7HT (071–631 4408) and from other outlets elsewhere in the UK.

A particularly useful booklet *Travel Information for Medical*

Practitioners published by the Department of Health in 1989, provides advice on a broad range of immunization and other prophylactic measures for overseas travel, including giving relevant addresses and telephone numbers for additional information. Copies are obtainable from the DOH Store, Health Publications Unit, No. 2 Site, Manchester Road, Heywood, Lancs OL10 2PZ (quoting reference EL(89) P/33).

REFERENCES

Anonymous 1974 An outbreak of scrumpox due to herpes simplex virus. Public Health Laboratory Service Communicable Disease Report no. 15: iv

Berg R, Ringertz O, Espmark A 1971 Australia antigen in hepatitis among Swedish trackfinders. Acta Path Microbiol Scand. 79B: 423–427

Engblom E, Ekfors T O, Meurman D H, Toivanen A, Nikoskelainen J 1983 Fatal influenza A myocarditis with isolation of virus from the myocardium. Acta Medica Scandinavia 213: 75–78

Goldberg D J, Wrench J G, Collier P W, Emslie J A N, Fallon R J, Forbes G I, McKay T M, Macpherson A C, Markwick T A, Reid D 1989 Lochgoilhead fever: outbreak of non-pneumonic legionellosis due to *Legionella micdadei*. Lancet 1: 316–318

Goodman J L, Holland E J, Andres C W, Homann S R, Mahanti R L, Mizener M W, Erice A, Osterholm M T 1990 Herpes gladiatorum at a high school wrestling camp—Minnesota. Morbidity & Mortality Weekly Report 39 no. 5: 69–71

Gunby P 1988 Boxing: AIDS? JAMA 259(11): 1613

Ilback N G, Friman G, Beisel W R, Johnson A J 1984a Sequential metabolic alterations in the myocardium during influenza and tularaemia in mice. Infection & Immunity 45: 491–497

Ilback N G, Friman G, Beisel W R, Johnson A J, Berendt R F 1984b Modifying effects of exercise on clinical course and biochemical response of the myocardium in influenza and tularaemia in mice. Infection & Immunity 45: 498–504

Loveday C 1990 HIV disease and sport. In: Payne S. Medicine, sport and the law. Blackwell Scientific Publications, Oxford 81–86

Ludlam H, Cookson B 1986 Scrum kidney: epidemic pyoderma caused by a nephritogenic *streptococcus pyogenes* in a rugby team. Lancet 2: 331–332

Montague T J, Marrie T J, Bewick B J, Spencer A, Kornreich F, Horacek B M 1988 Cardiac effects of common viral illnesses. Chest 94: 919–925

Porter J D, Ragazzoni H P, Buchanan J D, Waskin H A, Juranek D D, Parkin W E 1988 Giardia transmission in a swimming pool. American Journal of Public Health 78 no. 6: 659–662

Sharp J C M, Adam E I 1990 Scrumpox. Communicable Diseases Scotland Weekly Report 24 no. 17: 7–8

Shute P, Jeffries D J, Maddocks A C 1979 Scrumpox caused by herpes simplex virus. British Medical Journal 2: 1629

Torre D, Sampietro C, Ferraro G, Zeroli C, Speranza F 1990 Transmission of HIV-1 infection via sports injury. Lancet 1: 1105

Vittecoq D, Mettetal J F, Rouzioux C, Bach J F, Bouchon J P 1989 Acute HIV infection after acupuncture treatments. New England Journal of Medicine 320 no. 4: 250–251

11. Physiotherapy and strapping in injury management

'Physiotherapy' encompasses all phases of treatment from the acute injury to return to normal activity and it is important to stress the value of the liaison between physiotherapist and clinician in the diagnosis of the injured athlete and his subsequent rehabilitation and fitness testing.

REHABILITATION FOLLOWING SOFT TISSUE INJURY

Rehabilitation begins immediately after the rest phase of treatment of the acute stage, preferably with gentle active movement but most certainly with passive movement if this is not possible. None of the physical treatment modalities—heating, cooling, electrical etc.—are as effective as active movement. Early mobilization should be confined within relatively pain-free ranges. Some degree of discomfort may be experienced, but as the movement will be slow and voluntary, no further damage will occur. Movement increases circulation and venous return and reduces oedema and the risk of atrophy.

Joints do not tolerate immobilization well and care should be given to those joints which are immobilized but undamaged. Certain mechanoreceptors fail to function in immobilized joints (Wyke 1972) with resultant loss of coordination and abnormalities in posture. Enforced rest can result in a generalized atrophy as well as specific degeneration around the lesion. The aim therefore of a rehabilitation programme is to prevent atrophy in unaffected tissues without disrupting the healing of the lesion.

Giving the patient instructions to rest can be too vague and, depending upon motivation and level of competition, difficult to enforce. Ideally, a schedule should be made up of e.g. weight-training for unaffected muscle groups, stretching exercises, specific exercises in a pool where weight-bearing is eliminated. Use can also be made of an exercise cycle.

Specific exercises and numbers of repetitions should be stated. To say 'Do a few of these daily' is indefinite and vague. To a weekend sportsman this can mean two to ten repetitions. To an athlete of international standard it can mean several hundred.

Exercise in some form will help the athlete psychologically. He feels he is still training, maintaining fitness and losing the minimum amount of time in returning to full function. This can prevent an undesirable early return to competition.

Following active movement, gentle resistance should be applied to affected muscles or the muscles controlling an injured joint. This is best done by manual resistance because the range and direction of movement can be controlled. Resistance can be graduated throughout the range and can be halted if pain occurs. Supportive strapping may be used between treatments, which ideally should be short and frequent each day. Where this is impractical, the patient is taught the exercises and told how many repetitions are required daily. When full pain-free movement is achieved, resisted exercises can also be increased in range, weight and repetition.

After the early stage, consideration has to be given to the general requirements of most sports: flexibility, strength, endurance and coordination.

Flexibility

Flexibility is of primary importance and can be restored by stretching exercises. Without a full range of movement and full soft tissue extensibility none of the other factors can be recovered satisfactorily. Competing while flexibility is limited may result in further injury. Passive stretching by a trained person who can recognise different 'end feels' and their significance is useful but if carried out by a team-mate or other untrained person can be counterproductive if not positively dangerous. The most effective method is to teach the athlete the exercises which will be useful to him. They should be performed at least twice daily and incorporated in any subsequent warm-up routine. Static stretching exercises are safest and more effective than ballistic stretching exercises (De Vries 1962) especially in recovery from injury: 'Stretch very slowly to the end of the range, hold the position without bouncing, then slowly relax.' This is superior to ballistic stretching, in which a stretch reflex can be provoked and unstable positions occur during the movement. The stretch can be facilitated by contracting the antagonists to the muscle group being stretched.

Strength

Most sports require a balance between strength and endurance. Recovering strength requires relatively large resistance exercises with low repetitions. Isotonic exercise is more efficient than isometric because it produces functional movement. In the early stage, weight-and-pulley systems may be of more use than a bar and weights. The range and direction of pull can be controlled more easily and the weight can be dropped without danger.

Endurance

This is achieved by employing high repetitions against a low resistance. It assists the athlete to cope with the stresses of training and competition without sacrificing skills. When fatigue sets in poor technique can result. Long sessions of activities such as swimming, cycling and running at submaximal levels can maintain fitness. The work-load can be gradually increased as the injury resolves.

Coordination

This is defined as 'bringing parts and movement into proper relation'. A knowledge of the sport involved is useful at this point. The exercises must be task-specific, performed slowly until they can be carried out confidently and without hesitation.

Before returning to competition, fitness testing is recommended. All the previously mentioned parameters must be demonstrated without evidence of postural abnormalities. If you do not know the sport ask the coach to perform the practical session while you observe the patient. Ideally, progress should be uneventful but setbacks and frustrations are not uncommon. They are, however, less likely to occur if rehabilitation is correctly timed and, as far as possible, designed for each athlete's needs.

TREATMENT TECHNIQUES

The aim is to provide optimum healing conditions and reduce pain so that normal movement can be resumed. Physical and electrical methods are complementary to normal movement.

Heat

Several methods increase tissue temperature—hot water baths, gel packs, infra-red lamps, short-wave and microwave diathermy. While hot water and gel packs are self-explanatory the other modalities require explanation.

INFRA-RED HEAT

Infra-red lamps have a local heating effect due to increased cutaneous circulation. Infra-red heat is of value in inducing relaxation and reducing muscle spasm. Heat packs have similar effects.

SHORT-WAVE DIATHERMY (SWD)

This modality induces heat by the production of wireless waves, 11 m in length. The electrodes and tissues between act as a capacitor with the tissues acting as the dielectric. A rapidly alternating current produces field penetration to varying depths depending upon power output and the arrangement of electrodes. However, the field tends to concentrate in the subcutaneous fat, which has a low dielectric constant.

Short-wave diathermy can produce heat in deeper structures, such as the hip joint, but can irritate acute lesions like haematomas. Metal implants in or near the treatment area preclude its use because burns would be produced.

Indications for short-wave diathermy are:

1. Subacute or chronic lesions
2. Injuries to deeply placed structures
3. Low dosage can be used to encourage sinus drainage.

MICROWAVE DIATHERMY (WAVELENGTH: 1 CM–1 M)

In physiotherapy only two frequency setups are available, 2450 MHz and 433.92 MHz, giving wavelengths of 12.25 cm and 69 cm respectively. Since the depth of penetration is approximately 3 cm it is less suitable for deeply placed lesions. The main difference from short-wave diathermy is that microwaves tend to concentrate in tissues with a high fluid content, such as muscle. Microwave diathermy has a greater heating effect on muscle than short-wave diathermy, where the main heating effect is dissipated in subcutaneous fat.

Microwaves are most useful for the treatment of small, localized lesions, e.g. small joints, subcutaneous muscle lesions. They can irritate acute lesions. Protective goggles should be worn, since lenticular degeneration can occur. Microwaves should not be applied to the genitalia.

Ultrasound (20 kHz +)

The machines presently in use have frequencies ranging from 0.75 MHz to 3 MHz, delivering intensities from 0.5 W/cm^2 to 3 W/cm^2. The energy is dissipated in two main ways, absorption and scatter. Absorption is the conversion of mechanical energy into heat. The amount absorbed is dependent upon the absorption coefficient of the tissue insonated. The greatest coefficients are found in tissues with a high collagen content. The absorption coefficient of bone is ten times that of muscle, which in turn is two and a half times that of fat at a frequency of 1.0 MHz (Dunn et al 1969). The beam is therefore reflected from many tissues and tissue interfaces in its path. Such scatter of the beam by reflection results in reduction of the heating effect.

A continuous beam can produce heat in the range of 40–45°C, which is useful in the treatment of chronic lesions. Heating of tissues can be avoided by the use of a pulsed beam, which has an application in acute lesions where heat would not be advisable.

The biological effects of therapeutic ultrasound aid tissue repair. Reduction of chronic inflammatory processes and stimulation of protein synthesis associated with an increase in lysosomal permeability (Harvey et al 1975) have been observed. Changes in the diffusion rates of cell membranes have also been recorded, with relief of pain in chronic lesions related to the intensity of the beam.

Pulsed ultrasound does not have a thermal effect. It is indicated in acute lesions where agitation of the tissue fluid has been shown to increase the rate of phagocytosis, and this perhaps explains why early application of ultrasound is effective (Dyson & Suckling 1978). It improves absorption of extravasated fluid, reducing oedema and secondary effects of recent trauma. It will reduce pain and is extremely useful in treating small joints in the hand.

Massage

Massage has many applications in the treatment of soft tissue lesions, the most useful techniques being effleurage, petrissage and deep frictions, circular and transverse. Effleurage, a firm stroking motion only in the direction of the venous and lymphatic return, and petrissage, a localised kneading action, are said to relieve muscle spasm, induce relaxation and reduce oedema. Deep friction requires accuracy in applying the massage directly to the lesion. This is used to break down adhesions in muscle, tendons and ligaments and is especially useful in chronic lesions. In chronic tenosynovitis, for example, logic dictates that an overuse injury should be rested, but the pain can be relieved in some cases by applying transverse friction at 90° to the tendon on stretch. Although initially uncomfortable the pain often settles after treatment and if the part is then actively mobilized further adhesions may not recur. Despite its recent neglect, massage is still a form of effective treatment for some soft tissue problems.

Strapping

Strapping satisfies two objectives:

1. To provide physical support for the injured part, limiting pain, assisting or resisting specific movements and allowing an injured area to come into graduated use

2. To provide psychological support and relieve anxiety.

In general it allows normal movement distal and proximal to the lesion and prevents atrophy or abnormal postures.

ANKLE

The most common site of injury in the ankle is the lateral aspect of the joint capsule. In the acute situation, when swelling is present, compression may be applied by placing a horseshoe of adhesive felt or cotton wool around the malleolus then applying a double layer of Tubigrip® from the toes to the popliteal fossa (Fig. 11.1). When the swelling has subsided, the ankle can be strapped in slight eversion to ensure healing in a shortened position, avoiding subsequent laxity. This is done by using 25 mm non-elastic tape, beginning below the medial malleolus, bringing the tape under the foot, over the lateral malleolus, using the felt pad to fill the spaces around the malleolus, up to 50 mm below the head of the fibula.

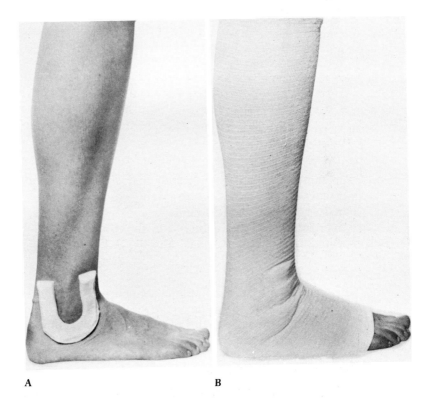

A   B

Fig. 11.1   Ankle strapping for control of swelling **A** Horseshoe of adhesive felt **B** Tubigrip®

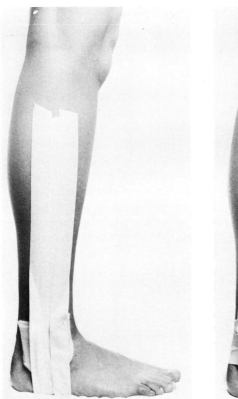
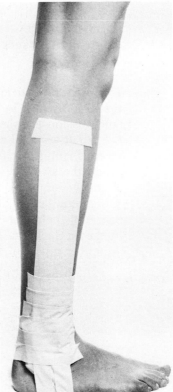

Fig. 11.2   Eversion ankle strapping

Repeat until there are three strands in position, each over-lapping its predecessor, place a fourth strand on top as a reinforcement then use small transverse strands to tape down the edges, especially over the lateral malleolus. This strapping (Fig. 11.2) may be repeated until the patient has returned to light training.

KNEE

To control swelling, a horseshoe-shaped pad of adhesive felt is applied around the patella and over the suprapatellar pouch. When the pad is in place, the joint is covered by a double layer of Tubigrip® extending from mid-calf to mid-thigh: Shaped Tubigrip® is preferable if available (Fig. 11.3). For medial or lateral ligament problems, the ligament is reinforced by 25 mm tape, applied fanwise, diagonally from superior to inferior. This allows enough supporting strands to be applied but avoids excessive skin tension. The strapping is then completed by circular strands to

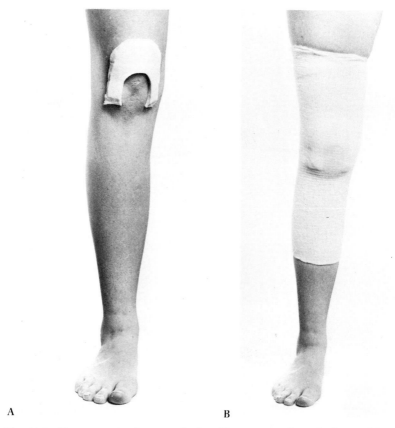

Fig. 11.3 Knee strapping for control of swelling **A** Horseshoe of adhesive felt **B** Tubigrip®

maintain the position of the longitudinal strapping (Fig. 11.4). Mild anterior cruciate strains may be allowed a graduated return to activity with a check strap in place to prevent hyperextension. The strap is formed by applying the adhesive surfaces of two pieces of 25 mm tape together. It is then placed behind the knee and secured by circular tapes above and below the joint (Fig. 11.5).

HAND

The basic strapping for thumb and fingers is the basket weave (Fig. 11.6). Use 12 mm tape, or cut the tape lengthwise to produce 6 mm tape for small joints. The tape is looped around the digit, the ends crossing each other diagonally, with a trip to secure the ends either at the base of the phalanx or around the wrist if the thumb is being strapped. Fingers may be strapped to each other for support

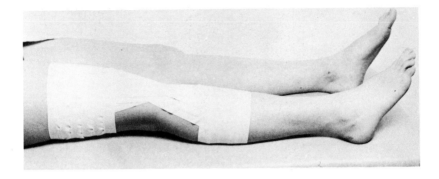

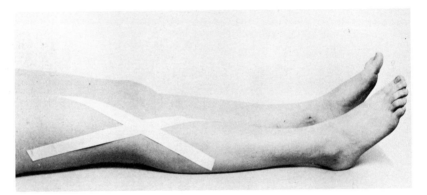

Fig. 11.4 Knee strapping for medial/lateral ligament problems

and a tongue depresser may be used between the fingers to prevent movement. A check strap can be employed to limit thumb extension and abduction to a pain-free range while still allowing the use of the hand (Fig. 11.7).

Useful as strappings are, allowing a degree of safety in returning to training, athletes using strappings should be discouraged from taking part in competitions, as further injury may occur.

Cold applications

The use of ice in the treatment of soft tissue injuries is now almost universal. The physical effects claimed are:

1. Local anaesthesia, produced by a reduction in the rate of conduction of sensory nerves
2. Decrease in metabolic rate in the area treated
3. Changes in the local circulation.

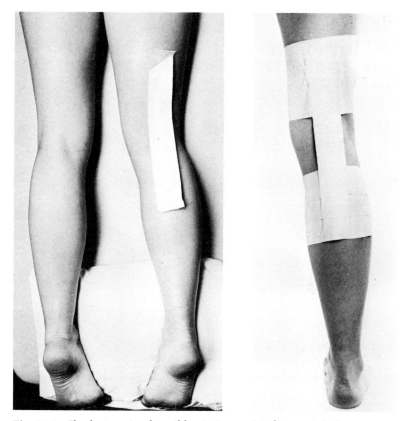

Fig. 11.5   Check strapping for mild anterior cruciate ligament strains

Ice produces cutaneous vasoconstriction, but this may be less important than its other effects. Clotting and vasoconstriction will already have begun in most injuries even when ice is applied promptly and there is no evidence that ice application produces increased muscle blood flow by reflex (e.g. in the quadriceps muscle) (Wyper & McNiven 1976, Knight & Londeree 1977, Knight 1976) thus increasing the extent of deep haematomas. Its most important effects appear to be the reduction of pain and diminution of the metabolic rate of the cells undamaged by the initial trauma which are at risk from hypoxia due to vascular disruption and vasoconstriction. They may then survive until the circulation improves. This would reduce the degree of secondary damage and a smaller lesion which can be more quickly resolved.

The use of ice at a later stage of rehabilitation is more dependent on its anaesthetic effect. The patient may be enabled to carry out

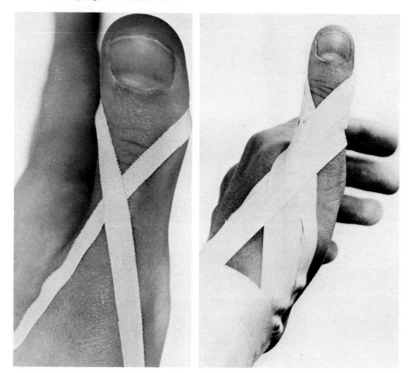

Fig. 11.6   Basket weave strapping for the thumb and fingers

active movement, which is the first major step in restoring normal function. The system of applying ice to numb the part, moving it actively then repeating the procedure three to four times, is known as cryotherapy or cryokinetics (Grant 1964, Hayden 1964). Sensation is reduced but not absent and the patient can halt the movement at any time.

There are several methods by which tissue temperature can be lowered. Ice itself may be applied, crushed to increase the cross-sectional area, in a wet towelling bag. Cold packs are commercially available in several forms and may be easier to use in many situations; however, some are not re-usable and all are more expensive than ice. Cold water is a good alternative when neither of the others is available. Either immerse the part or wrap it with a wet towel or bandage which can be applied under a compression bandage.

The effectiveness of ice as a treatment for soft tissue injuries lies not only in its physical effects but also in the ease and simplicity of its use. The athlete can also carry out the treatment himself, which is always an advantage in the treatment of sports injuries since

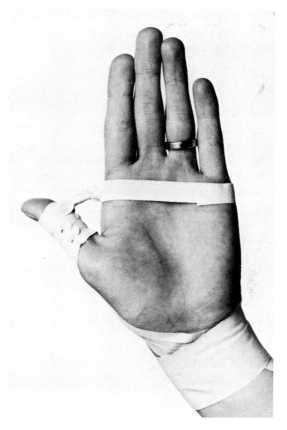

Fig. 11.7 Check strap to limit extension and abduction of the thumb

many cannot rely on the services of trained staff daily. There is little risk of overdose and the materials are inexpensive.

TREATMENT OF ACUTE SOFT TISSUE INJURIES

The use of ice, compression and elevation is already well-documented. Early application of an ice pack, gel pack or cold water can minimize secondary damage. The cooling effect relieves pain and, by decreasing the metabolic rate in those cells on the periphery of the lesion, may reduce its eventual size.

Compression, applied by tubular or elastic bandage or by an air splint applied from below to above the lesion avoiding constriction, decreases bleeding and inflammatory exudate.

Elevation allows drainage of oedema by gravity. This in turn produces pain relief. At this stage also, pulsed ultrasound may prove valuable since phagocytosis is more effective in tissue fluid which is being gently agitated.

In the first 24 hours treatment aims to reduce inflammatory exudate and subsequent secondary damage. Relative rest is indicated, movement being within the limits of pain, since activity may further aggravate the lesion. If the lesion is large the flow of exudate can increase for 4–5 days. It is therefore recommended that cold applications should be continued for the first 48 hours and that compression is maintained for 48–72 hours.

After the first 24 hours gentle, non-weight-bearing exercises should be initiated. Such early contraction is thought to influence the direction in which collagen fibres are laid down. However, since subsequent contraction will otherwise occur, accompanied by shortening, the patient should be taught stretching exercises which must be performed daily and incorporated into warm up/ warm down procedures for at least a year. Supportive strapping in the early stages assists active mobilization while preventing excessive movement. Prompt treatment prevents the risk of secondary damage and may accelerate primary healing.

TREATMENT OF CHRONIC SOFT TISSUE LESIONS

Unfortunately, chronic problems frequently present. Most are overuse injuries which have been shrugged off only to recur until participation in sport is impossible. It is at this stage that the patient presents. Why has the lesion not healed? Causes other than simple or recurrent trauma must be excluded, but these are rare in sport. In many instances the institution of acute primary care, as described, will allow resolution of symptoms.

Where symptoms are due to continued overstretching of scar tissue, strapping may limit movement within a pain-free range. If the pain is persistent, immobilization in a plaster-of-Paris splint may be necessary. Heating may also be beneficial—applied in the form of SWD, microwave or ultrasound depending on the nature and the extent of the lesion. Transverse friction often proves beneficial in specific conditions such as chronic tenosynovitis.

When the problem begins to resolve, rehabilitation follows the same guidelines as in the acute stage, with emphasis on regaining length by static stretching exercises.

REFERENCES

De Vries H A 1962 Evaluation of static stretching procedures for improvement of flexibility. Research Quarterly 33: 222–229

Dunn F, Edmonds P D, Fry W J 1969 Absorption and dispersion of ultrasound in biological media. Biological Engineering, McGraw-Hill, New York

Dyson M, Suckling J 1978 Stimulation of tissue repair by ultrasound—a survey of the mechanisms involved. Physiotherapy 64: 105

Grant A E 1964 Massage with ice (cryokinetics) in the treatment of painful conditions of the musculoskeletal system. Archives of Physical Medicine and Rehabilitation 45: 233–238

Harvey W, Dyson M, Pond J B, Grahame R 1975 The in vitro stimulation of protein synthesis in human fibroblasts by therapeutic levels of ultrasound. Proceedings of the 2nd European Congress on ultrasonics in medicine. Excerpta Medica, International Congress Series 363: 10–21

Hayden C 1964 Cryokinetics in an early treatment program. Journal of the American Physiotherapy and Therapeutics Association 44: 990–993

Knight K L 1976 The effects of hypothermia on inflammation and swelling. Athletic Training 11: 7–10

Knight K L, Londeree B R 1977 Comparison of blood flow in normal subjects during therapeutic applications of heat and cold and exercise. Medicine, Science, Sports 9: 62

Wyke B 1972 Articular neurology—a review. Physiotherapy 58: 3: 94–99

Wyper D, McNiven D R 1976 Effects of some physiotherapeutic agents on skeletal muscle blood flow. Physiotherapy 62(3): 83–85

12. Injury in sport

INCIDENCE

Many sports-related injuries show a tendency to spontaneous healing, some are treated by the athlete himself or his coach and relatively few therefore present for medical opinion. In fact only about half of all injured sportspeople will see a doctor for advice (Hogan & Hoerer 1981). The difficulties thus created in collecting injury data are further compounded, in Great Britain, by the absence of a comprehensive registration system for sports-related injuries. The recent upsurge of interest in and growth of sports medicine is therefore welcome. As public demands for higher safety standards in travel and at work will doubtless soon be transferred to the sports field, the medical profession must be prepared for this to happen and make efforts to establish an accurate data collection system so that effective audit can be undertaken (McLatchie 1989).

Contact team sports have the highest injury rate, followed by fencing, cricket and cycling. The traditional combat sports, such as boxing and judo, have a low injury rate, but when an injury occurs it tends to be more serious and produce a longer lay-off time than the other sports (Weightman & Browne 1975) (Figs 12.1 and 12.2).

There is little difference between the injury rate in men and women, although regional variations occur. However, unfit women are more prone to knee and ankle injuries than men (Whiteside 1980). Boys and girls also show similar patterns (Shively et al 1981), but over 14 years of age boys are three times more commonly injured than girls of the same age (Watson 1984).

In some contact sports as many as 25% of all injuries are due to foul play, so the potential for prevention of such trauma by tighter control is vast (Jorgensen 1984, Davies & Gibson 1978).

NATURE OF INJURY

Soft tissue lesions account for over 80% of sports injuries (McLatchie 1982) and most of the bone injuries incurred can be adequately managed in the Accident and Emergency Department of the local hospital, although in sports such as skiing osseous

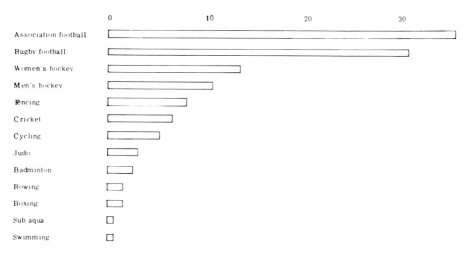

Fig. 12.1 Number of injuries per 10 000 man-hours of play in selected sports (Weightman & Browne 1975)

trauma is a major problem. Nevertheless, specialized orthopaedic care is infrequently required for most sports injuries.

Up to 10% of patients attending their general practitioner do so because of symptoms relating to the soft tissues—musculo-skeletal inflammatory disorders and soft tissue injuries. Lesions

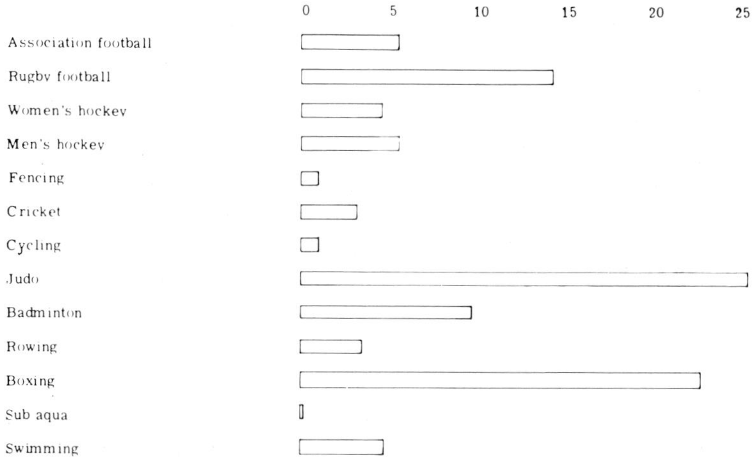

Fig. 12.2 Median days off play per injury during the season in selected sports (Weightman & Browne 1975)

of tendons and their sheaths, fascial disorders, bursitis, inflammation of the tendoperiosteal junction are common in all age groups and often occur in the absence of systemic disease. Common causes include repetitive low grade trauma, direct injury or unaccustomed use. The extent of the problem is enormous. Although mostly self-limiting, which is reassuring for both the patient and practitioner, they can lead to loss of time from work [up to 11 million days annually (Hazlemann 1989)] or play.

Reasons for treating patients with soft tissue injuries (there are several million people injured each year):

1. Time may be lost from work
2. Time may be lost from sport
3. Self treatment may lead to chronic injuries
4. The 'headache' phenomenon (most go away but we prefer relief as soon as possible)

The financial, physical and psychological consequences are therefore considerable. Fortunately, most can be diagnosed and successfully treated by the general practitioner.

SITE OF INJURY

The lower limbs are the area of the body most frequently injured, followed by the upper limbs, the head and trunk, in that order (Fig. 12.3).

In running sports almost all injuries occur to the lower limbs.

CLASSIFICATION

Injuries may be classified according to their cause. In effect there are three causes—direct trauma, overuse and environmental factors (Fig. 12.4). These factors may interact as, for instance, overuse achilles tendonitis is more liable to occur during a football match on a cold day if the tendon has already been injured in a tackle.

Most traumatic injuries occur in contact and combat sports. Overuse injuries are commoner in aerobic activities where there is repetition of a movement over a long period of time. They also tend to occur at specific sites, such as the tendons around the ankle, knee, hip, shoulders and wrist. The management of overuse injuries, too, may be more difficult, for the athlete is likely to carry on performing the causative action. This increases the risk of both chronicity and recurrence.

Environmental injury is caused by extremes of temperature, immersion in water, altitude and depth. The problems produced by each particular environment are discussed in Chapter 13.

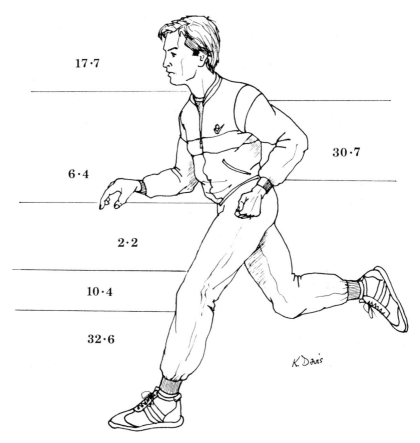

17·7

30·7

6·4

2·2

10·4

32·6

K. Davis

Fig. 12.3 The anatomical sites of injury in sport (percentages) (n = 1600) (McLatchie 1984 A 3-month prospective study of patients with sports injuries attending a city A & E department. Glasgow Royal Infirmary, unpublished observations.)

As in all branches of medicine it is important to establish the cause of injury by accurate history taking. Often, in sport, there will be many contributors to the picture. Nevertheless, the doctor must decide whether he is dealing with the type of injury which requires treatment in hospital immediately, or later the same day (i.e. whether the player can return to his home town if he is injured at an away game), or not at all. If the third option is chosen the doctor should treat the injury himself or give clear guidelines to the patient and his coach as to how to proceed with treatment and rehabilitation.

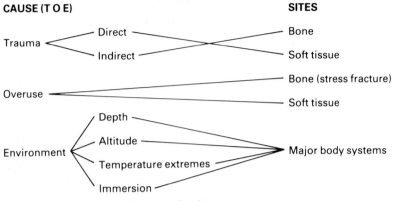

Fig. 12.4   Classification of sports-related injuries

PATHOPHYSIOLOGY OF SOFT TISSUE INJURIES

Neither biopsy nor surgery are commonly used in the management of soft tissue injury and therefore the relevant pathology is poorly understood and histological data is scanty. Recent interest has centred on the role of prostaglandin synthesis and release in response to soft tissue injury due to either trauma or overuse. Prostaglandins derive from arachidonic acid within the cell membrane phospholipids. After injury there is a prostaglandin 'cascade'. This biochemical reaction occurs secondary to tissue damage. Prostaglandins, especially of the E series, are synthesized and prostaglandin E_2 (PGE_2) is especially incriminated in the production of hyperalgesia (Ferreira 1978). This prostaglandin acts synergistically with other inflammatory mediators such as histamine, serotonin and bradykinin to potentiate both swelling and pain (Fig. 12.5). Theoretically, at least, anti-inflammatory agents should block part of this reaction and therefore decrease the pain and oedema associated with soft tissue injury.

TREATMENT OF SOFT TISSUE INJURIES

Traditional treatment involves the use of physical modalities such as cooling, heat therapy or ultrasound at one end of the scale to interventional techniques like local injection with steroid and anaesthetic to surgical decompression at the other. The management spectrum of soft tissue injuries comprises:

- Do nothing! They tend to heal spontaneously. Reassure the patient!

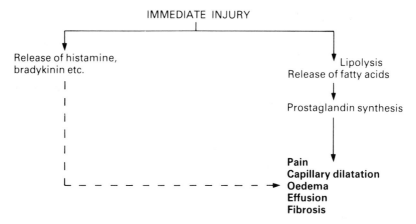

Fig. 12.5   Stages in the pathophysiology of inflammation after soft tissue injury (after Muckle 1980)

- Selective rest
- Splinting, e.g. tenosynovitis of wrist
- Pendular exercises, e.g. acute shoulder
- Heel raises/arch support—TA lesions, planter arch strain
- NSAIDs—widely used for all conditions
- Local anaesthetic/steroid injection
- Surgery. Reserved for soft tissue emergencies, reconstruction and chronic problems

The use of non-steroidal anti-inflammatory drugs (NSAIDs) for minor soft tissue lesions and injuries is widespread and is becoming increasingly common especially in the case of acute soft tissue injuries such as occur in sport or work (Gardiner 1983). It has been known for many years that these drugs have anti-inflammatory, analgesic and antipyretic properties. These effects are the result of the inhibition of prostaglandin production considered to be a mediator of the inflammatory response (Vane 1971). This simple concept has been challenged more recently since other inflammatory mediators have been identified as playing a part in the inflammatory process and the prostaglandins themselves shown to have other actions—perhaps as immuno-modulators which regulate antibody production in lymphocytes and collagenase in macrophages. They may also have positive roles to play in the metabolism of bone and therefore by implication may have an effect on the tendo-periosteal junction (Ceuppens et al 1982, Tornkvist et al 1984). Numerous clinical studies have been carried out but few have been double blind or with a placebo group.

Table 12.1 NSAIDs: deaths related to ingestion

Estimate:	More than 4000 per annum
Perspectives:	Self-poisoning (regarded as a modern epidemic) also causes around 4000 deaths per annum

Table 12.2 Oral NSAIDs: the two ends of the spectrum

Protagonists	Antagonists
General practitioners	Surgeons (GI bleeds)
Rheumatologists	Pathologists (post-mortem confirmation)

In those utilizing a placebo group almost 70% showed that NSAIDs were superior but support for a quicker recovery using NSAIDs is not uniform (Almekinders 1990). The controversy may be resolved however by more standardized and objective studies in the future.

Treatment with NSAIDs can be associated with side-effects, especially gastric irritation leading in some patients to haematemesis and melaena. The incidence of death from NSAID medication has been compared to self poisoning (around 4000 per year) (Table 12.1, Table 12.2) and a CSM update (1986) quoted deaths per million prescriptions in patients on oral anti-inflammatory medication as ranging from 0.7 to as high as 77.8. The search for an effective agent with minimal side-effects in the treatment of self-limiting conditions is therefore justified.

Topical anti-inflammatory agents

In Europe, especially France, topical anti-inflammatory/analgesic agents have been prescribed for many years. Their main indications are in tendinitis, trauma and peripheral joint arthropathies. Large numbers are available over the counter (OTC) and most are salicylate based. Many patients receive a combination of oral and topical therapies for soft tissue rheumatism but unfortunately there are no major controlled studies to demonstrate the efficacy of such a combination of agents.

MODE OF ACTION

When applied to the intact skin overlying inflamed tissue diffusion of topical agents depends on the permeability of the epidermis and can be accelerated by using occlusive dressings or in the presence of local hyperaemia or irritation. Joints distant from the site of application are exposed to the drug by transport in the blood and there is considerable evidence that several of these drugs (e.g. ibuprofen, felbinac, indomethacin) can reach therapeutic levels in synovial fluid and muscle. Some only achieve a small percentage of the plasma concentration compared to oral dosage (e.g. ibuprofen). This is enticing and may reduce the incidence of unwanted systemic side-effects (Wagener 1989). Recent studies with felbinac demonstrated similar efficacy with a significantly lower incidence of drug related toxicity compared to oral therapy in patients with localized arthritis and penetration to deeper tissues has been demonstrated with a more favourable synovial and muscle tissue to plasma ratio than was observed with oral therapy (Anako 1986, Bolten et al 1986). However, multiple applications may be necessary to maintain these therapeutic levels.

In clinical studies however felbinac gel (Traxam), piroxicam (Feldene), diclofenac (Voltarol) and ibuprofen (Proflex) have demonstrated efficacy in the management of both soft tissue injuries and extra-articular rheumatism (McLatchie et al 1989, Hazelmann 1987, Kroll et al 1989, Peters et al 1987).

WHY USE A TOPICAL AGENT?

Apart from the possible advantage of reduced risk to the patient are there are other reasons why topical agents might be attractive? We have observed from our involvement in sports medicine over many years that rubs are popular among sports players. One only has to visit a football, rugby or even ladies' hockey changing room to experience the smell of prematch embrocations. Further, in our studies of several different topical NSAIDs since 1986 we have noted an exceptionally high compliance rate (90%) in groups of young fit patients who did not show the same compliance in respect of oral agents. Topical agents may, then, represent a form of self-treatment or even shared treatment (when a partner applies the gel). Whatever the reason—whether their local physical effect, self application or ease of use—they remain popular with patients of all ages suffering from a wide range of musculo skeletal disorders. Reasons for using a topical agent include:

- Rubs are popular, e.g. embrocation in sport
- It is a form of self or shared therapy
- It has a local physical effect
- It may have reduced systemic side-effects? Reduced risk?

WHO ARE THE POTENTIAL PATIENTS?

- Patients with acute tissue trauma especially sports players
- Patients with extra-articular rheumatism
- Patients with OA or RA

From the available evidence topical agents would appear to be appropriate particularly in patients with soft tissue trauma (especially sports participants) who are likely to be indisposed for 5–20 days but who have no major soft tissue disruption. A further group might include those with extra-articular rheumatism and possibly those with osteoarthrosis or rheumatoid arthritis in combination with oral therapy.

CONCLUSIONS

- All can cause problems
- Few clinical trials are large enough to establish accurate incidences of side-effects
- Post marketing surveillance (PMS) may provide useful data

The studies published to date suggest that topical therapy has a significant role to play in the management of patients with common soft tissue problems. Furthermore, the studies cited have been used as the criteria for assessment of these new agents by the statutory authorizing body (the CSM). The conditions which these studies have satisfied are:

1. The topically applied agent is unequivocally effective in the claimed indication
2. The substance has minimal local toxic or allergic effects
3. The substance reaches the target tissue in sufficient amounts
4. The concentrations in plasma do not lead to undesirable dose related side-effects
5. The metabolism and excretion of the substance must be similar to those occurring when the drug is given parenterally (Wagener 1989)

Based on these criteria the new topical agents described have been accepted and granted product licences. While it is inevitably true that few clinical trials have the power to establish or refute differences in the incidence of side-effects useful data must therefore come from the concept of pharmaco-epidemiology. That is we should all be involved in post-marketing surveillance of new drugs and accurately report adverse reactions in conjunction with the major reviews carried out by the pharmaceutical companies (and as part of our clinical contract).

RECOMMENDATIONS

- Beware the elderly—is the NSAID really necessary?
- Avoid their use in minor conditions
- Do not prescribe for 'at risk' patients
- Consider an alternative—?topical agent
- Consider use with protective drugs, e.g. H2 antagonists

Topical therapy may be especially helpful in patients who dislike injections or oral therapy and appears to be better tolerated with appreciably less morbidity than other treatments (Hazlemann 1989). It represents an attractive alternative to the first line use of systemic agents to manage mild or moderate localized soft tissue injury, extra-articular rheumatism and may provide an adjuvant effect in patients with osteoarthrosis or rheumatoid arthritis. Topical agents may also be appropriate for OTC sales giving more choice to the patient and decreasing NHS costs (McLatchie 1992).

MUSCLE INJURY

About 15% of all injuries will be injuries to skeletal muscle (Newman et al 1969). They can occur because of factors within the muscle itself or from external trauma. When a muscle ruptures it does so near the muscle–tendon junction. Tears, strains and pulls all describe degrees of partial rupture.

Muscle injuries are associated with bleeding to a greater or lesser degree and interstitial haematomas form when the muscle fascia is ruptured. The blood leaks into the interstitial spaces. Intramuscular haematomas produce marked pain and loss of function because the blood remains within the muscle (epimysium intact). Repair involves the formation of non-contractile collagen with scarring. The muscle scar is at its strongest after 2–3 months (Douglas 1966). This is important clinically. The doctor should forewarn his patient that some flexibility may be lost. It is important to include stretching exercises in the rehabilitation programme.

Regeneration of muscle has been demonstrated in animal models (Carlson & Gutmann 1972) and it is probable that this happens in all species of mammalian skeletal muscle. The process is slow, however, and is less likely to occur efficiently in the presence of extensive crushing with haematoma formation or superadded infection.

Rest after an injury should be as brief as possible. Endurance capacity and strength are reduced by more than 25% with prolonged rest (up to 21 days—Saltin et al 1968, Booth 1977), so post-injury activity within the limits of pain must be encouraged.

SPECIFIC INJURIES

Haematoma

This is a collection of blood within a space—usually the soft tissues of the thigh, around the eye or subcutaneously on the shin.

More sinister sites are within the thoracic, abdominal or cranial cavities.

TREATMENT

Haematomas should be aspirated under aseptic conditions. A compressive dressing should then be applied to prevent re-accumulation and to protect the area from further injury. Hyaluronidase can be used to increase the absorption of residual blood (O'Donoghue 1976). We have only rarely used this technique.

Blisters

These are caused by shearing forces on the skin, usually of the hands or feet. Their formation is more likely in hot, humid atmospheres such as the interior of a sports shoe, especially when it fits poorly (Brazin 1979).

TREATMENT

The fluid should be aseptically aspirated or drained as often as it accumulates. The roof of the blister should be left. It acts as a biological dressing and allows healing to occur more rapidly (Cortese et al 1968). The area should then be covered with barrier cream or a dressing to prevent further damage.

Burns

Burns in sport are usually generated by friction rather than physical heat, though the latter kind do occur in motor sport. 'Mat' burns are commonly seen in wrestlers and judoka. 'Grass' burns are a group of injuries associated with playing on synthetic turf.

TREATMENT

The affected area should immediately be cooled with tap water or an ice pack. Unless extensive, when hospital care is needed, this and an analgesic is all that is required.

Fungal infections

A persistent moist environment created by recurrent perspiration predisposes to tinea infections such as 'athlete's foot' and 'jock itch'. The role of showers and swimming pools as reservoirs for these conditions is well known. Up to 37% of tinea pedis sufferers use a club shower facility (Gentles et al 1975). Using the same towel all week, sharing towels and wearing dirty underwear all contribute to infection.

PREVENTION

Adequate foot care is essential. Regular washing, without soaking, and careful drying, especially between the toes, prevents infection. Socks should be changed daily.

TREATMENT

Once the feet are dry, miconazole cream is indicated for acute infections (of foot or groin). When there is toe wet maceration, aluminium chloride 20%, an astringent, is useful for drying the wet spaces.

Strain

Strains affect muscles. Grade 1 and 2 involve fibre damage only (sheaths intact); Grade 3 describes a partial rupture of fibres and sheath; Grade 4 involves complete rupture (Ryan 1969).

TREATMENT

Minor grades need cooling and compression accompanied by early anti-inflammatory medication. Activity should be encouraged within the limits of pain. Grade 3 and 4 may require hospital treatment. Working on the principle that regeneration is more likely to occur in incised rather than torn muscle we prefer to repair major tears surgically. In all cases controlled early mobilization is the key to successful rehabilitation.

Ligamentous injuries—sprains

A sprain is an overstretch injury of a ligament. It may affect only a few fibres or involve complete rupture. For this reason three grades are described, covering varying degrees of severity. In all there is pain, swelling and local tenderness.

TREATMENT

It is important clinically to decide upon the extent of injury. Complete ruptures should be treated by surgical repair and, contrary to popular belief, may be relatively painless because tension within the joint is dissipated by tracking of the haematoma and effusion. It is extremely important to suspect in such cases that there has indeed been a complete rupture. The examination will detect abnormal or excessive movement and a gap may be felt. This is a soft tissue emergency. Best results are seen with early repair.

Partial tears, by contrast, may be exquisitely painful. While radiological investigation in hospital may be needed to confirm anatomical integrity, most of these injuries respond to cooling, strapping and early treatment with anti-inflammatory drugs. If there is a haemarthrosis it should be aspirated. This is one injury for which rest is indicated—best achieved in a plaster-of-Paris splint for 2 weeks.

Tendons

Each tendon is surrounded by a paratenon and, in sites where movement occurs around bone, is further enclosed in a fibrous sheath. Most tendon injuries are due to overuse.

Rupture may be complete or partial. Complete rupture is associated with loss of function and a gap may be felt clinically. Again, this must be considered as a soft tissue emergency. We advocate early surgical repair in most instances.

Partial ruptures also present with sudden pain but no gap can be felt and after a short period limited function returns. Pain is the most clamant feature. Its relief allows early return of movement. However, these injuries should be treated by immobilization for at least 7–14 days.

TENDONITIS/PERITENDONITIS

In these conditions either the tendon or its coverings become inflamed and swollen. While early surgical decompression is effective, many cases respond to relative rest, heel raising (in Achilles tendonitis) and anti-inflammatory drugs. It is important to aim for early resolution of symptoms. Chronic peritendonitis may respond only to surgical decompression.

Tendo-vaginitis. This condition occurs in sites where there is no synovial sheath, e.g. the anterior tibial tendons as they traverse the front of the ankle joint. The sheath becomes inflamed and there is crepitus and pain on movement (tendo-vaginitis crepitans).

Treatment. The condition settles with immobilization in a plaster-of-Paris splint. Other measures include early treatment with anti-inflammatory drugs.

BURSITIS

Bursae are found where tendons or muscles move over bony prominences, e.g. retrocalcaneal, trochanteric. They may also be subcutaneous, e.g. olecranon, prepatellar. When acutely inflamed there is marked swelling, tenderness and pain. Bursae may also become infected.

Treatment. Acute bursitis responds well to anti-inflammatory drugs. Antibiotics are indicated only when there is infection. Chronic inflammation of a bursa responds best to surgical excision.

COMPLICATIONS OF SOFT TISSUE INJURIES

Infection

Infection is always a risk when a wound is contaminated. After careful cleaning, tetanus toxoid 0.5 ml should be given intra-muscularly as soon as possible, but certainly within 24 hours of injury. Immunity should then be kept up to date by regular booster injections. If the patient is already immunized a booster dose will maintain protection.

Bacterial infection in the form of cellulitis or abscess formation may also complicate injuries. In cases of cellulitis a broad spectrum antibiotic such as flucloxacillin or an augmented penicillin such as Augmentin® is effective. Abscess formation is best treated by surgery. Adequate drainage of the abscess with Milton packing of the cavity is the treatment most often advocated. This method is superior to drainage with primary closure and antibiotic cover (Simms et al 1982).

Infection is an uncommon complication of muscle injury and is only likely to occur when there is also a skin laceration.

Cyst formation

When a large muscle haematoma fails to reabsorb, a fluid-filled sac may remain in the muscle. This is not a true cyst in that its membrane is developed by compression of surrounding tissues. Clinically, there is a soft fluctuant swelling which may be demonstrable both by ultrasound and by soft tissue radiology.

TREATMENT

Surgical drainage of the cyst fluid under sterile conditions is indicated.

Myositis ossificans (traumatica)

This is a post-traumatic soft tissue ossification which commonly complicates elbow injuries but is also seen as a complication of muscle injuries (e.g. quadriceps haematoma). It can occur without bony injury. There is invasion of the haematoma by osteoblasts, which are probably derived from the damaged periosteum. Movement, instead of increasing, lessens and there is pain and increasing stiffness.

Myositis ossificans may simulate the early stages of osteogenic sarcoma both radiologically and histologically. The history should therefore not be completely ignored and the cause of the lesion should be carefully investigated over a 10–14 day period when there is doubt.

TREATMENT

Soft tissue radiology will demonstrate the ectopic calcification/ ossification. Exercise should be strictly avoided, because this may accelerate further ossification. It may take several weeks or months for symptoms to subside. Frequent soft tissue films at 10-day periods should be taken. This will allow the doctor to decide if the process is extending or 'burning out'. Once it appears to be quiescent, gentle active exercise can begin again but always within the limits of pain. Passive stretching should be avoided for up to 6 months.

In the early stages surgery should not be considered. However, a mature exostosis may be removed several months after injury.

PREVENTION

Where possible, muscle haematomas should be aspirated and passive stretching avoided. Massage of thigh injuries may predispose to myositis, so coaches should be discouraged from this practice.

REFERENCES

Almekinders L C 1990 The efficacy of non-steroidal anti-inflammatory drugs in the treatment of ligament injuries. Sports Medicine 9: 137–142

Anako T 1986 Clinical evaluation of topical L–141 in osteoarthritis of the knee—a comparative study with indomethacin ointment. Jpn. Pharmacol. Ther. 14: 397–416

Bolten W, Goldmann, Inone Y, Kitamma M, Lawrence G 1986 A randomised study of 2 dose levels of BPAA gel (felbinac) and Fenbrufen (an oral prodrug) to compare systemic levels and local tissue to plasma ratios. In: Proceedings of the Fourth International Seminar on the Treatment of Rheumatic Diseases, Jerusalem

Booth F W 1977 Time course of muscular atrophy during immobilisation of thin limbs in rats. Journal of Applied Physiology 43: 656–661

Brazin S A 1979 Dermatologic hazards of long distance running. Journal of American Military Dermatology 5: 8–9

Carlson B M, Gutmann E 1972 Development of contractile properties of minced muscle regenerates in the rat. Experimental Neurology 36: 239–249

Ceuppens J L, Rodriguex M A, Goodwin J S 1982 Non-steroidal anti-inflammatory agents inhibit synthesis of IgM rheumatoid factor in vitro. Lancet 1: 528–531

Cortese T A Jr, Fukuyama K, Epstein W L 1968 Treatment of friction blisters. Archives of Dermatology 97: 717–721

Davies J E, Gibson T 1978 Injuries in rugby union football. British Medical Journal ii: 1759–1762

Douglas D M 1966 Wound healing. J & A Churchill, London

Ferreira S H 1978 Participation of prostaglandins in inflammatory pain. Advances in Pharmacology and Therapeutics. Proceedings of 7th International Congress of Pharmacology

Gardiner P F 1983 Anti-inflammatory medications. Physician and Sportsmedicine 11: 71–73

Gentles J C 1975 Efficacy of miconazole in the topical treatment of tinea pedia in sportsmen. British Journal of Dermatology 93: 79–84

Hazlemann B 1989 Topical analgesic/anti-inflammatory agents: what indications/patient types? Medical Dialogue 233

Hazlemann B 1989 Soft tissue rheumatism: what are the pros and cons of today's treatment options? Medical Dialogue Weekly 231

Hazlemann B L, Bolton W, Lawrence G P, McDonald M, Lisai, P, Fugimori M 1987 Flebinac—an overview of the European experience. Xl European Congress of Rheumatology

Hogan Dean C, Hoerner E F 1981 Injury rates in team sports and individual recreation. In: Vinger P F, Hoerner E F (eds) Sports injuries—the unthwarted epidemic, PSG Publishing, Littleton, Mass, ch 5

Jorgensen U 1984 Epidemiology of injuries in typical Scandinavian team sports. British Journal of Sports Medicine 18 2: 59–63

Kroll M P, Wiseman R I, Guttadamia M 1989 Clinical evaluation of piroxicam gel: An open comparative trial with diclofenac gel in the treatment of acute musculoskeletal disorders. Clinical Therapeutics 11: 382–391

McLatchie G R 1982 Risk factors in sport. Proceedings of Royal Medico-Chirurgical Society. Scottish Medical Journal 27: 189

McLatchie G R 1989 The incidence and nature of sport related injuries. Sports Medicine and Soft Tissue Trauma 1: 4–5

McLatchie G R 1992 Local NSAIDs—A Topical Issue. Rheumatology Now. In press

McLatchie G R, McDonald M, Lawrence G F, Rogmans D, Lisai P, Hibbard M 1989 Soft tissue trauma: a randomised controlled trial of the topical application of felbinac, a new NSAID. British Journal of Clinical Practice 43: 277–280

Muckle D S 1980 Non-steroidal antiinflammatory agents in soft-tissue injuries. Medisport 2(2): 54–57

Newman P H, Thompson J P S, Barnes J M, Moore T M C 1969 A clinic for athletic injuries. Proceedings of the Royal Society of Medicine 62: 939–941

O'Donoghue 1976 In: Treatment of injuries to athletes, 3rd edn. W B Saunders, Philadelphia, ch 4, p 48

Peters H, Chlud K, Berner G, Wagener H H, Staab R, Melchiar E, Zimmermann P 1987 Zur perkutanen Kinetik von ibuprofen. Aktuelle Rheumatologie 12: 208–211

Ryan A J 1969 Quadriceps strains, rupture and charley horse. Medicine and Science in Sports 1: 106–111

Saltin B, Blomquist C, Mitchell J H, Johnson R L, Wildenthal K, Chapman C B 1968 Response to exercise after bedrest and after training. Circulation, Supplementum 7

Shively R A, Grana W A, Ellis D 1981 High school sports injuries. Physician and Sportsmedicine 9/8: 46–50

Simms M H, Curran F, Johnson R A, Oates J, Givel J C, Chatloz R, Alexander-Williams J 1982 Treatment of acute abscesses in the casualty department. British Medical Journal 284: 1827–1829

Tornkvist H, Lindholm S, Netz P, Stromberg L, Lindholm T C 1984 Effect of ibuprofen and indomethacin on bone metabolism reflected in bone strength. Clinical Orthopaedics and Related Research 187: 255–259

Vane J R 1971 Inhibition of prostaglandin synthesis as a mechanism for aspirin-like drugs. Nature: New Biology, 231: 232–235

Wagener H H 1989 Topical analgesic/anti-inflammatory agents: what is the pharmacokinetic evidence? Therapy Express 4

Watson A W S 1984 Sports injuries during one academic year in 6799 Irish school children. American Journal of Sports Medicine 12 1: 65–71

Weightmann D, Browne R C 1975 Injuries in eleven selected sports. British Journal of Sports Medicine 9 3: 136–141

Whiteside P A 1980 Men's and women's injuries in comparable sports. Physician and Sportsmedicine 8 3: 130–140

13. Sudden death and injury in selected sports

In times of prosperity such as we live in the range of available sports and leisure activities is wider and more easily accessible to most people. It thus becomes a matter of some importance that the possible risks involved in participating in sport should be identified and, if possible, measured. As we have stated previously, data on injuries, and even on death, in many sports is sadly lacking and uncorroborated statements about risk potential, in the absence of scientifically collected facts, often present an ambiguous picture of the dangers involved in sport.

Many deaths in sport are natural. Every golf club has lost some elderly members who have died on the course due to ischaemic heart disease and cerebrovascular disease. This natural end may even be interpreted as an acceptable form of voluntary euthanasia. Each year, too, elderly football spectators die due to ischaemic heart disease, often on cold days, as the excitement mounts during a game.

Such deaths are acceptable and predictable. However, there is increasing concern about the number of sudden deaths occurring in young athletes. Some, but not all, of these are due to congenital heart disease like hypertrophic cardiomyopathy (HCM); others may be attributed to the intrinsic dangers attached to particular sports. These will be considered in more detail.

COMBAT SPORTS

BOXING

Once extremely popular both as a spectator sport and among participants, boxing has largely given way in recent years to other growing sports. Nevertheless about 7000 bouts take place in Britain each year. There are two types—amateur and professional. In amateur boxing, bouts of up to five rounds are permitted, although in practice three rounds even at international level is the rule. In professional boxing the fight may last from 10 to 15 rounds.

The target of attack (the head) and the instruments of attack (the hands) are most often injured—indeed injury to other parts of the body is rare.

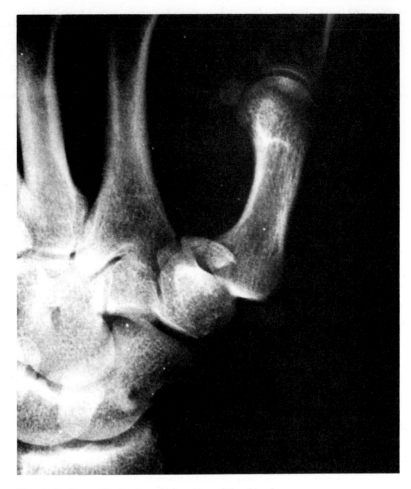

Fig. 13.1   Bennett's fracture dislocation of the thumb

Hand injuries

Sixty per cent of all boxing injuries are to the upper limb. Of these, 83% are to the hand (Montanaro & Francone 1966). One common injury is fracture or fracture dislocation (Bennett's fracture) of the base of the metacarpal of the thumb (Fig. 13.1). This occurs, as a result of poor punching technique, because the thumb is housed in its own separate compartment in the glove. Such injuries require manipulation and/or internal fixation, with immobilization in a plaster-of-Paris splint for 3–4 weeks.

The heads of the fifth and second metacarpals are those next

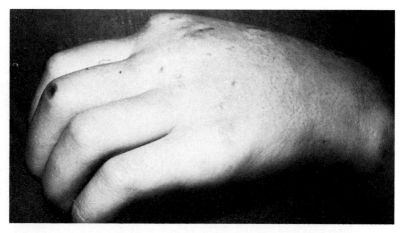

Fig. 13.2   Clinical appearance of fracture of second metacarpal

most commonly fractured (Figs 13.2 and 13.3). They should be reduced if displaced to prevent deformity and future disability for the boxer. Immobilization for up to 3 weeks is required.

Fractures of the metacarpal shafts are usually spiral. They cause only slight shortening, with virtually no long-term disability. Active movements should be encouraged, but actual punching should be discontinued for at least 3 weeks.

Head injuries

Forty per cent of boxing injuries are to the face and head (Fig. 13.4). Head injuries, however, are the commonest cause of death in the sport. The cumulative effects of recurrent head injuries also give cause for concern. The British Medical Association recommendation that boxing should be banned is based on the inherent dangers of both ocular and cerebral damage (British Medical Journal 1984).

RULES REGARDING KNOCKOUT

Following any knockout, the boxer is not permitted to fight again for 4 weeks. Professional boxers are also required to have an electroencephalogram (EEG). A medical examination is mandatory before returning to the ring. If an amateur boxer sustains more than three knockouts in a year he is suspended indefinitely pending further medical examination, which is clinically based with an EEG if this is deemed necessary. A minimum of 3 months suspension applies to the professional boxer.

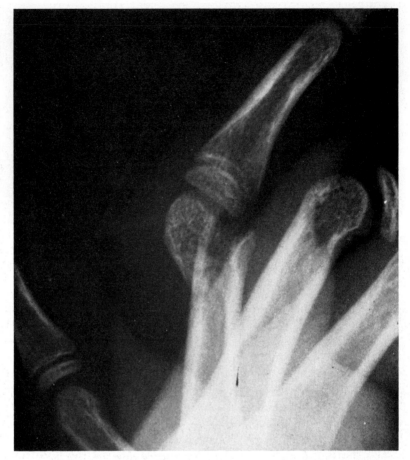

Fig. 13.3 Radiological appearance of a displaced fracture of the second
metacarpal

DEATH DUE TO HEAD INJURY

Subdural haemorrhage, usually into one of the middle cranial
fossa, is the commonest cause of death (Green 1978a). The current
theory of causation is that prolonged battering produces repeated
minor deceleration forces with tearing of dural emissary veins.
Diffuse brain injury and extradural haemorrhage are less common
causes of death due to head injury.

CHRONIC SEQUELAE OF HEAD INJURY

Boxing can produce irreversible cerebral damage (traumatic encephalopathy, punch drunkenness—Roberts 1969, Corsellis et al

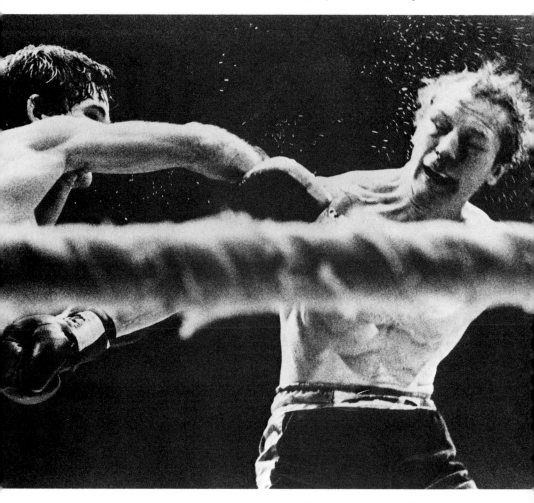

Fig. 13.4 Forty per cent of injuries sustained in boxing are to the head

1973). The fully developed syndrome presents with progressive premature dementia, dysarthria and ataxia. Alcohol tolerance is poor and the mood is labile. In pathological terms there is loss of cortical tissue with scarring of the cerebellum. The septum pellucidum becomes fenestrated and there is degeneration and depigmentation of the substantia nigra. Brain mass is lost (Fig. 13.5).

When such symptoms present it is already too late for that boxer. The aim should be to prevent the syndrome altogether or to forewarn boxers of early changes which may be detected by computerized axial tomography (CT scan—Casson et al 1982) or by a

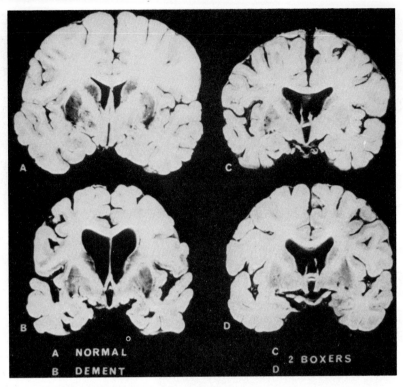

Fig. 13.5 Boxer's brain—comparison between normal and damaged subjects

combination of clinical and psychometric evaluation with EEG (McLatchie et al 1987, McLatchie 1990).

Injuries to the face

THE EYE

The periorbital area is frequently injured. Hyphaema, dislocation of the lens and retinal detachment have all been reported (Rugg-Gunn 1965). These complications are, however, common in other contact and combat sports than boxing (Whiteson 1984).

Retinal detachment in this sport tends to be of a central type caused by repeated minor trauma which leads to macular cyst formation.

Corneal abrasions are common, and the importance of cleaning the gloves of a boxer who has touched the canvas should be stressed to the referee. Local anaesthetic instillation relieves the

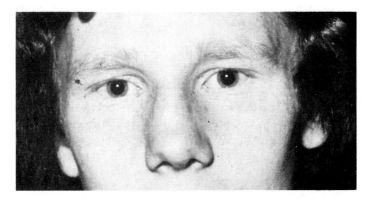

Fig. 13.6 Pugilist's nose

pain of corneal abrasions and the fight should be stopped. Antiseptic cleaning is required.

Periorbital lacerations are also common. They should be carefully approximated by sutures to prevent excessive scarring.

NASAL AND AURAL INJURY

'Pugilist's nose' is the result of frequent encounters. There is septal deviation with old or recent bony or cartilaginous fracture. Repair should be deferred until the fighter has retired. If there are breathing problems, however, it should be carried out immediately. Boxing can be resumed after 6 months (Fig. 13.6).

THE EAR

'Cauliflower ear' is considered the trademark both of the prop forward and of the boxer. It is a complication of haematoma formation. Treatment should be immediate. The haematoma should be aspirated and hyaluronidase (3000 IU) in local anaesthetic injected.

THE MANDIBLE

Fracture of the mandible is rare due to the protection afforded by the gumshield. The presentation and management are discussed in Chapter 17.

Prevention of injury

Strict medical control; education of boxers, coaches and referees on the implications of head injury; and the use of sprung flooring are essential to the prevention of primary acute and chronic brain injury. Protective headgear reduces the number of knockouts (Schmid et al 1968) but may not protect the fighter against cumulative brain damage. The increased availability of thorough neurological examination and psychometric testing may allow the detection of early changes. By the time CT scan changes appear atrophy is well-established (McLatchie et al 1987).

The measures just listed add to the protection afforded to fighters. However, the really decisive role will probably be played by the experienced ringside doctor. His jurisdiction should be extended to stopping the fight when a boxer has, in his view, taken excessive punishment.

KARATE

According to the Martial Arts Commission in London, 60 000 people practise karate in the United Kingdom. Injuries occur both during training and competition but tend to be more severe in competition (Birrer & Birrer 1983). Training injuries often go unreported because of the stoical attitude of those taking part. In competition, an injury will occur once in every 15 fights (Mc-Latchie 1984). Most are to the limbs and digits (60%) with the head and face next in order of frequency and then the trunk.

Digital sprains and dislocations are common, as is bruising of the limbs. Knockouts occur infrequently because strict control is mandatory and facial lacerations are reduced in number when fighters wear protective mitts.

Neuropraxia effects the radial nerve in the upper arm, the ulnar nerve at the elbow and its deep branch in the hand (damaged by striking objects with the hypothenar eminence). The superficial peroneal nerve may be injured during sweeping manoeuvres.

The commonest trunkal injury is acute 'winding' caused by a kick or punch to the solar plexus (coeliac plexus). However, major organic rupture or cardiac dysrhythmia can occur. These injuries are rare, but were the cause of three deaths during karate bouts in the 1980s.

Prevention of injury

Since 1974 the injury rate in karate, in the UK, has been reduced from 1 injury per 4 contests to 1 per 15 contests. The standards achieved in the sport have been maintained—Great Britain were world champions 1983–1984 and Scotland the European champions in the same year (McLatchie 1984). These results have been achieved through concentration on the following safety precautions:

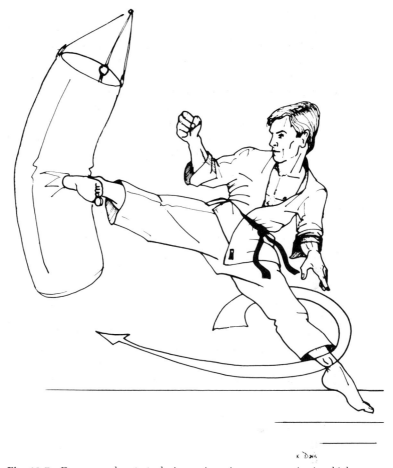

Fig. 13.7 Dangerous karate technique—jumping reverse spinning kick

1. Protective padding and gumshields
2. Insistence on opponents having equivalent body weights
3. Padded or sprung flooring
4. Reduction of emphasis on the breaking of blocks of wood
5. Coach, referee and participant education in BASIC injury management (BASIC—Basic Athletic/Sports Injury Care). This is a scheme launched by the British Association of Trauma in Sport in co-operation with the Phoenix Orthopaedic Center, Phoenix, Arizona, USA
6. Stricter refereeing
7. Medical cover at all competitions
8. Outlawing of dangerous techniques (Fig. 13.7)

GRAPPLING SPORTS

WRESTLING, JUDO AND AIKIDO

Joint injuries are one of the main risks in grappling sports, and symptoms relating to the menisci of the knee and the rotator cuff of the shoulder are common. Deaths are rare and are mainly due to ischaemic heart disease in older competitors. Cervical injury is a risk in Eastern Europe (Gabashvili 1971).

Strangling holds in judo are not permitted in the lower weight classes in juveniles. Although this ruling is quite illogical there are no reports of the punchdrunk syndrome in judoka. It is a sport, however, which might repay systematic investigation. In all the grappling sports 'mat burns' are frequent. They are painful but eminently manageable, and the prognosis is good.

Prevention of injury

Equivalent weight classes apply in competition. Pre-fight medical examinations are a prerequisite in international wrestling. The fighters must also have short hair and well-trimmed nails. Neck injury in the United Kingdom is prevented by adequate strengthening exercises (Fig. 13.8) and strict rules regarding the breaking of a wrestlers' bridge. In the United Kingdom the bridge can only be broken by flexion of the neck (Fig. 13.9), whereas in the USSR it is within the rules to apply downward pressure to the bridge itself.

The foregoing safety principles also generally apply to judo and aikido.

FENCING

The Amateur Fencing Association (AFA) has 3 500 paid-up members but estimates that there are about ten to twelve thousand people fencing in the country at any one time (Crawford 1989).

The AFA has required the reporting of all fencing accidents since April 1984. During the period April 1984–September 1989 30 accidents were notified giving an overall accident rate of 6 per year or 1–1.2 accidents per 100 000 fencing sessions, which is considerably less than the 7.5 injuries per 10 000 fencing hours reported by Weightman and Browne (p. 141). Although under-reporting of injuries inevitably occurs this appears to be at the less serious end of the range. Further, a retrospective questionnaire carried out by medical students on Scottish University fencers disclosed only a small number of relatively minor injuries among a representative group of fencers.

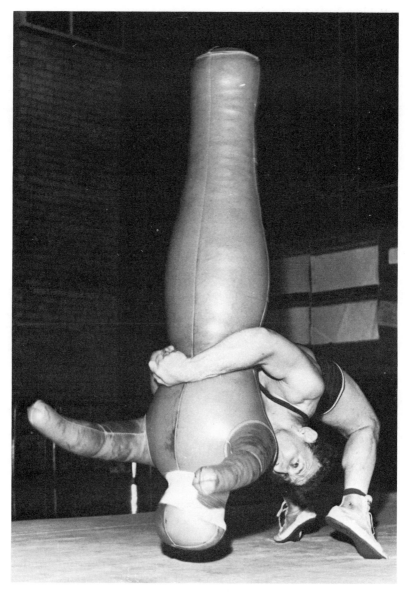

Fig. 13.8 Neck-strengthening exercises. The wrestler's forehead contacts the mat as he throws the dummy

Fatalities

Only one death has been reported in British fencing, in 1983, and the death of a top Russian fencer in 1982 caught media attention.

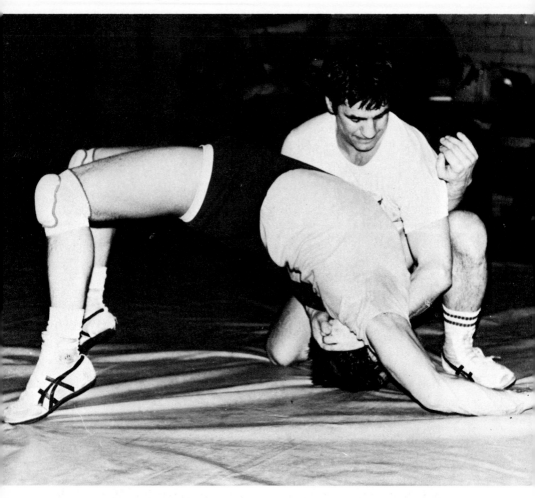

Fig. 13.9   Flexion of the bridger's neck is the safe method of breaking the wrestler's bridge

His death resulted from a penetrating orbital injury after his opponent's foil had broken. The potential for prevention is emphasized by such examples but fencing appears to be considerably safer than other combat sports.

CONTACT SPORTS

SOCCER, RUGBY FOOTBALL, HOCKEY

The incidence of injury in soccer is 37–40 injuries per 10 000 player hours (Jorgensen 1984, Weightman & Browne 1975). Over

80% affect the lower limbs. Of these the ankle and foot are most frequently injured, followed by the knee, quadriceps and calf strains and inguino-crural injury. Goalkeepers are at greatest risk, and foul play may be responsible for as many as 25% of all injuries.

Serious head injuries are uncommon (Tysvaer & Storli 1981), despite the fact that a footballer may head a ball several thousand times throughout his career and it is frequently blasted at him with great force. Nevertheless, a condition resembling the punchdrunk syndrome has been observed in some football players (Corsellis 1974) due to recurrent minor head injuries sustained from heading the ball.

Both osteitis pubis and sacroiliitis are well recognized long-term problems of footballers and the incidence may be as high as 70%. These conditions may be caused by the use of lighter boots which expose the player to the risk of side skids, with twisting of the sacrum and pelvis.

RUGBY FOOTBALL

The number of people playing rugby is estimated at around 200 000 in England, New Zealand, France and South Africa and 100 000 in Japan and the USA. Wales has approximately 35 000 adult players and Scotland 14 000. The game is controlled by the International Rugby Football Board which takes advice on player safety from the Medical Advisory Committee established by the Board in 1977.

The incidence of injury is reported to be 30 injuries per 10 000 rugby playing hours (Weightman & Browne 1975) but in a 30-match season one in 10 regular players will be sufficiently injured to leave the game (Walkden 1975). The leg is the most common site of injury. Neck injuries are more likely to occur when play is static or on wet pitches (Davies & Gibson 1978). Injuries to the face, head and neck account for about 30% of the total with the shoulder girdle and upper limb being affected in 25% of cases (MacLeod 1991).

The number of injuries sustained in tackles has increased, particularly among schoolboys whose technique may be poor. The incidence of serious cervical injury is, however, low. In a 30-year period 67 players were treated in a major regional centre (Silver 1984). Reports from New Zealand confirm this low incidence (Burry & Gowland 1981) and reveal no increase in injury over the study period (see Chapter 20, Injuries to the neck and spine). The risk of injury is similar in rugby league (Patel et al 1984).

One of the commonest injuries is a simple cut. Many of these are minor and do not significantly interfere with playing or training but may have more sinister implications in terms of tetanus infection or contamination of other players (AIDS and Hepatitis—see 'Infection in Sport', Chapter 10).

Serious injuries can also occur in mini-rugby, in particular traumatic dislocation of the hip. This unusual injury may have serious consequences, among which avascular necrosis, osteoarthrosis and recurrent dislocation predominate. Children tend to adopt a 'knee–elbow' position after a fall which predisposes to posterior dislocation (Rees & Thompson 1984).

Overall, foul play may be implicated in as many as 31% of rugby football injuries (Davies & Gibson 1978).

Prevention of injury

Recognizing the risk factors, the Rugby Football Union has banned deliberate collapsing of the scrum and intensified efforts to educate players, especially schoolboys, in the importance of good technique and observation of the rules. Emphasis has also been placed on players staying on their feet, if possible, and avoiding pile-ups. There should additionally be better use of substitutes. The fact that up to 31% of injuries in rugby and 25% in soccer are thought to be due to foul play is a sad indictment on both games. If official control is not tightened it may be left to the players themselves to sue for compensation (see Chapter 1).

FIELD HOCKEY

The injury incidence is 15 injuries per 10000 hours of play in women's hockey and only slightly fewer in men's. Most injuries are to the lower limbs, but the stooped position adopted when playing also predisposes to low-back pain.

Serious injuries are dislocation of the knee (Ambeganonker & Dixit 1971), facial cuts and nasal injury (Oliver et al 1977). The first is caused by loss of balance when swerving, the other two by blows from the stick. More recently, serious ocular injuries have been observed, with blindness resulting in the injured eye (Elliot & Jones 1984). All such injuries were inflicted by the follow-through stroke of the stick.

Prevention of injury

Before 1982, players were penalized for raising the stick above shoulder height. This rule was inexplicably withdrawn in that year, yet in ice-hockey a 'high sticks' rule, introduced in 1975, reduced serious ocular injuries.

Hockey is an aggressive field sport and the shape of the stick allows orbital penetration. Yet facial protection is worn only by the goalkeeper.

RACKET SPORTS

SQUASH AND BADMINTON

In both squash and badminton injury can be produced by either the racket or its projectile—the ball or shuttlecock.

Ocular hazards exist in both sports but the incidence is uncertain. Both projectiles, however, fit very snugly into the orbit and are therefore capable of producing extensive injury and legal blindness (Fig. 13.10) (Chandran 1974). (See Chapter 18, Injuries to the eye and orbit.)

Approximately 70% of all injuries are to the lower limb. They are usually minor and take the form of strains and sprains.

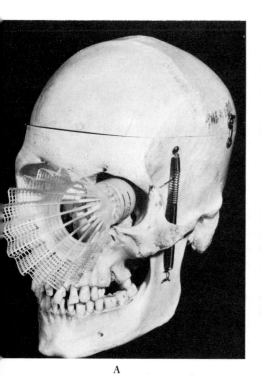 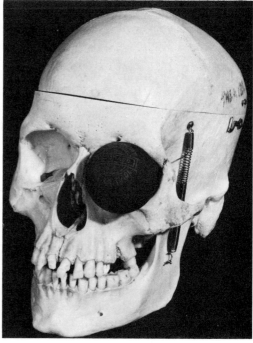

A   B

Fig. 13.10 A The shuttlecock fits snugly into the orbit **B** The squash ball, when cold, cannot penetrate the orbit. When warm, however, it is malleable and fits into the orbital cavity

Dental injury is a risk wherever rackets are being swung, and juniors especially should be forewarned of this danger.

More recently, squash has been incriminated as one of the high-risk sports producing cardiac death. Abnormal cardiac rhythms have been detected during matches (Northcote et al 1983). Players who are unfit or older than 40 are at greatest risk. The number of deaths attributable to this cause is still small; nevertheless unfit people should be forewarned of this danger.

Prevention

Improved coaching techniques in young people will reduce the risk of injury. Eye and dental injuries can be prevented by wearing suitable protective equipment, and this should be encouraged through educational posters in club changing rooms.

WATER SPORTS

WATER SKIING

This sport is limited by weather conditions but is popular during the summer months. Serious injuries are not common but with speeds of 40 km/h and greater there is a real risk. Most injuries are strains, sprains and soft tissue facial lacerations. Falling at speed may also cause tympanic membrane rupture.

The most serious injuries are cervical dislocation associated with high-speed falls or collisions with other craft. Two types of injury associated typically with waterskiing are propeller injuries and perineal douching. Both are preventable.

Prevention

Propeller injuries are almost always caused by foolhardiness and ignoring safety regulations. They can lead to traumatic amputation, head injury and drowning. The rules are clear: the tow rope must be over 21 m (70 ft) in length and an adult observer must accompany the boat driver. Abstinence from alcohol is obviously recommended.

Rectal and vaginal douching can both follow sudden squat positions while skiing. Vaginal laceration, salpingitis or urethritis can result. Rectal tears and rupture of the recto-sigmoid junction are also real risks. If a wet suit is worn the skier is completely protected.

SUB-AQUA DIVING

The main risk to sub-aqua divers is from sudden changes in pressure. Atmospheric pressure is doubled at 10 m of depth and increases by an atmosphere (101 kPa) for every 10 m descended. A rapid ascent can therefore lead to overdistension of the lungs and air-spaces such as the paranasal sinuses and middle ear. The diver may also suffer from 'the bends' if decompression is too rapid or 'nitrogen narcosis' if descent is too great.

Pulmonary barotrauma

If the diver holds his breath or has laryngeal spasm on ascent the lungs become overdistended due to the falling atmospheric pressure. This is followed by hypoxia caused by displacement of blood from increased pulmonary air pressure. There may also be rupture of alveoli, with chest pain and subcutaneous emphysema of the face, head and neck. Haemoptysis is common. Air embolism may also occur after exhaling at the surface (Malhotra & Wright 1960).

Nitrogen narcosis

This is more a commercial than a sports diving problem. In the North Sea, for example, air diving is not permitted at depths greater than 50 m (165 ft). Symptoms are due to the narcotic effect of nitrogen as its dissolved proportion in tissues increases at depth. Described by Jacques Costeau as *l'ivresse de la profonde* this condition does indeed cause the diver to exhibit the mannerisms, euphoria and lack of coordination of a drunk man. There is loss of judgement and sometimes generalized numbness. As exposure to depths is increased divers adapt and this strange narcosis becomes less evident. Why nitrogen should have such effects is unknown.

'The bends'

The name 'bends' is derived from the posture adopted by the affected diver. He becomes fixed in a flexed position because of pain in the large joints. During decompression, nitrogen bubbles are released from solution into the circulation. These block capillaries and cause pain, especially in joints but also in the skin, larynx (producing 'chokes') and lungs. The use of gradual decompression for divers is the major prevention factor.

'The bends', its complication, caisson disease of bone (aseptic necrosis), which is produced by repeated exposure to compression and rapid decompression, and nitrogen narcosis are uncommon in amateur scuba divers. They are, however, a major consideration in professional, industrial and exploratory (historical sea-bed research) diving.

PREVENTION

The British Sub-Aqua Club has stringent safety precautions for sports divers. Sadly, however, anyone can buy diving equipment and is subject to no restrictions if he wishes to dive without instruction or education into the dangers. We believe that sales of sub-aqua equipment should be restricted to affiliated members of recognized clubs.

MARATHON SWIMMING

The major risk in long-distance swimming is of hypothermia. Human beings are not equipped for long periods of immersion, although marathon swimmers differ from other athletes in that they develop a higher percentage of body fat compared to speed swimmers (22% as opposed to 10%—Pugh et al 1960). This provides a degree of insulation.

Prevention

Adequate preparation is vital. Many marathon swimmers spend more than 6 hours per day in the water and even longer when a long swim is imminent. Not surprisingly, many of the outstanding long-distance swimmers are women, who benefit from their naturally high percentage of body fat.

SWIMMING

There are few hazards associated with public swimming pools. Most accidents which result in drowning relate to private swimming parties held either at home or at the seaside. The Registrar General reports about 300 recreational drownings per annum, which makes recreational swimming by far the commonest cause of death in sport and leisure.

Prevention

Prevention depends on forewarning the public of the dangers involved, and local authorities should provide suitable weather warnings (e.g. red flags) on shore in adverse conditions. The provision of lifeguards and safety boats is also important. Despite efforts to prevent accidents many people drown every year. It would indeed be difficult for legislation to take into account the stupidity and lack of common sense which figure substantially in many leisure drownings.

DIVING

Most of the dangers involved in diving come into play when the diver hits the water, often at high velocity. Common injuries are to the soft tissues of the shoulder and thigh. The competitive diver may also sustain head injuries as well as eardrum rupture and wrist fractures. Cervical dislocation is not common in competitive high-diving, presumably because such divers use good technique and the water is always deep enough. In leisure swimming, however, cervical dislocation is well-recognized and is usually associated with 'high spirits' (often in the form of alcohol intoxication) and diving into shallow water.

Prevention

Good diving technique is essential to avoid injury. Flexibility of the trunk and limbs is also a prerequisite to obtain a good piked position in the air.

Leisure diving accidents will continue to happen because of the factors listed above. We can only continue to warn swimmers about dangerous sports and dangerous circumstances such as diving into water that is too shallow. Bars are standard around seaside resorts and beaches. Should we perhaps promote the use of gimmick rhymes, such as STAY ALIVE! IF YOU DRINK, DON'T SWIM OR DIVE!?

AERIAL SPORTS

PARACHUTING

The British Sports Parachuting Association (BSPA) reports less than three deaths per year. Most are due to equipment malfunction followed by the incorrect response from the parachutist, e.g. failure to release the reserve parachute.

The risk points are: 1, exit from the plane; 2, parachute release and its development; 3, landing (Green 1978).

Exit

In most aircraft the door is completely removed, so the risk of striking the tail or becoming caught in the undercarriage or fuselage is small, although bizarre cases have been reported (Flight International 1975). The term 'flat spin' is applied to an accident consisting of a rapid rotation of the trunk about its long axis. This is a risk of free fall and produces disorientation.

Parachute development

Packing errors are the commonest causes of equipment failure. They can lead to unretarded deployment, rope burns or perineal tears. A split canopy will produce a descent at 190 km/h. The reserve parachute has then to be deployed manually with the risk of facial injury.

Landing

Stress is laid on being 'tucked up' on landing, where most injuries occur. Fractures of the lower limbs are common. After high-speed descents multiple fractures are seen. There are often extensive injuries to the musculoskeletal system and to the intra-abdominal and thoracic organs—usually they are detached from their pedicles due to the rapid deceleration on striking the ground. We have queried the sense of using heavy helmets (Chapter 8). These can produce severe cervical flexion, with rupture of the sternum and atria.

Prevention

At least 10 hours of ground training is required before jumping. Since most accidents are due to human error in reacting when things go wrong it will be difficult to reduce their number. Nevertheless even more careful packaging of parachutes and the vetting of candidates regarding their physical and mental suitability to jump may save a few more lives.

RUNNING EVENTS

There are three main areas of concern in the field of running event injuries—injuries which occur to the lower limbs and are almost always related to overuse, and symptoms referable to the gastrointestinal and urinary tracts. In long-distance running environmental injury also becomes a major consideration.

Injuries to the lower limbs

The knee is most often injured, followed by the ankle, hip and groin (James et al 1978). These injuries are adequately discussed in Chapters 24–26.

Gastrointestinal symptoms

Abdominal cramping and bloating are frequent complaints of long-distance runners. Frank diarrhoea and melaena may also present following an increase in mileage or even during a race.

One runner in our experience became incontinent of faeces during a fast marathon run.

The cause of these symptoms is believed to be gut ischaemia related to changes in regional blood flow during submaximal exercise. These are more pronounced in less well-trained runners and symptoms tend to diminish with increased training (Fogoros 1980). The symptoms have also been ascribed to hypovolaemia, hyperthermia and the 'caecal-slap syndrome'. In this condition the posterior wall of the caecum impacts against the anterior producing bleeding and bruising (Porter 1982). This hazard may be analogous in its cause to the mechanism described to explain the haematuria and bladder contusions seen in long-distance runners (Blacklock 1977).

INVESTIGATIONS

While it is safe to reassure most runners, persistent bleeding or diarrhoea must be fully investigated if symptoms continue or increase over a 3-week period in spite of symptomatic treatment and a modified training regimen.

Prevention

Graded preparation before an event is the key to prevention. Runners should train on tracks or level parkland using well-fitting equipment. If there are injuries then early presentation and treatment will prevent chronicity.

Sports haematuria

This condition, although not exclusive to running events, was first described in long distance runners but has also been observed in boxers, hockey players, rowing, lacrosse, football, swimming and aerobics. It may be non-traumatic or traumatic, renal or non-renal in origin.

In non-traumatic cases the haematuria, microscopic or macroscopic, relates to changes in renal haemodynamics during exercise. At rest in the supine position renal blood flow is approximately 20% of cardiac output (1200 ml per minute). Renal plasma flow is 700 ml per minute of which 15% is filtered through the glomeruli (glomerular filtration rate—GFR). Exercise, which demands increased blood flow in the heart, lungs and skeletal muscle may cause a decrease in renal plasma flow from 700 ml to 200 ml per minute. The decrease is proportional to the intensity of the exercise undertaken. Therefore, during prolonged exercise the nephron may suffer relative hypoxic damage leading to increased permeability of the glomerulus and increased excretion of erythrocytes and protein in the urine. Renal vasoconstriction also probably occurs affecting the efferent glomerular arterioles more than the afferent which results in increased filtration pressure.

In cases of haematuria due to trauma the pathophysiology of the conditions relates to shaking or agitation of the kidneys during sport. It can also, of course, be caused by direct renal trauma. Traumatic haematuria is also related to the degree and length of exertion. For example, in one early study only 50% of football players (start–stop activity) had haematuria compared to 80% of swimmers (prolonged intensive activity) (Alyea and Parish 1958).

When haematuria originates from the bladder the single factor involved is trauma. Cystoscopic findings after exercise in long distance runners confirm loss of the urothelium and lesions of the trigone and interureteric bar due to repeated impact of the flaccid posterior wall against the bladder base analogous to the caecal slap syndrome (Blacklock 1977).

Sports haematuria is usually self-limiting but it may in rare cases be associated with acute renal failure due to renal damage and may also contribute to the phenomenon of sports anaemia (McSearraigh et al 1979, Carlson & Mawdslay 1986).

When faced with an athlete with reddish discolouration of the urine both march haemoglobinuria and exercise myoglobinuria should be excluded. These conditions are due to the excretion of haemoglobin and myoglobin molecules due to traumatic haemolysis or breakdown of muscle cells. More importantly pre-existing renal disease may present as haematuria making the investigation of renal function necessary in athletes with recurrent episodes (more than two within a week—rule of thumb). The doctor should also warn patients with a previous history of renal disease that there may be serious risks associated with strenuous exercise (Abarbanel et al 1990).

ENVIRONMENTAL INJURY

Hypothermia and hyperthermia are both recognized complications of long-distance running. (See Chapter 14, Cold injury) Yet they seem to occur only rarely in the sense that few patients have symptoms. Although the rectal temperature in marathon races has been recorded in a range of 35.6–39.6°C, few runners complain of discomfort and most recover after administration of simple measures such as warm or cool drinks and cover as required (Maughan et al 1982).

Even on hot days the problem of hyperthermia is not as great as might be predicted. As few as 5% of runners will present at first-aid stations because of such constitutional problems (Nicholl & Williams 1983). It appears that runners now take note of weather conditions and alter their pace accordingly.

Treatment of heat collapse

The diagnosis of heat collapse is confirmed in any runner with a rectal temperature $> 38\,°C$ who is collapsed or feels unwell. The treatment of uncomplicated heat collapse involves tepid sponging, oral fluids and elevation of the legs. Intravenous fluids are indicated in collapsed runners. Either Hartmann's solution or alternate saline/dextrose infusion should be given. Any collapsed runners should be transported quickly to hospital for specialist investigation.

Hypothermia

Rectal temperatures of less than $35\,°C$ are frequently associated with cerebromuscular dysfunction. Acid–base regulation is disturbed and the blood sugar falls. At first there may be slowing of pace, cramps or stumbling. Later, confusion and euphoria may present. Such people must not be left alone. They should receive warm drinks, shelter and a change of clothing as quickly as possible. Shelter from the wind, using any means available, reduces cooling and could be achieved using a shared sleeping bag. When safety is reached rapid rewarming in a hot bath restores the body temperature.

If there is any risk of circulatory collapse removal to hospital is essential.

Frostbite

Frostbite is due to exposure to cold and is a risk undergone by mountaineers and overland explorers in Arctic conditions. Pathologically, there is vessel-wall damage followed by exudation and oedema. Extremities such as the nose, ears, fingers and toes are first affected. The condition presents with painful extremities and later with gangrene.

TREATMENT

If there is no gangrene the affected parts should be slowly rewarmed and dressed with cotton wool dressings. Narcotic analgesics will relieve pain and hyperbaric oxygen may also be of value. Gangrenous extremities require conservative amputation.

PREVENTION

Prevention is by protecting vulnerable areas.

Immersion injury

A fall into cold water near freezing point may be fatal within 15 minutes. Even at temperatures of 5 °C death will occur in about an hour. Extra clothing will delay heat loss by both conduction and convection. The immersed person should remain as still as possible, because swimming promotes heat loss.

PREVENTION

The use of wet and dry suits in combination with life-jackets reduces the risk of death from immersion. The ideal situation is to ensure early rescue, a change of clothing and warm drinks (not alcohol).

REFERENCES

Abarbanel J, Benet A E, Lask D, Kimche D 1990 Sports haematuria. Journal of Urology 143: 887–890

Alyea E P and Parish H H Jr 1958 Renal response to exercise: urinary findings. Journal of the American Medical Association 167: 807

Ambeganonker S D, Dixit N D 1971 Acute and sub-acute injury: field hockey. In: Lawson L A (ed) Encyclopaedia of sports sciences and medicine. Macmillan, New York

Birrer R B, Birrer C D 1983 Unreported injuries in the martial arts. British Journal of Sports Medicine 17 2: 131–134

Blacklock N J 1977 Bladder trauma in the long distance runner—10 000 metres haematuria. British Journal of Urology 49: 129–132

British Medical Journal 1984 Annual report of Council. Appendix II: Report of the board of science and education working party on boxing. British Medical Journal 288: 876–877

Burry H C, Gowland H 1981 Cervical injury in rugby football—a New Zealand survey. British Journal of Sports Medicine 15(1): 56–59

Carlson D L and Mawdslay R H 1986 Sports anaemia: a review of the literature. American Journal of Sports Medicine 14: 109–112

Casson I R, Sham R, Campbell A, Tarlau M, Didomenico A 1982 Neurological and CT evaluation of knocked-out boxers. Journal of Neurology, Neurosurgery and Psychiatry 982: 45: 170–174

Chandran S 1974 Ocular hazards of playing badminton. British Journal of Ophthalmology 58: 757–760

Corsellis J A N 1974 Personal communication: Brain damage in sport. Lancet (i): 401–402

Corsellis J A N, Bruton C J, Freeman-Browne D 1973 The aftermath of boxing. Psychological Medicine 3: 270

Crawford R 1989 Injuries in fencing. Personal communication

Davies J E, Gibson T 1978 Injuries in rugby union football. British Medical Journal ii: 1759–1762

Elliot A J, Jones D 1984 Major ocular trauma: a disturbing trend in field hockey injuries. British Medical Journal 289: 21–22

Flight International 1975 (20 November) Private flight, p 748

Fogoros R 1980 'Runner's trots'. Gastrointestinal disturbances in runners. Journal of the American Medical Association 243: 1743–1744

Gabashvili I 1971 Death of sportsmen in the Georgian SSR 1955–1970 In: Abstracts of the XVIIIth World Congress of Sports Medicine, British Association of Sports Medicine, London, p 57

Green M A 1978a In: The pathology of violent injury. Edward Arnold, London, ch 15, p 256

Green M A 1978b In: The pathology of violent injury. Edward Arnold, London, p 268–271

James S L, Bates B T, Osternig L R 1978 Injuries to runners. American Journal of Sports Medicine 6: 50–60

Jorgensen U 1984 Epidemiology in injuries in typical Scandinavian team sports. British Journal of Sports Medicine 18 2: 59–63

Malhotra M S, Wright H C 1960 Air embolism during decompression underwater and its prevention. Journal of Physiology (London) 151: 32–35

Maughan R J, Light I M, Whiting P H, Miller J D B 1982 Hypothermia, hyperkalaemia and marathon running. Lancet 11 Dec: 1336

Montanaro M, Francone A 1966 Roentgenicinematographic study of the hand in boxing. Proceedings of the 6th Amateur International Boxing Association Medical Congress, Rome

MacLeod D A D 1992 Risks and injuries in rugby football. In: The Soft Tissues: Trauma, Rheumatism and Sports Injuries. McLatchie G, Lennox C (eds) Butterworth Heinemann, Oxford (in press)

McLatchie G R 1984 Injuries in karate—the Scottish competition register. Report presented to the Scottish Karate Board of Control

McLatchie G R et al 1987 Clinical, neuropsychological, EEG and CT scan examination of amateur boxers. Journal of Neurology, Neurosurgery and Psychiatry 50: 96–99

McLatchie G R 1990 Combat sports: common injuries and their treatment. In Payne S (ed) Medicine, sport and the law. ch 17, 210–229 Blackwell Scientific Publications, Oxford, London, Edinburgh, Boston

McSearraigh E T M, Kallmeyer J C, Scluff H B 1979 Acute renal failure in marathon runners. Nephron 24: 236–241

Nicholl J P, Williams B T 1983 Injuries sustained by runners during a popular marathon. British Journal of Sports Medicine 17 1: 10–15

Northcote R J, MacFarlane P, Ballantyre D 1983 Ambulatory electrocardiography in squash players. British Heart Journal 50: 372–377

Oliver J H, MacKasey D, Percy E C 1977 Experience of the Canadian medical team at the 21st Olympiad. Canadian Medical Association Journal 117: 609–612

Patel M K, Burt A A, Bradbury J A 1984 Are spinal injuries more common in rugby union than in rugby league football? British Medical Journal 288: 1308

Porter A M W 1982 Marathon running and the caecal-slap syndrome. British Journal of Sports Medicine 16 3: 178

Pugh L G C E et al 1960 A physiological study of channel swimming. Clinical Science and Molecular Medicine 19: 257–273

Rees D, Thompson S K 1984 Traumatic dislocation of the hip in mini rugby. British Medical Journal 289: 19–20

Roberts A H 1969 Brain damage in boxers. Pitman, London

Rugg-Gunn A 1965 Eye injuries in boxing. In: Medical aspects of boxing. Pergamon Press, Oxford, p 9011

Schmid L, Hajik E, Votipka F, Teprik O, Blonstein J L 1968 Experience with headgear in boxing. Journal of Sports Medicine and Physical Fitness 8: 171–173

Silver J R 1984 Injuries of the spine sustained in rugby. British Medical Journal 288: 37–43

Tysvaer A, Storli O 1981 Association football injuries to the brain—a preliminary report. British Journal of Sports Medicine 15 3: 163–166

Walkden L 1975 The medical hazards of rugby football. Practitioner 205: 201–206

Weightman D, Browne R C 1975 Injuries in eleven selected sports. British Journal of Sports Medicine 9 3: 136–141

Whiteson A 1984 Boxers' brains. British Medical Journal 288: 1007

14. Cold injury

INTRODUCTION

Cold can produce a variety of systemic, local and indirect effects on humans but the severity of the cold stress at any particular time depends on the interaction of absolute temperature, 'wind-chill' (wind or draughts) and moisture (rain, mist or damp).

SYSTEMIC COLD INJURY

HYPOTHERMIA

Hypothermia has been reported during marathons and on the mountains, in caving and canoeing, at work on land and at sea, and in and underwater. Geographically, hypothermia has in fact been recorded from most parts of the world even at low altitudes in the Sahara and from tropical Kampala.

DEFINITION

To allow for the diurnal variation in core temperature of 1 to 2°C, and the marked, environment dependent, variation of the temperature of the superficial tissues ('shell'), *hypothermia* can only be diagnosed when the temperature of the deep ('core') tissues of the body is below 35°C. Even with this definition, hypothermia is not a diagnosis but merely a gradation of degrees of severity.

To provide a useful classification it is necessary to consider changes which occur during the development of hypothermia viz. the state of energy balance, fluid balance and intercompartmental fluid shifts.

Fluid balance in the cold

Cold induced vasoconstriction shunts blood into the deep capacitance vessels, and the relative excess of volume is removed by a diuresis. Even with total body dehydration, exercise causes an increase in the intravascular fluid volume, thus increasing the diuresis and worsening the dehydration. Respiratory moisture loss is increased by exercise especially in cold dry air, e.g. in the polar regions and at high altitude. Also cold air is dry, evaporation is rapid and even 1–2 litres/day sweat loss may be unnoticed.

During exposure to cold, fluid also shifts from the intravascular into the intracellular space. During rewarming the fluid shifts reverse and the circulating blood volume increases, up to 130% of the value prior to cooling, depending on the potential volume of fluid available, which in turn is related to the duration of cooling.

The fluid status of any hypothermic individual will depend on the relative importance of these two responses.

Classification of hypothermia

1. In a very rapid, acute, 'immersion' hypothermia, the cold stress is so great that the core temperature is forced down despite the heat production of the body being at or near the maximum possible. However since the heat generating capacity of the body remains unimpaired, there will be very little difficulty in rewarming once the person has been removed from the severe environment. The shifts of body fluids will be minimal.
2. In subacute or 'exhaustion' hypothermia the cold stress is moderate and the core temperature only falls because, through exhaustion, the supply of heat has failed. Thermal protection must consider every avenue of heat loss however small the absolute quantities, because this may make the difference between life and death. There is also the probability of complications due to variable fluid shifts and losses.
3. In slow or 'subclinical chronic' hypothermia, the exposure to cold, while relatively mild, has been prolonged. The core temperature has remained normal (35°C or above) possibly for days, weeks or even months before drifting or being precipitated into hypothermia, e.g. by a fall. The energy reserves will be very variable, but there will be large intercompartmental fluid shifts.

The different types can only be distinguished by the case history. For example the commonest cause of immersion hypothermia is falling into cold water. However if a climber in a snowstorm is disabled by a broken leg, the shock of the injury will increase the rate of heat loss, and the fracture will prevent heat generation through muscle activity. He or she will probably cool as rapidly as if immersed. Similarly a diver, at pressures equivalent to 150 m of water or deeper, may suffer 'immersion' hypothermia even in a dry pressure chamber because the heat transfer capacity of the compressed oxyhelium gas breathing mixtures produces such a tremendous respiratory heat loss. On the other hand a swimmer lost overboard in relatively warm water is a candidate for 'exhaustion' hypothermia like mountaineers or hill walkers. A middle-aged man or child with severe malnutrition is likely to develop 'subclinical chronic' hypothermia, usually found in the elderly,

Table 14.1 Signs and symptoms at different levels of hypothermia (from Lloyd 1989 Science in Progress, Oxford 73: 101–116)

°C	
37.6	'Normal' rectal temperature
37	'Normal' oral temperature
36	Increased metabolic rate in attempt to balance heat loss
35	Shivering maximum at this temperature. Hyperreflexia, dysarthria, delayed cerebration
34	Patients usually responsive and with normal blood pressure, lower limit compatible with continued exercise
33	Retrograde amnesia ⎫ Pupils dilated.
32	Consciousness clouded ⎬ Most shivering ceases
31	Blood pressure difficult to obtain ⎭
	⎧ Progressive loss of consciousness
30 ⎫	⎪ Increased muscular rigidity
29 ⎬	⎨ Slow pulse and respiration
28 ⎭	⎪ Cardiac arrhythmia develops
	⎩ Ventricular fibrillation may develop if heart irritated
27	Voluntary motion lost along with pupillary light reflex, deep tendon and skin reflexes. Appear dead
26	Victims seldom conscious
25	Ventricular fibrillation may appear spontaneously
24 ⎫	
23 ⎪	Pulmonary oedema develops. 100% mortality in shipwreck victims in
22 ⎬	Second World War
21 ⎭	
20	Heart standstill
18	Lowest *accidental* hypothermic patient with recovery
17	ISO-ELECTRIC EEG
9	Lowest artificially cooled hypothermic patient with recovery
4	Monkeys revived successfully
1 to – 7	Rats and hamsters revived successfully

whereas a fit 70-year old out walking in the hills probably has 'exhaustion' hypothermia.

The importance of the differential diagnosis is that inappropriate treatment may kill a potential survivor. Collapse during rewarming is almost unknown during rewarming from immersion hypothermia whereas it is relatively common in exhaustion hypothermia. In subclinical chronic hypothermia, if rewarming is too rapid, the volume of fluid returning to the circulation may cause an overload and result in cerebral and/or pulmonary oedema.

SYMPTOMS AND SIGNS (see Table 14.1)

The early signs and symptoms of hypothermia are indistinguishable from those of hypoglycaemia, exhaustion, incipient heat stroke and even a minor cerebral stroke. Also individuals show a great range of responses, e.g. one person was unconscious at 33 °C while another person was still conscious at 24.3 °C. Similarly though shivering has been recorded at a core temperature of 24°C, many mountain rescue cases never shiver, and cooling can occur without shivering.

Death and revival

Profound accidental hypothermia may show a clinical picture very difficult to distinguish from death and the only certain diagnosis of death in hypothermia is failure to recover on rewarming.

People, especially children, known to have been totally submerged in very cold water, can recover even after periods of 15 to 40 minutes (normal submersion survival is about 3 minutes), but survival depends on resuscitation being started immediately.

Methods of rewarming

In the field (pre-hospital) the only practical methods are surface heating, spontaneous rewarming and airway warming.

Surface heating is often used because the rescuers feel that they must do something active. The hot bath is the fastest method but it is only of real benefit within 20 minutes of rescue, is only available where there is human habitation, and the supply of hot water may be inadequate. Surface warming has been associated with rewarming collapse. Also cold blood carries less oxygen than warm blood and the oxygen carried may be inadequate for the increased demand of the warmed superficial tissues, producing a dangerous metabolic acidosis. Finally if there is no circulation (or very little) through the skin, surface warming is ineffective and may cause burning even at 'baby bath' temperatures.

As soon as the victim is found, the body surface, including the head, should be insulated, and the patient allowed to *rewarm spontaneously*. Any available material can be used, but the 'space blanket', though often recommended, was shown on theoretical grounds and in experiments, to be no better than a similar thickness of polythene, which is much cheaper. Insulation includes shelter from the wind, e.g. a hut, a survival bag or behind a large boulder. However heat production may be insufficient to compensate for continued heat loss, and the patient may fail to rewarm, or may continue to cool.

Even with perfect surface insulation the patient is still losing heat through breathing. *Airway warming* (AW) stops this by providing warmed, humidified air to breathe. AW should only be used with adequate body surface insulation. AW produces a significant increase in the rate of rewarming, and a marked improvement in cardiorespiratory function, cerebral function, conscious level and

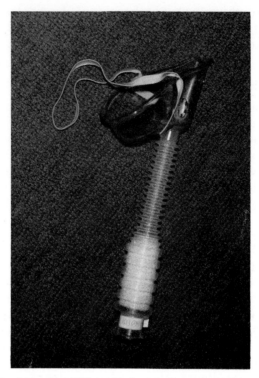

Fig. 14.1 Condenser humidifier with face mask attached. This can be used in the emergency treatment of accidental hypothermia. The end of the humidifier should be under the clothing next to the skin and the whole device, including mask, covered with a scarf

patient morale. Shivering is inhibited, but, despite the decreased oxygen consumption, rewarming is not slowed. In young patients with acute or subacute hypothermia, AW has a lower mortality than spontaneous or hot bath rewarming. However AW should not be used in the elderly unless they are being treated in an intensive care unit. There is a variety of designs of equipment including electrically operated humidifiers (not nebulizers), a design which utilizes the chemical reaction between soda lime and carbon dioxide, and a condenser humidifier attached to a face mask (Fig. 14.1).

In hospital there are a variety of other rewarming methods which have been used successfully. However the results suggest that almost any method may be safe provided the patient is treated using *intensive care* management.

Other treatment

Cardiac drugs are ineffective, and the effects of other drugs are unpredictable. Any medication should be given intravenously. *Oxygen* can be given but, if it is too cold, it may cause cardiac arrest. *Corticosteroids* are worth considering *in extremis*. *Glucose* may be required in exhaustion hypothermia to allow heat generation. If *intravenous fluids* are given they must be warmed.

Cause of death after rescue

During the infamous Dachau experiments the Nazis noticed that, after the person had been removed from cold water, the rectal temperature continued to drop for a while before starting to rise again, and they called this phenomenon the 'afterdrop'. Because death often occurred at about the time the afterdrop was at its lowest, it was postulated without any actual evidence, that the afterdrop caused the death through ventricular fibrillation. The afterdrop is in fact the result of normal physics of temperature equilibration, and this theory should now be relegated to history.

The cause of death following rescue is almost always due to an imbalance between the circulating blood volume and the capacity of the active vascular bed. Death would occur either if the vascular bed became too large for the actual circulating blood volume (hypovolaemic shock) or if the reversal of the fluid shifts was too great overloading the circulation and resulting in cerebral and/or pulmonary oedema. Death may still occur from ventricular fibrillation if the hypothermic patient is handled roughly.

Late effects of hypothermia

Most patients have no after-effects following rewarming, but some may develop diffuse intravascular coagulation with thrombosis leading to stroke.

OTHER CONDITIONS

Familial cold urticaria is a genuine *allergy* to cold, transmitted as a genetic dominant. The clinical features are malaise with shivering, aching joints, generalized urticaria, and local wheals and rashes. Lesions may even be produced by cold drinks or in an indoor swimming pool. Proper counselling and prevention of exposure to cold may save the life of a susceptible person, since some deaths which occur within a few minutes of entering cold water may be due to anaphylaxis in a person with previously unsuspected cold urticaria.

LOCAL COLD INJURY

FROSTBITE

Frostbite is most commonly associated with northern latitudes but may also occur in unexpected parts of the world, e.g. in the Sahara desert at night.

Precipitating factors

Skin freezes at – 0.5°C but true frostbite occurs when there is sufficient heat loss in the local area to allow ice crystals to form in the extracellular spaces.

The risk is increased in smokers, in peripheral vascular disease and Raynaud's syndrome, and by a previous episode of frostbite, by dehydration, alcohol, excess tiredness, altitude, and by a lowered deep body temperature. Negroid people are more susceptible than Caucasians.

Though the ears, nose and the distal extremities of the limbs are most commonly affected, the site of frostbite is influenced by physical immobility, position, pressure, lack of insulating fat, liability to wetting (including overflow incontinence), or by contact with cold metal, e.g. penile frostbite from metal zips. Anything which restricts the circulation, e.g. too tightly laced training shoes, increases the risk and worsens the outcome. Inadequate or tight clothing worn during skiing or running in extreme cold can also produce penile freezing.

Classification of cold injury

In *frostnip* the exposed skin, which has been painful, blanches and loses sensation, but remains pliable. In *frostbite* the part is insensitive, wooden and grey-purple or marble white (Fig. 14.2). Because tendons are less sensitive to cold and the associated muscle groups are distant from the injury, the part can still be moved voluntarily even in deep frostbite. The initial assessment of depth and severity is inaccurate but in practice the treatment is not determined by the severity of the damage.

Thawing

Frostnip can be rewarmed by placing the affected part in the armpit or under clothing. The part tingles, becomes hyperaemic, and within a few minutes sensation is restored and normal working can be resumed. There may be some skin desquamation several days later.

No attempt should be made to thaw frostbite if the part may be

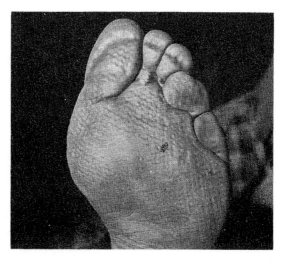

Fig. 14.2 A cold rigid forefoot without sensation or digital motion. Tissue compression and sock marks are obvious

refrozen, because refreezing causes much more damage than continuous freezing. It is possible, and better, to walk to safety on frozen feet; one man did for 74 hours.

Frostbite should be rewarmed by immersion of the part or the whole person in a whirlpool or bubble bath (38–41°C) until the distal tip of the thawed part flushes. The best prognosis is if clear blebs develop over the next 48 hours (Figs 14.3, 14.4). If the part remains cyanotic and cold and blebs do not develop (Fig. 14.5), there is no chance of tissue recovery (Fig. 14.6). Gradual spontaneous thawing should be used if the part has been thawed previously, and is probably satisfactory for superficial frostbite but not for deep injury. Delayed thawing or using ice or snow rubbing often results in marked tissue loss. The worst results follow thawing with excessive heat (Figs 14.7–14.9) at or above 50°C, i.e. temperatures produced by diesel exhausts, stoves or wood fires, or scalding water.

Blebs should be protected but drained if infected. Dislocations should be reduced immediately the part has been rewarmed but fractures are treated conservatively. Since the gangrene of frostbite is much more superficial than it appears, debridement or amputation should be delayed up to 90 days till mummification and tissue demarcation is complete. After the blackened areas have separated, the underlying tissue is raw, shiny, tender and unduly

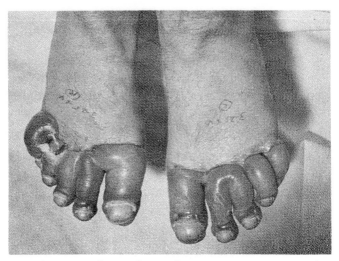

Fig. 14.3   36 hours post-thawing by rapid rewarming in warm water showing clear blebs reaching to the end of the toes. Patient complained of severe pain

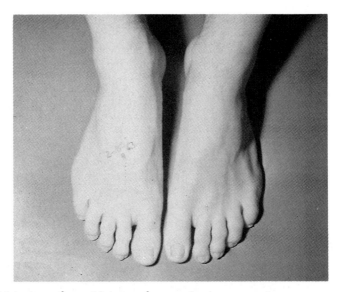

Fig. 14.4   4 months post injury and rewarming in warm water. Epithelialization is complete and the anatomy has been preserved, but the changes of deep injury included volar fat pad loss, early IP joint contracture, nail changes, hypaesthesia and hyperhydrosis, and some are obvious. At the end of 1 year the extremity had adequate sensation, there was mild subcutaneous loss and interphalangeal contracture, with a few interphalangeal subarticular lesions present on X-ray. Increased sweating was still present.

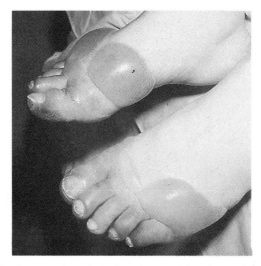

Fig. 14.5 The feet are approximately 5 days post-freezing and 48 hours post thawing, which was by rubbing with ice and snow. A very poor prognostic sign is evident. The blebs are all proximal and are dark, while the toes and distal tissues are without blebs or blistering, and are dusky, oedematous, painless and insensitive. Phalangeal amputation is generally unavoidable with this pattern and may be predicted as early as 24 hours post thaw. (See Fig. 14.6).

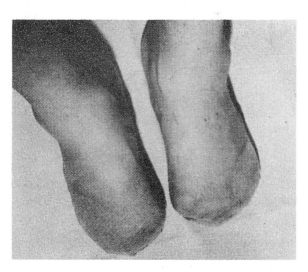

Fig. 14.6 Amputation at the distal metatarsal level. Despite this the patient was back in the Arctic the following winter and continued trapping and hunting for many years.

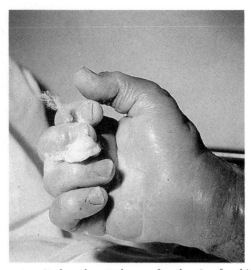

Fig. 14.7   The extremity less than 24 hours after thawing frostbite by using excess heat (boiling water in this case). The hand is cyanotic, painful and foul smelling and there are no blebs (see Fig. 14.8).

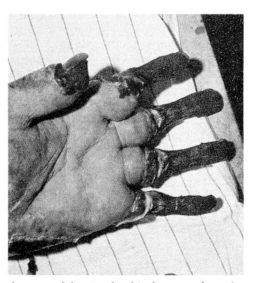

Fig. 14.8   Another case of thawing frostbite by excess heat. At approximately 5 weeks the digits show tissue death, being hard and rigid with the soft tissue completely mummified. There is evidence of infection, superficial only, at the area of tissue demarcation

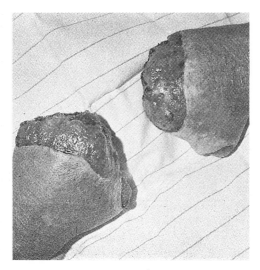

Fig. 14.9 Spontaneous amputation at the MP junction at 6 weeks. This is typical of the extent of tissue loss and the hopelessness for recovery when gangrene is caused by 'cooking' frozen tissues with excessive dry or wet heat

sensitive, and there may be abnormal sweating. This should return to normal in 2–3 months.

Other measures

The treatment of hypothermia, if present, takes precedence. Rehydration with warmed fluids is very important. Sedatives and analgesics should be given as required. Smoking is prohibited because of its vasoconstrictor effect. Digital exercises are encouraged throughout the day and, for the lower limbs, Buerger's exercises four times daily.

TRENCH FOOT (NFCI)

Cold can also cause tissue damage without freezing: 'Trench Foot', 'immersion injury', 'non-freezing cold injury' (NFCI). There is sometimes confusion between frostbite and NFCI, though NFCI is likely to be present proximal to areas of frostbite. NFCI was frequent during the wars, among soldiers living in wet trenches, and among sailors after long periods spent in lifeboats. Even in the Falklands campaign in 1982, NFCI accounted for 20% of the men received on the hospital ship Uganda. Prolonged trekking through boggy terrain in northern countries could result in NFCI.

Running barefoot on frozen ground, though painless during the run due to cold-induced neuropathy, has resulted in considerable loss of tissue on the soles of the feet.

Risk factors

NFCI requires longer exposure than does frostbite, and develops when the legs are exposed to the wet and cold above 0°C, though wet conditions are not absolutely necessary. If the part is wet, tissue damage may occur even with skin temperatures up to 29°C. As in frostbite (and hypothermia) predisposing factors include dehydration, inadequate nutrition, fatigue, stress, intercurrent illness or injury. Damage is more likely to occur and be more extensive if the limb is dependent, immobile or is constricted by footwear. If footwear has been soaked in sea water the incidence of NFCI is higher because the salt crystals attract water, and in the mountains, NFCI can develop if the boots are impervious to water because the build-up of sweat inside the boot is the equivalent to immersion.

SIGNS AND SYMPTOMS

Numbness ('walking on cotton wool') is replaced on rewarming by paraesthesia and/or pain, sometimes very severe. On re-use, e.g. weight-bearing, the initial almost unbearable pain is gradually replaced by numbness on re-exposure to cold. The typical case has cold, swollen and blotchy pink-purple or blanched feet which feel heavy and numb. This is succeeded by hyperaemia, with hot, red, swollen feet, and pain which may be severe. This phase may last for days or weeks. There may be bleeding into the skin and severe injury is indicated by large blisters. The damage may progress to gangrene which tends to be deeper than in frostbite.

TREATMENT

Remove the person from the hostile environment, give analgesics for the pain, and bed rest. Unfortunately at present there is no satisfactory treatment for the many late manifestations of NFCI.

After-effects of local cold injury

There may be nerve damage, viz. vasomotor paralysis, analgesia and paraesthesia, which may be permanent, and hyperhydrosis. Muscle damage may leave weakness. Damage to cartilage and bone may include toe rigidity and fallen arches, and osteoporosis, though new bone formation usually restores the normal X-ray appearance. Epiphyseal damage and eroded joints predispose to osteoarthritis. There may be hardening and atrophy of soft tissues. Some victims suffer permanently from intermittent local ulceration of the skin with fissuring and chronic infection. Obliterative endangiitis may occur and Raynaud's syndrome, with the feet in particular tending to develop a marked and persistent vasospasm when presented with cold stimuli, and the vasospasm persists long after the cold stimulus has been removed. This cold hypersensitivity of the feet may persist for years or even be permanent, and re-exposure to cold is very liable to cause relapse. Finally there may be weakness and deformity because of muscle damage and/or amputation.

Prevention of local cold injury

The most useful preventive measures are:

1. to limit the time the person is exposed to the hazardous environment
2. taking a hot drink whenever possible—of thermal and hydration benefits
3. adequate foot care to keep the feet as dry and abrasion free as possible
4. 'buddies' can keep a close watch on each other for early signs, e.g. disappearance of pain, or total anaesthesia on attempting to move the fingers and toes.

OTHER CONDITIONS

Conjunctivitis due to cold, and cold injury to the cornea, have been seen in downhill skiers and ice skaters unprotected by goggles.

INDIRECT DANGERS

MUSCLE TEARS

AETIOLOGY

In the cold, joints are stiff. Muscles are also stiffer especially in response to rapid or large movements. Cold slows nerve conduction, increasing the risk of incoordination. It is therefore not surprising that muscle tears are much more common in the cold.

PREVENTION

1. Clothing must be appropriate for the environment, the activity, and the person. Unfortunately in many team sports the macho image, which the participants want to project, may override

commonsense, e.g. it may be difficult to persuade a rugby wing threequarter that he should wear a thermal vest, to keep warm and alert, and thermal tights, to reduce the risk of a muscle tear.

2. The warm-up, including correct stretching techniques, must be active and should be taken to the point where the athlete is almost sweating. A hot bath is not a substitute. Following an active warm-up the cellular metabolism of the relevant cells, including muscles, is at maximum efficiency and the blood vessels in the active muscles are functioning to their maximum capacity bringing oxygen and nutrients and removing carbon dioxide and other waste products.

OTHER DANGERS

Sudden immersion

Sudden entry into very cold water produces marked cardiorespiratory responses which may cause death or unconsciousness or incapacity, and therefore drowning, through a stroke, a myocardial infarction, or because of uncontrollable hyperventilation. Swimming is impossible in very cold weather and even Olympic class swimmers become incapacitated probably because of the effect of cold on nerve and muscle function. Water in the ears and/or nose may cause a vagal reflex with instantaneous cardiac and respiratory arrest.

Cardiovascular

Angina is increased when the exercise is in the cold, and the effects of cold may cause heart attacks, strokes and heart failure.

Raynaud's phenomenon

This is an over-reactive arterial vasoconstriction in response to a cold stress whose severity does not affect normal people. It may be idiopathic, an indicator of underlying autoimmune disease, or secondary to exposure to arsenic or the hand vibration syndrome from using pneumatic drills or driving snowmobiles. It may cause great difficulties in cold environments.

Respiratory

Breathing cold air triggers *asthma* with some people being very susceptible. The mucosal responses to cold may explain some of the paradoxes in the transmission of the *common cold*, and if divers breathe cold oxyhelium under pressure they may drown in their own secretions. Cold, interacting with hypoxia, is probably a factor in the aetiology of *high altitude* pulmonary oedema and high altitude pulmonary hypertension.

Nervous system

The effect of cold on nerves, muscles and joints impairs manual performance. Cold impairs the higher senses and slows reaction times. Incoordination develops and mistakes are more frequent. Accidents are therefore more likely. One of the earliest signs of incipient hypothermia is a change in personality, and impairment of cerebration may develop to misinterpretations or hallucinations. Some sufferers have even paradoxically undressed while exposed to the cold.

ACKNOWLEDGEMENTS

Figures 14.2–14.9 were taken by Dr W J Mills, Jnr of Anchorage, Alaska, and are reproduced by kind permission of Dr Mills. They were previously published in Mills 1973 Alaska Medicine 15: 22–27

FURTHER READING
General dealing with the field covered and closely related areas
Lloyd E L 1986 Hypothermia and Cold Stress. Croom Helm, London
Maclean D, Emslie-Smith D 1977 Accidental Hypothermia. Blackwell Scientific Publications, Edinburgh
Ward M P, Milledge J S, West J B 1989 High Altitude Medicine and Physiology. Chapman and Hall, London

Physiology of cold exposure
Alexander G 1979 Cold thermogenesis. In Robertshaw D (ed.) Environmental Physiology III. University Park Press, Baltimore, pp 43–155
Bligh J 1984 Temperature regulation: a theoretical consideration incorporating Sherringtonian principles of central neurology. Journal of Thermal Biology 9: 3–6
Enander A 1984 Performance and sensory aspects of work in cold environments—a review. Ergonomics 27: 365–378
Horvath S M 1981 Exercise in a cold environment. Exercise, Sports and Science Review 9: 221–263
Keatinge W R 1969 Survival in Cold Water. Blackwell Scientific Publications, Edinburgh

Hypothermia and its treatment
Hayward J S, Eckerson J D, Kemna D 1984 Thermal and cardiovascular changes during three methods of resuscitation from mild hypothermia. Resuscitation 11: 21–33
Lloyd E L 1990 Airway warming in the treatment of accidental hypothermia: a review. Journal of Wilderness Medicine 1: 65–78
Lloyd E L 1991 Equipment for airway warming. Journal of Wilderness Medicine 2 330–350

Pozos R S, Wittmers L E (eds) 1983 The Nature and Treatment of Hypothermia. Croom Helm, London

Steinman A M 1986 Cardiopulmonary resuscitation and hypothermia. Circulation 74, Suppl IV: IV–29–32

Frostbite and NFCI

Foray J, Salon F 1985 Casualties with cold injuries; primary treatment. In Rivolier J, Ceretelli P, Foray J, Segantini P (eds) High Altitude Deterioration, Karger, Basel, pp. 149–158

Francis T J R 1984 Non-freezing cold injury; a historical review. Journal of the Royal Naval Medical Service 70: 134–139

Francis T J R, Golden F St C 1985 Non-freezing cold injury; the pathogenesis. Journal of the Royal Naval Medical Service 71: 3–8

Killian H 1981 Cold and Frost Injuries. Springer-Verlag, Berlin

Lloyd E L 1992 Cold: injuries and risks In McLatchie G, Lennox C M E (eds) The Soft Tissues: trauma, rheumatism and sports injury. Heinemann, London. In press.

Mills W J 1973 Frostbite. A discussion of the problem and a review of an Alaskan experience. Alaska Medicine 15: 27–47

Mills W J 1983 Frostbite. Alaska Medicine 25: 33–38

Oakley E H N 1984 The design and function of military footwear: a review following experiences in the South Atlantic. Ergonomics 6: 631–637

Schmid-Schonbein H, Neumann F J 1985 Pathophysiology of cutaneous frost injury; disturbed microcirculation as a consequence of abnormal flow behaviour of the blood. Application of new concepts of blood rheology. In Rivolier J, Ceretelli P, Foray J, Segantini P (eds) High Altitude Deterioration, Karger, Basel, pp. 20–38

Other effects of cold

Elsner R, Gooden B 1983 Diving and Asphyxia. Cambridge University Press, Cambridge

Lahti A 1982 Cutaneous reactions to cold. Nordic Council for Arctic Medical Research Rep. No. 30: 32–35

15. Immediate care of the injured

INTRODUCTION

The necessity for the provision of the best possible trauma care is emphasized by the types of injury sustained in the high risk sports of motor racing and horse trials (eventing). While equestrian competition is mercifully free of the dreaded hazard of fire, the kinetic energies of impact are considerable. For example, it can involve the half-ton weight (500 kg) (Miles 1970) of a horse landing on the rider in a fall (Fig. 15.1). The kick from a steel-shod hoof can deliver ten kilonewtons of energy (Firth 1985) and involve competitor, groom or bystander. Consequently, with these mechanisms of injury, severe head, neck and maxillofacial injuries are

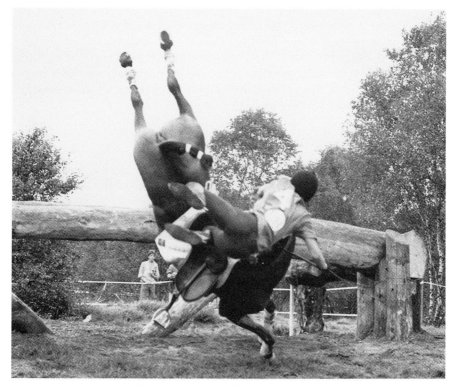

Fig. 15.1 After the impact of the fall, the horse may land on the rider.

seen. Life threatening emergencies such as tension and haemo-pneumothorax or ruptured spleen, liver and disruption of the pelvic ring occur and may rapidly induce shock from hypovolaemia and/or hypoxia.

MEDICAL COVER

The aim of medical cover is to rapidly provide the means and ability to tackle the immediate threat, commence lifesaving treatment where indicated and, with necessary careful immobilization, promptly transport the seriously injured patient to the pre-arranged accident and emergency service. The vital opportunity of the Golden Hour has been highlighted by the report of the Royal College of Surgeons of England, (Royal College of Surgeons 1988).

The planning for such contingencies must begin early and involves liaison with the appointed voluntary aid societies such as the British Red Cross Society, St Andrews Ambulance Association, St John Ambulance or a paramedic unit. If necessary, provision should be made to implement the proposals of the Gibson Report (1990) following the Hillsborough Football Stadium disaster. Large competitions will require a team of medical units with an appointed Chief Medical Officer who has local knowledge of people and terrain. The necessary medical skills to be recruited must include experience in trauma management and will be obtained from the various disciplines of anaesthesia, accident and emergency, surgery and general practice.

COMMUNICATION

The standard of communication must be of the highest order. It will entail the identification of each member of the medical team by individual introduction and the wearing of easily visible apparel. The availability of adequate radio handsets must be guaranteed with facilities for replacing failing batteries, together with dedicated external telephone lines and radiophones. Radios should never be left unattended and it is mandatory that explicit instructions on their use are properly understood. The opportunity should be taken to evaluate the standard of emergency care available and to instigate a policy of injury management with due provisions for any weaknesses exposed. It is essential to have both briefing and debriefing sessions on the day of the competition. The provisions of suitable transport and navigational guides for the Doctors and Ambulance Units must be negotiated from the outset.

PERSONAL EQUIPMENT

It may be necessary to prepare individual small field kits for the use of doctors not normally equipped for their emergency role. These should include oro-pharyngeal airways, pocket mask or face shield, one unit of intravenous fluid such as Haemaccel, an administration set, cannulae, tourniquet, adhesive dressings, syringe and sample bottle, Tuf-cut scissors, disposable gloves and haemo-static compression bandages. (The Laerdal First Aid Kit is excellent and will continue to serve its purpose on future occasions.)

Equipment provided for individual medical officers at Burghley Horse Trials

1 Holdall sponsored by Hoechst UK
1 Laerdal Pocket mask with one-way valve
1 each of oral airways 2, 3 and 4
1 Haemaccel (500 ml)
1 blood administration set
1 14G IV cannula
1 16G IV cannula
2 Mediswabs
1 Tourniquet
1 Syringe (20 ml)
1 Plain blood tube
1 Vecafix dressing
1 Micropore (2.5 cm)
1 Crepe bandage (7.5 cm)
1 Syringe (2 ml)
1 21G Needle
1 Medium ambulance dressing
1 Pack sterile gauze swabs (7.5 × 7.5 cm)
1 ampoule of analgesic—issued to individual doctor on day
1 'DOCTOR' Tabard
1 Patient report form and pen

EMERGENCY DRUGS

The field kits will not contain emergency drugs for which provisions must be made. The Misuse of Drugs Regulations, 1985 must be adhered to for controlled drugs such as diamorphine, morphine and pethidine. This will be the responsibility of individual doctors but the appropriate measures may require explanation for those less familiar with their role. Normally, the drugs

Table 15.1   Drugs for emergency use

	Strength	Volume	Dose	
*Adrenaline	1:10 000	10 ml	10 ml	Small increments in anaphylaxis
*Atropine	1 mg	10 ml	1–2 mg	
*Lignocaine	2% 100 mg	5 ml	100 mg	
*Morphine	20 mg	2 ml	5 mg	Increments
Diamorphine	10 mg powder		2.5 mg	Increments
Cyclimorph	10 mg 1 ml morphine 50 mg 1 ml cyclizine		5 mg	Increments
*Naloxone	0.4 mg	1 ml	0.1 mg	Increments
Midazolam	10 mg	2 ml	2.5–5.0 mg	Increments
Diazemuls	10 mg	2 ml	10–20 mg	Increments
Ketamine	100 mg	10 ml	25–50 mg	
Cyclizine	50 mg	1 ml	50 mg	
Meto-clopramide	10 mg	2 ml	10 mg	
Salbutamol	0.5 mg	1 ml	0.25 mg	
Salbutamol nebulizer	0.1%	2.5 ml	2.5–5 ml	
*Frusemide	80 mg	8 ml	20–50 mg	
*Dextrose	50% w/v	50 ml	25–50 ml	

*Available in pre-filled syringes (International Medication Systems)

to be used in such circumstances must be given intravenously although adrenaline, atropine and lignocaine in the management of cardiac arrest may be given in twice the normal intravenous dose through an endotracheal tube. Poorly perfused subcutaneous tissue and muscle in hypovolaemic patients renders the subcutaneous and intramuscular route unreliable and inadequate. It must be anticipated that analgesia will be necessary despite the use of 50% nitrous oxide: 50% oxygen (Entonox, Nitronox) and increments of a suitable opioid, e.g. diamorphine, may be administered intravenously in aliquots with antiemetics in the same syringe (Steggles 1986). Naloxone should be available in the event of opioid-induced respiratory depression but is short-acting and may need to be repeated. Small doses of Midazolam to relieve anxiety may reduce the dose of opiate required and in rare instances, such as entrapment, a benzodiazepine may be followed by Ketamine (in analgesic dosage) (Baskett 1989).

Cardiac arrest or dysrhythmia may require the administration of adrenaline, atropine or lignocaine. Diazemuls may be required for grand-mal epileptic fits while adrenaline and salbutamol should be available for acute anaphylactic reactions.

Table 15.1 lists commonly used drugs for intravenous administration with suggested dosages.

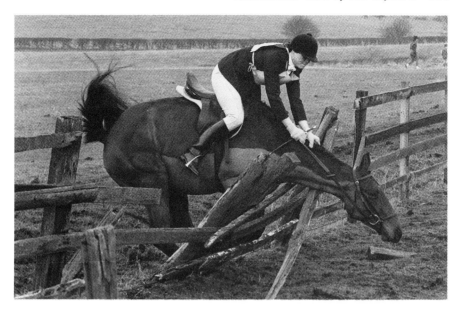

Fig. 15.2   The head forward position in riding leads to the same posture when the rider falls forward to hit the ground

ABC

Undoubtedly, the standard of trauma care will depend upon the speedy and correct application of the core skills in the ABC (Airway, Breathing, Circulation) of management together with an accurate appraisal of the injuries or the likelihood of certain injuries in the absence of immediate signs. For instance, the head forward stance (Becker 1959) adopted in horse riding (Fig. 15.2), motor cycle racing or driving should always arouse the suspicion of head or neck injury. If the person is rendered unconscious there is a high association of head injury with proven spinal cord injury (Silver et al 1980) with an overall incidence of cervical spine injury in 10–15%. The history of the accident must always be clearly obtained, if the event has not been witnessed by the doctor, and passed onto the receiving hospital.

Airway

The fundamental basis for successful resuscitation in severe trauma is control of the airway, but firstly the safety of approach to the injured is established (the second injury to patient or rescuer must be avoided at all costs) and others alerted of the need for

assistance. The level of consciousness can be rapidly ascertained—**A** (Alert), **V** (responding to Voice), **P** (responding to Pain),
U (Unresponsive)—(Advance Trauma Life Support 1988) while
ensuring the patency of the airway. If necessary the head and neck
is stabilized, the airway is cleared by chin lift and then head tilt
(10%) (even when cervical spine injury is suspected) and the
removal of any obstruction or debris from the mouth by finger
sweep. Trismus may be encountered and overcome by either the
crossed finger manoeuvre, the fingers behind the teeth or the insertion of a naso-pharyngeal airway (Safar & Bircher 1988) (Size 6 or
7); the latter technique is very useful but often overlooked.

Breathing

Placing one's face close to that of the competitor and looking along
the line of the chest towards the feet will reveal chest expansion or
flail movement. The triad of look (chest movement), feel (exha-
lation of air) and listen (sounds of breathing or obstruction) must
be employed.

If breathing is inadequate or absent then basic life support
begins with the rescuer giving two breaths by the mouth-to-mouth,
mouth-to-face shield (Blenkarn et al 1990) or mouth-to-mask technique. The patient's chest must be noted to rise during the applied
inspiration.

Circulation

At this point, palpation of the carotid pulse will establish the
integrity of the circulation. In the absence of pulsation, external
chest compression (ECC) should commence. Fifteen compressions to a depth of 4–5 cm at a rate of 80/minute are applied. A
ratio of 15 compressions : 2 ventilations is continued unless a
competent assistant is available, in which case the responsibility
is shared with one applying five chest compressions then interrupted by one breath applied by the other. The patency of the
airway must be constantly checked.

ADVANCED LIFE SUPPORT

Advanced life support begins with the use of the appropriately
sized oropharyngeal airway. Its insertion must not be attempted in
those with intact upper airway reflexes to avoid provoking laryngeal spasm or vomiting. Guedel airways and a Laerdal Pocket

---

Fig. 15.3 Cardiopulmonary resuscitation card (Reproduced by permission of
Laerdal Medical Ltd)

ADVANCED CARDIAC LIFE SUPPORT

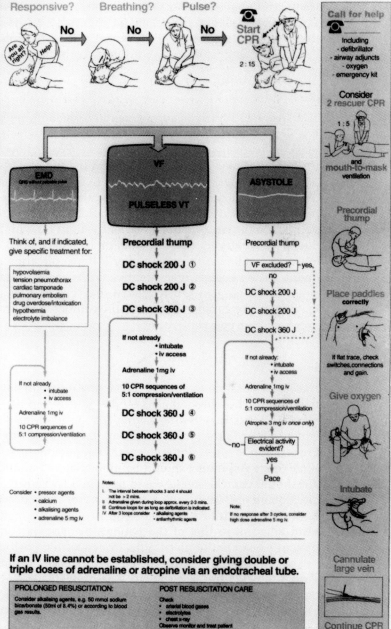

Guidelines for Advanced Cardiac Life Support.

European Resuscitation Council 1992.

Reference: Resuscitation, 24 (1992), 3 - 121.

Presented with the compliments of

Laerdal
helping save lives

P 6275

Laerdal Medical Ltd.
Laerdal House
Orpington, Kent BR6 OHX
Tel. 0689 876634
Fax. 0689 873800

If an IV line cannot be established, consider giving double or triple doses of adrenaline or atropine via an endotracheal tube.

European Resuscitation Council and Resuscitation Council (UK)

© European Resuscitation Council 1992

Mask may be usefully carried in the pocket or field kit. Naso-pharyngeal airways, such as the Linder (Cambmac) with its non-traumatic bubble-tip, may prove a necessary alternative. In cardiac arrest, the sequence illustrated in Figure 15.3 (the chart of the Resuscitation Council (UK) for ventricular fibrillation, asystole or electro-mechanical dissociation) must be initiated immediately.

Oxygenation

The adequate supply of supplemental oxygen from a gas cylinder is a first-step priority. It may be administered by connection to a mask or bag-valve-mask resuscitator at a high flow rate (10–15 l/min) and it must be emphasized that the use of 24 or 28% fixed performance masks is inappropriate. Expired air contains 16–17% oxygen while a mask (e.g. Laerdal) with oxygen supplement will provide about 50%. It is very important to attach an oxygen reser-voir bag to the resuscitator in order to supply the higher levels of 60–90%. However, the resuscitator bag may not deliver 600–800 ml if inadequately squeezed or if the application does not ex-clude mask leak. Consequently, a two-person technique is suggested (Campbell). It is crucial that hypercarbia and hypoxia leading to increased intracranial pressure be forestalled and this may require hyperventilation.

Intubation

If it is not possible to control the airway or adequately oxygenate the patient by these means endotracheal intubation may be required. This may be life-saving for the unprotected and inad-equate airway but should only be attempted by skilled personnel. Preparation is vital. Portable suction apparatus (e.g. Vitalograph Emergency Aspirator) should be immediately to hand. An assist-ant should control the head and neck in a neutral in-line position and cricoid pressure (Sellick's manoeuvre) applied. Under certain circumstances, intubation may require lying full length with one's head adjacent to that of the patient, or even by controlling the patient's head with one's thighs from a sitting position and lean-ing backwards to visualize the laryngoscope at the entrance to the glottis, albeit from a distance. It is as well to remember spare batteries and bulbs for the laryngoscope and a commercially avail-able endotracheal tube holder may overcome the difficulty of securing it in place with tape. Endotracheal tubes should be pre-cut in accordance with the appropriate chart supplied with them e.g. 22/23 cm length for size 8 mm tube and 24 cm for size 9 mm tube. Correct placement of the endotracheal tube must always be ascertained by confirming that the tube passes through the vocal cords, and the use of a gum elastic bougie may prove essential in the most difficult situation. Auscultation should then be performed to check that inadvertent right main bronchus intubation has not occurred. The FEF End-tidal CO_2 Detector may prove to be of value in difficult situations. There are alternative techniques using the (Brain) Laryngeal Mask Airway or the Pharyngo-Tracheal Lumen Airway (Silverston 1989b) which are currently being evaluated in the emergency field, but cannot yet be recommended and have similar problems to endotracheal intubation.

Cricothyrotomy

Inability to intubate the trachea is the only indication for creating a surgical airway (Advanced Life Support 1988). This may occur in severe maxillo-facial injury or when the normal anatomical landmarks are obscured or distorted. Cricothyrotomy will involve the incision of the cricothyroid membrane in the supine patient. This is identified by palpating the thyroid cartilage between thumb and middle finger of the left hand and sliding the index finger caudally in the mid-line from the thyroid notch to the depression immediately above the cricoid cartilage. A horizontal 2–3 cm incision is made through the skin and then the membrane. The opening may then be enlarged by the use of a tracheal spreader, or the handle of a scalpel rotated through 90° to allow insertion of a cuffed 6 mm tracheostomy tube. An assistant may have to steady the larynx and bleeding may well add to the difficulty of the task.

The Melker Emergency Cricothyrotomy Catheter Set (Cook Critical Care) (Fig. 15.4) utilizes the Seldinger technique to achieve tracheal access after a vertical stab incision over the cricothyroid membrane. The passage of a dilator then allows the use of a 6 mm emergency airway which will permit spontaneous breathing or positive pressure ventilation. Catheter-over-needle cricothyrotomy and ventilation may be required temporarily for patients in extremis prior to formal cricothyrotomy. It is also the necessary procedure in children and may buy vital time for up to 45 minutes. A 12 or 14 gauge over-the-needle catheter is inserted at 45° caudally with a Luer-Lok attachment for the tube from an oxygen cylinder when available. The use of a Y-tube connector will enable jet insufflation with the thumb placed over the open end of the Y connector for 1 second and then removed for 4 seconds repetitively (oxygen flow 6 l/min, 2 l/min for children). Once the adequacy of the airway and ventilation is established then a vigilant watch is undertaken of the patient's colour, pulse and breathing. A semi-automatic external defibrillator (e.g. Laerdal

MELKER EMERGENCY CRICOTHYROTOMY CATHETER SETS

SET COMPONENTS

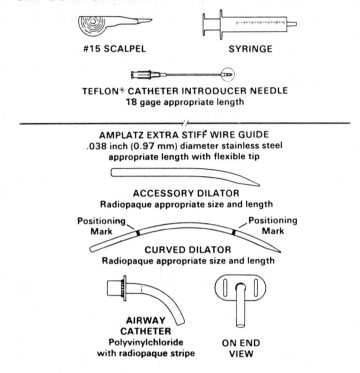

#15 SCALPEL   SYRINGE

TEFLON® CATHETER INTRODUCER NEEDLE
18 gage appropriate length

AMPLATZ EXTRA STIFF WIRE GUIDE
.038 inch (0.97 mm) diameter stainless steel
appropriate length with flexible tip

ACCESSORY DILATOR
Radiopaque appropriate size and length

Positioning Mark   Positioning Mark
CURVED DILATOR
Radiopaque appropriate size and length

AIRWAY
CATHETER
Polyvinylchloride
with radiopaque stripe   ON END
VIEW

SET CONSISTS OF ITEMS SHOWN ABOVE AND CLOTH
TRACHEOSTOMY TAPE STRIP FOR FIXATION OF
AIRWAY CATHETER.

Patent Number 4,677,978

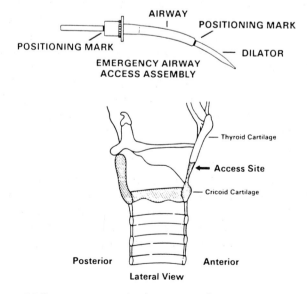

AIRWAY
POSITIONING MARK
POSITIONING MARK
DILATOR
EMERGENCY AIRWAY
ACCESS ASSEMBLY

Thyroid Cartilage

Access Site

Cricoid Cartilage

Posterior   Anterior
Lateral View

Fig. 15.4 Melker emergency cricothyrotomy catheter sets

Heartstart 3000) can be used to monitor the rate and rhythm of the heart, a sphygmomanometer for blood pressure and pulse oximeter to measure and monitor the oxygen saturation of arterial blood (Silverston 1989a).

It must be remembered, however, that pulse oximeters are notoriously inaccurate in shocked or hypovolaemic patients and close clinical observation is far more reliable.

Chest injury

Where chest injury is observed or anticipated then a search for a flail chest with associated pulmonary contusion, an open pneumothorax or tension pneumothorax must be instigated immediately. There is a strong association between sternal and spinal injuries.

Tension pneumothorax

One will be alerted by the marked deterioration of the patient and the presence of pain, dyspnoea, cyanosis and a respiratory rate of more than 20/minute together with tracheal displacement, reduced chest movement, hyper-resonance on the affected side and a reduction in air entry. Unfortunately, the clinical features of pneumothorax and haemothorax (dullness to percussion) are often very difficult to detect in these situations, as for instance, hypovolaemia may preclude the important clinical sign of distended neck veins. Pressure may be relieved by the insertion of a 14 gauge intravenous cannula into the second intercostal space, in the mid clavicular line, just above the third rib to avoid damaging the artery and vein that shelter under the protection of each rib. The second rib is joined to the sternum at the sternal angle. The release of air into the attached syringe used for local anaesthetic will confirm the diagnosis. A chest drain (adult 28 FG, 40 cm) is then inserted at the same site or, if the situation allows, into the 4th–5th intercostal space just anterior to the mid-axillary line. The percutaneous Thal-Quick Chest Tube Set (Cook Critical Care) utilizes the Seldinger technique for introduction of the chest tube after a small incision in the skin that is slightly larger than the diameter of the tube.

The Portex or Vygon Chest Drainage Sets also require the addition of local anaesthetic, antiseptic wipes and a clamp. It is necessary to make a 2–3 cm horizontal incision through skin and subcutaneous fat and to insert a 2.0 purse string suture around the incision; local anaesthetic (1% plain lignocaine) should be used initially and infiltrated down to the pleural layer. Further incision of muscle and then blunt dissection with finger and blunt forceps or scissors will reach the pleura which is breached with a minimum of force to insert the drain. Look for fogging of the tube or listen for breath sounds and then connect the tube to the drainage bag and secure in position both by suture and taping. Unfortunately, in the presence of blood a Heimlich Valve may obstruct. An open wound should be closed with Opsite or Tegaderm (Carney 1990) or possibly a defibrillator pad, although there is then the potential for a tension pneumothorax.

Cardiac tamponade is usually due to a penetrative injury and may be recognized by the failure to resuscitate haemorrhagic shock. Beck's triad of distended neck veins (not in hypovolaemia), decline in arterial blood pressure and muffled heart sounds may not be detected in clinical practice.

SHOCK

Shock, which has graphically been described as a pause in the act of dying, is the circulatory abnormality that leads to inadequate organ perfusion. The majority of cases will be due to hypovolaemia although cardiogenic and even neurogenic shock may have to be considered. Its early recognition is of the essence and it must be remembered that in previously fit individuals up to 30% of the circulating volume may be lost before the systolic blood pressure falls. The arousal of the sympathetic response, increasing the pulse and respiratory rate, may provide a vital clue with cutaneous vasoconstriction causing pallor and coldness.

CONTROL OF HAEMORRHAGE

Direct pressure should be used to control blood loss from visible external wounds. Femoral shaft fractures and more importantly disruption of the pelvic ring can be formidable, for the blood loss can exceed 2000 ml. The use of pneumatic anti-shock garments is recommended by some authorities for the control of severe haemorrhage in the abdomen or from the pelvis and lower limbs. In the latter cases, the garment will also act as a splint for fractures. However, there are drawbacks of which inappropriate or precipitous removal is a major hazard. They should not be applied if diaphragmatic rupture is suspected and their use with normal blood volumes may cause an increase in intracranial pressure. Their application should not exceed two hours and volume replacement should be established from the outset (Baskett 1989).

Intravenous infusion is established through the largest and most readily accessible vein (usually in the forearm or ante-cubital fossa). The external jugular may be considered in emergency for the supine patient; the site of entry is at the midpoint between the angle of the jaw and the clavicle. The vein may be lightly compressed just above the clavicle to aid cannulation, but it is a flat vein and requires a low angle of approach (Zideman 1991). A short large bore cannula should be used as the flow is directly related to the fourth power of the radius and inversely related to its length. At least a 14 gauge cannula which has a water flow rate of 270 ml/min for the 45 mm catheter length, is required and two carefully secured and splinted (e.g. Arm-lok, E.M.S.) lines are preferable. It is recommended that the blood administration set is warmed using an Infupak (Denley Instruments) and a pressure infusion device (e.g. Biocuff, Cambmac) used for rapid replacement. Alternatively, a very high flow rate can be elegantly achieved using an Arrow peripheral emergency infusion device (Kimal) or an existing peripheral cannula can be replaced utilizing an Arrow Rapid Infusion Catheter Exchange Set. An initial bolus of 1–2 litres is then reviewed in the light of the patient's response. The 1:1 ratio of crystalloid solution to colloid is a general rule for replacement but it does have exceptions. Table 15.2 gives the classification of haemorrhagic shock and suggestions for intravenous replacement of blood loss.

SPINAL INJURY

The cervical spine, initially manually immobilized, may be partly stabilized by a rigid cervical collar (e.g. Stifneck, Vertebrace). However, it is an adjunct to manual in-line immobilization without traction which must be continued even during transportation. The collar must fit and a range of sizes are available, usefully taken to the scene as a nest of collars carried on the forearm. The recognition of spinal injury requires a high index of suspicion from the circumstances (Fig. 15.5), although a conscious patient may have pain in the neck or back. Bizarre symptoms should not be dismissed as hysterical e.g. burning sensation or a feeling that the position of the body is that which pertained before the accident. It is inexcusable to make a competitor sit up or stand up until this very serious injury can be excluded. Early information is valuable and the Medical Equestrian Association (Zideman, personal communication), has produced a pocket-sized aide-memoire Spinex Card as illustrated in Figure 15.6. Its interpretation may be helped by considering a rule of fours:

Table 15.2 Classification of haemorrhagic stock. Suggestions for intravenous replacement of blood loss

	Class I	Class II	Class III	Class IV
Blood loss	< 750 ml	750–1500 ml	1500–2000 ml	> 2000 ml
% Blood volume	< 15%	15–30%	30–40%	> 40%
Systolic blood pressure	Normal	Normal	Decreased	Very low
Diastolic blood pressure	Normal	Raised	Decreased	Very low or unrecordable
Pulse	< 100/min	> 100/min	> 120 thready	> 140 very thready
*Capillary refill	< 2 secs	> 2 secs	> 2 secs	Undetectable
Respiratory rate	Normal 14–20	Normal 14–20	Increased > 20	Increased > 20
Skin colour	Normal	Pale	Pale	Very pale, cold
Mental state	Minimal anxiety	Anxious or aggressive	Anxious, aggressive or drowsy	Confused, drowsy or unconscious
**Fluid replacement	Self compensatory not required	Crystalloid or colloid	Colloid, crystalloid and blood	Colloid, crystalloid and blood
Initial volumes	Not required	1–1.5 litres	1–1.5 litres colloid then 1 litre crystalloid	1–1.5 litres colloid then 1 litre crystalloid

* Detect by pressure on the fingernail or the hypo-thenar eminence. (Not applicable in hypothermia)
** Crystalloids such as Hartmann's Solution (Compound Ringer's Lactate)
    Colloids such as Haemaccel, Gelofusine

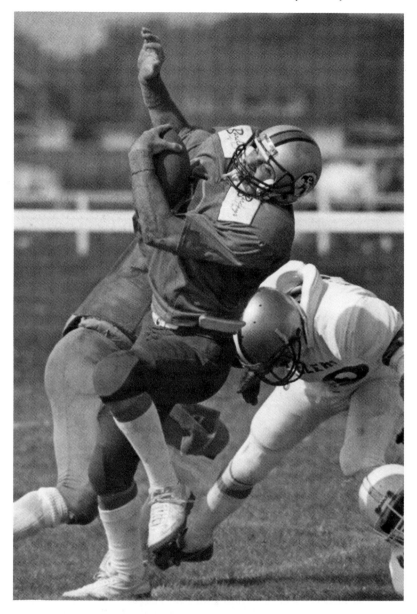

Fig. 15.5 Axial loading of the cervical spine is about to occur in the tackler on the right. This predisposes to cervical injury

1. 60% of spinal cords lesions are incomplete
2. All four limbs are examined as to
3. Four motor and
4. Four sensory functions

MEDICAL EQUESTRIAN ASSOCIATION

SPINEX CARD

SPINAL CORD INJURY CARD

> THE LEVEL AT WHICH SENSATION IS ALTERED
> OR ABSENT IS THE LEVEL OF INJURY.

> IT IS VITAL TO CARRY OUT MOTOR AS WELL AS
> SENSORY EXAMINATION AS THE PATIENT MAY
> HAVE MOTOR DAMAGE WITHOUT SENSORY
> DAMAGE AND VICE VERSA.

SENSORY EXAMINATION
1. EXAMINE BY:
    A. Light touch.
    B. Response to pain.
2. USE:
    The forehead as the guide
    to what is normal
    sensation.
3. EXAMINE:
    A. Upper limbs and hands.
    B. Lower limbs and feet.
4. EXAMINE:
    Both sides.
5. T.4 EXAMINATION:
    Must be carried out in
    the MID–AXILLARY
    line, NOT the MID-
    CLAVICULAR line, as
    C2, C3 and C4 all supply
    sensation to the nipple line.

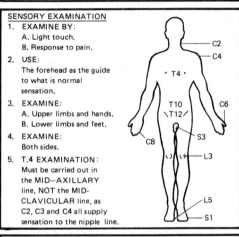

> IT IS IMPORTANT TO CARRY OUT ALL THE ABOVE
> AS A VARIETY OF SENSORY CHANGES MAY OCCUR.

*The production of this card has been made possible by the
financial support of Duphar Veterinary Limited, suppliers
of The Duvaxyn RiderCard obtainable from veterinary surgeons.*

Fig. 15.6   Spinex card

MOTOR EXAMINATION

> THE LEVEL AT WHICH WEAKNESS OR ABSENCE OF
> MOVEMENT IS NOTED IS THE LEVEL OF INJURY.

MOTOR EXAMINATION: EXAMINE BOTH SIDES

UPPER LIMB		LOWER LIMB	
ASK PATIENT TO:		ASK PATIENT TO:	
A. Shrug Shoulders	*C4	A. Flex Hip	*L1 & L2
B. Bend the Elbow	*C5	B. Extend Knee	*L3
C. Push Wrist back	*C6	C. Pull Foot up	*L4
D. Open/Close Hands	*C8	D. Push Foot down	*L5 & S1

> THORACIC AND ABDOMINAL MOTOR EXAMINATION :
> LOOK FOR ACTIVITY OF INTERCOSTAL &
> ABDOMINAL MUSCLES

DIAGNOSIS OF SPINAL CORD INJURY
IN THE UNCONSCIOUS PATIENT

A. Look for paradoxical
    respiration, as in
    quadriplegia the loss of
    use of the intercostal
    muscles means the
    diaphragm must be used
    to breathe.
B. Flaccid limbs.
C. Loss of response to
    painful stimuli below the
    level of lesion.

D. Loss of reflexes below
    the level of lesion.
E. Erection in the
    unconscious male.
F. Low B.P. (systolic less
    than 100) associated with
    a normal pulse or brady-
    cardia indicates patient
    may be QUADRIPLEGIC

> IF YOU DON'T THINK ABOUT A SPINAL CORD
> INJURY YOU WILL MISS IT!!!

TREATMENT: 1. A.B.C.
2. Immobilise injured part.
3. Lift patient in one piece in position found
4. Only move the patient when it is necessary

*We are indebted to Dr. J. Toscano for his original concept and
his kind permission to reproduce this card.*

The level of injury is at the last (highest) fully intact dermatome and myotome. If ventilation is required then atropine 0.3 mg intravenously should be given before the insertion of an airway, suction or intubation. It may be given prophylactically if the pulse rate has slowed to 50 as asystole from a trivial stimulus is an ever present threat due to unopposed vagal activity. The fluid requirements of an isolated cord lesion are low and 500 ml may be adequate to restore systolic blood pressure to 90 mm Hg.

POSITIONING THE UNCONSCIOUS ON TO THE SIDE

To prevent possible aspiration, it is mandatory to turn the unconscious patient carefully on to their side provided breathing is adequate. The side position has been the subject of considerable debate and a suggested position is shown in the accompanying illustration (Figures 15.7A–E) (Medical Equestrian Association). If there is no assistant to control the head and neck a very simple method, which requires later adjustment for stability, is to place the patient's arm that is nearest to the rescuer in the extended position as in the back-crawl at swimming. The near knee is bent so that the sole of the foot is brought into contact with the ground. Then controlling the patient's head on the extended arm the body is rolled slowly towards the rescuer by tugging on the clothing at the furthest hip. Any method is obviously attempting to minimize neck movement and this is best achieved with assistance in applying a cervical collar, then maintaining manual in-line immobilization in the neutral position.

LIFTING THE PATIENT

The lifting of a patient requires five assistants under the control of the most responsible member supporting the head and neck (this may be reduced to three if trained in special skills) (Baker 1989).

However, a scoop stretcher or Donway Lifting Frame should be utilized when available to transfer the minimum distance to a vacuum mattress (e.g. Evacumat (see Fig. 15.8) Paraid). Care must be taken to remove sharp objects and to protect any pressure points. Extremes of temperatures must be avoided.

SPLINTING OF FRACTURES

Pain relief and reduction of blood loss from a fractured shaft of femur may be considerably enhanced by the application of a traction splint. Entonox is given and then an assistant applies gentle traction at the ankle to align the leg. The Sager Splint is easy to use and has the advantage of immobilizing both limbs which may be necessary in serious traffic accidents, for example. The Donway Traction Splint is supplied for the use of UK racecourse medical officers and its technique of application is quickly learned.

Entrapment may prove a hazardous experience for everyone. The ABC priority of care will be essential and the use of analgesics considered. In the context of sporting competition such as motor racing and equestrian cross country jumping, facilities for the release of a competitor must be planned and, ideally, rehearsed.

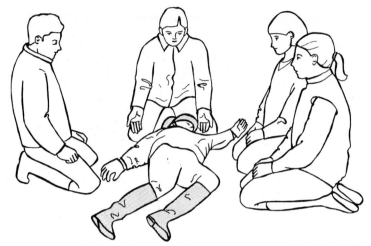

Fig. 15.7A–F Method for positioning the unconscious on to the side. **A** The disposition of the unconscious (?neck-injured) patient as found

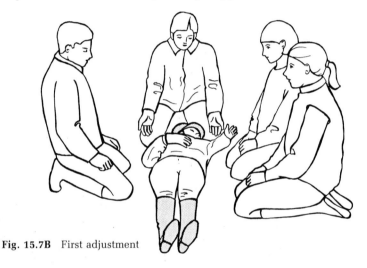

Fig. 15.7B First adjustment

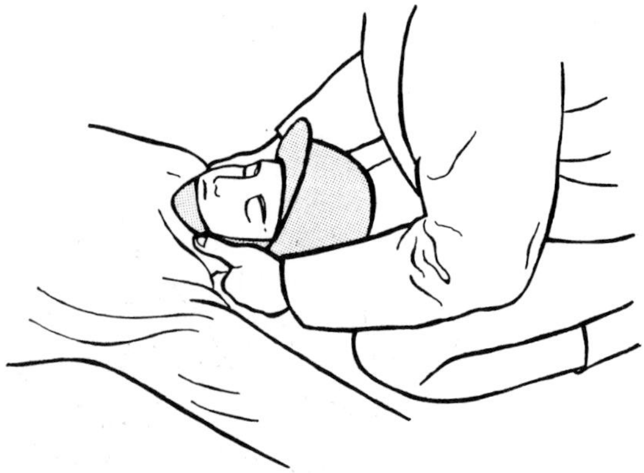

Fig. 15.7C Immobilizing the head and neck (do not apply traction)

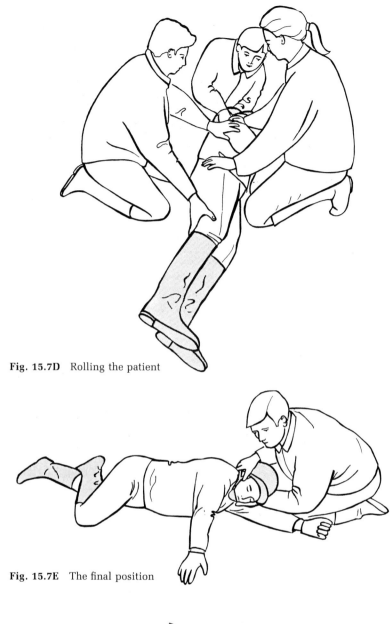

Fig. 15.7D Rolling the patient

Fig. 15.7E The final position

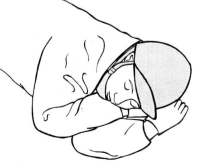

Fig. 15.7F Another suitable final position

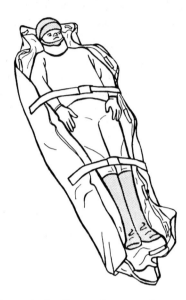

Fig. 15.8   Patient in cervical collar on Evacumat for transport

CONCLUSION

The provision of skill in trauma management is an essential for high risk sports although one day even the less hazardous may produce a life-threatening emergency.

It is within the experience of all those concerned in sports medicine that there are present shortcomings. Future standards will depend upon the enthusiasm of the appointed medical officers and the cooperation of the governing bodies. The training and funding of the voluntary aid organizations is a very important aspect of this, demanding considerable support from the medical profession, the participants and the general public alike.

It will be an exciting decade in the emergency field and it is notable that the Royal College of Surgeons of England now provide formal training in advanced trauma life support (ATLS) and that there is a Diploma in Immediate Medical Care examination of the Royal College of Surgeons of Edinburgh. The Royal Scottish Colleges include such practical skills in their examination for the Diploma in Sports Medicine. We should all develop our abilities in the ABC of trauma management to the best of our endeavour but this requires constant revision and dedication.

APPENDIX: TECHNIQUE OF INSERTION OF THE MELKER EMERGENCY CRICOTHYROTOMY TUBE

The set has been designed to establish emergency airway access when endotracheal intubation cannot be performed. Access to the airway is achieved via the cricothyroid membrane using the percutaneous Seldinger technique. The emergency airway can be passed after the tract and tracheal entrance site have been dilated.

Note: An emergency airway with a 6 mm internal diameter permits positive pressure ventilation to be used and also allows adult patients to breathe spontaneously.

INDICATIONS

Airway obstruction above the level of the larynx. Examples include:

- Obstruction of the airway at the level of the epiglottis or vocal cords by foreign body (commonest)
- trauma to the face and neck
- burns obstructing the upper airway
- infectious diseases such as epiglottitis
- obstruction of the upper airway due to anaphylaxis

ANATOMICAL LANDMARKS

The thyroid cartilage is easily palpable in the midline of the neck distal to the mental symphysis (chin). Proceeding distally the thyroid ring (cricoid cartilage) is encountered. The space between the thyroid cartilage and the cricoid cartilage is the cricothyroid space which is covered by the cricothyroid membrane. Distally are the tracheal rings. In females these may be palpated proximally towards the cricothyroid space if the thyroid cartilage is not easily identified.

PROCEDURE

1. Identify the cricothyroid membrane between the cricoid and thyroid cartilages.
2. Palpate the membrane. Stabilize the cartilages and make a vertical incision in the midline with the No. 15 short handle scalpel blade. Make this big enough to admit the dilator.
3. Attach the 18 gauge Teflon catheter introducer needle to the 6 cc syringe and advance it through the incision into the airway at an angle of 45° to the frontal plane proceeding candally.

(Aspiration of air in the syringe ensures the correct siting in the airway).

4. Remove the syringe and catheter leaving the Teflon needle in place.
5. Advance the soft, flexible end of the guide wire through the Teflon catheter and into the airway several centimetres.
6. The dilator is then placed through the breathing tube with the distal end of the breathing tube level with the black ring on the dilator. Apply a little sterile lubricant to the end of the dilator.
7. The tapered end of the dilator is then advanced over the wire until the proximal stiff end of the wire is visible at the blunt proximal end of the dilator. This ensures adequate wire within the airway for passage of the tube and allows the operator to control and prevent further advancement of the guide wire.
8. The dilator is advanced with a twisting motion into the airway at the level of the black line.
9. The breathing tube is then advanced along with the dilator in a firm circular motion and is passed over the dilator into the airway. As this is being done the dilator and guide wire are removed leaving the tube in place.
10. The tube is then fixed with the tracheostomy type strip in standard fashion.
11. The tube has a standard 15–22 adaptor which may now be connected to an ambu bag or ventilator.

REFERENCES

Advanced Trauma Life Support 1988 Core Course, American College of Surgeons, Chicago

Baker J H E 1988 The first aid management of spinal cord injury. Ambulance UK 3 1: 7

Baker J H E 1989 The first aid management of spinal cord injury. Seminars in Orthopaedics 4 1: 10

Baskett P J F 1989 In: Resuscitation Handbook. Gower Medical Publishing. p 106

Becker T 1959 Das Stumpfe. Als Sportunfall Mschs. Unfallheidelkd 62: 179

Blenkarn J F, Buckingham S E, Zideman D A 1990 Prevention of transmission of infection during mouth to mouth resuscitation. Resuscitation 19: 151–157

Campbell J E In: Basic Trauma Life Support, 2nd edn. ch. 3, p 61

Carney C J 1990 The management of chest injuries at the roadside. BASICS Monograph No. 1 on Immediate Care 2nd edn, British Association for Immediate Care, Ipswich, Suffolk

Firth J R 1985 Equestrian Injuries. In: Schneider R C, Kennedy J C, Plant M L, Fowler P J, Hoff J T, Matthews L S (eds) Sports injuries, mechanisms prevention and treatment. Williams and Wilkins, Baltimore

Gibson Report 1990. The Football League, Lytham St Annes, Lancashire

Johnston I G, Restall J 1989 The laryngeal mask-airway. Journal of the British Association for Immediate Care 12 1: 3–4

Medical Equestrian Association. The Medical Commission on Accident Prevention, Royal College of Surgeons, London

Miles J R 1970 The Racecourse Medical Officer. Journal of the Royal College of General Practitioners 19: 228

Royal College of Surgeons 1988. Report of the working party on the management of patients with major injuries

Safar P, Bircher N G 1988 Cardiopulmonary cerebral resuscitation 3rd edn., W B Saunders, USA p 26

Silver J R, Morris W R, Otfinowski J S 1980 Associated injuries in patients with spinal cord injury. Injury 12: 219–224

Silverston P 1989a The pharyngeal-tracheal lumen airway. Journal of the British Association for Immediate Care 12 1: 4–5

Silverston P 1989b Pulse oximetry in immediate care. Journal of the British Association for Immediate Care 12 2: 38–39

Steggles B 1986 Advanced life support in general practice. In: Evans T R (ed.) ABC of Resuscitation. British Medical Journal, p 20

Zideman D A 1991 personal communication

16. General principles of investigation

There are some practical differences between the clinical investigation of the acutely ill patient and that of the acutely ill sportsman or woman. Usually the examination of a patient is performed in the privacy of a hospital or clinical examination room with trained staff in attendance. By contrast, the doctor at a sports event may often have to make both examination and decision in public, perhaps in front of thousands of spectators, and without the assistance of either specialized equipment or staff. For these reasons one important decision must always be made by the doctor: *Can the player play on?*

The decision is vital. If a serious injury is suspected the player must be removed from the field of play, despite all protestations, for private examination or hospital care. If the injury is not thought to be severe then reassurance should be given and basic first aid carried out. Any player who returns to the field of play should be carefully observed thereafter, both by the referee and by the doctor.

THE INVESTIGATION OF 'ON THE FIELD' INJURIES

1. WITNESS THE EVENTS LEADING TO THE INJURY

It is of great value at major competitions to know exactly what has happened. Club doctors should therefore be sure that they understand their sport and know its risks.

2. ASK RELEVANT QUESTIONS

The injured person should be questioned: 'Do you remember what happened?' 'Where is the pain?' etc. Although simple, these questions will permit an early decision to be made regarding the wisdom of allowing the player to continue. Confused players, for instance, should not play on nor should those with suspected fractures or extensive tendon or ligamentous injury.

3. EXAMINE THE INJURED PART

Having determined whether or not the player can use the injured part it should then be examined. Before touching the patient look for deformity. Then carry out a brief clinical examination noting whether pain or abnormal movement is elicited. You should then decide if it is possible for the player to continue.

Initial exposure to large crowds of spectators can be threatening and inhibiting. The doctor has a responsibility, however, to the patient, the injured player, and although confidentiality may be disrupted by the presence of a large crowd this should not be allowed to influence clinical judgement. As in all areas of medicine this must remain unbiased.

INVESTIGATION OF ELECTIVE PATIENTS

Many injured sportsmen and women will present to the club doctor on the day of or within days of their injury. Others will try to manage their own problems and present late with chronic symptoms.

Avoid being cornered in the club changing room or bar. The ideal is to be able to examine the patient in comfortable, well-lit surroundings such as a club first-aid room, hospital or clinic department.

STANDARDS OF PRACTICE

We recommend that you maintain full and annotated records of each patient seen. This includes his or her name and date of birth with brief details of occupation and best performances. It is important to note the name of the patient's general practitioner who should receive information concerning your examination and findings.

Part of the sports-specific information required is details of training regimes, their frequency and intensity and the type of sport involved, i.e. whether anaerobic or aerobic. The remainder of the record is standard and covers the patient's past medical history including inoculations and patient idiosyncrasies such as asthma or epilepsy. Previous sport-related injuries and their treatment are also important when assessing a current injury. An example of the format we have used ourselves is given in Fig. 16.1.

The examination of the locomotor system is often the main area of interest. The injured area or joint must be tested through its range of mobility and compared to the normal on the other side.

LABORATORY INVESTIGATIONS

Where indicated, biochemical or haematological details may assist in making a diagnosis. In patients with vague symptoms such as polymyalgia or general malaise, blood should be taken for viral studies, especially of the Coxsackie A and B group and the

Page 1

Patient Details:

NAME: D.O.B.:   SEX:

ADDRESS: OCCUPATION:

SPORT/SPORTS:

STANDARD: **(club, county, international)**

NAME AND ADDRESS OF GENERAL PRACTITIONER:

Training Details:

AEROBIC: ANAEROBIC:

TRADITIONAL PATTERN OF TRAINING:

Winter: Summer:

DETAILS OF WARM UP:

Medical History:

PAST MEDICAL HISTORY:

SOCIAL AND DRUG HISTORY:

Smoker: Yes/No ⎫ If yes, how much:
Alcohol: Yes/No ⎭

DIETARY HISTORY:

IMMUNISATION RECORD:

Page 2

Current Injury:

DATE OF INJURY: ACUTE
                        CHRONIC

PREVIOUS SPORT-RELATED-INJURIES: Yes/No
                                 If yes, details:

TIME LOST FROM TRAINING: **Hours/days/weeks**

FULL DETAILS OF DISABILITY AND CLINICAL EXAMINATION LISTED HERE:

This part may be added to with continuation sheets.

Page 3

General Clinical Examination:

The general clinical examination should include demographic data such as height and weight of the patient and should be supplemented by a systemic examination of the body systems e.g. ENT, CVS, RS, GIT, CNS, locomotor system and flexibility.

Page 4

Treatment: Date: ⎛Tick treatment⎞
                                             ⎝ given   ⎠

R.I.C.E

NSAID   —   Dose

PHYSIOTHERAPY

SWD

Ultrasound

Cryotherapy

Massage

Infra-red

STRAPPING   —   Site

Fig. 16.1 Sports injury record. The record takes the form of a 4-page booklet

influenza viruses. Special investigations may also be required for conditions such as the zoonoses if there has been exposure to animals. If there is a suspicion of rheumatic disease, serochemical tests are indicated. Urine should be tested for sugar or ketones coupled with appropriate blood levels if diabetes is suspected.

RADIOLOGY

X-ray confirmation of clinical findings is often required and there is a high correlation between clinical and radiological diagnosis for fractures and dislocations (Morgan et al 1980). X-rays should be used whenever there is a suspicion of fracture or dislocation of the spine or of the skull, although it must be remembered that the spinal cord and brain can be damaged in the absence of any bony injury. Even if a skull fracture is present there is no definite evidence that it is an important consideration in predicting the seriousness of a head injury. Nevertheless, there is a slightly increased risk of an extradural haemorrhage occurring if the skull is fractured and such patients, even though they appear otherwise normal, should be observed in hospital for at least 24 hours. Radiological confirmation of other fractures is obviously important from the patient's point of view. It should be requested when fractures are suspected of the scaphoid bone in the wrist, where serial radiography may be necessary coupled with scintigraphy; of the ribs, where pneumothorax may be a complication; and in all other sites where there is marked deformity of an injured part. X-rays, however, are only of value in picking up 30% of stress fractures, especially in the early stages (when symptoms persist for several weeks over half of all stress fractures will be detected by straight X-ray; Greaney et al 1983).

If there is a suspicion of major ligamentous damage stress films are required to demonstrate abnormalities such as talar tilt or knee joint disruptions. Macroradiography may also be used in detecting stress fractures. In this investigation the resultant film is magnified many times.

Protocol for radiological investigation

1. Straight X-ray of the affected part
2. If the X-ray is negative or equivocal, some specialized form of radiography should be requested such as bone scan, stress films, arthrography or peroneal tenography.
3. If a specialized investigation is then negative it is unlikely that a major disruption of joint or ligament has taken place or that a stress fracture exists.

Soft tissue radiology

Soft tissue radiology can be used to detect myositis ossificans and to plot its course over a period of weeks or months. Follow-up films can be used to assess progression or whether the condition is becoming burned out. This may involve several X-rays over a period of months.

More recently, as a result of advances in imaging techniques most of the tissues of the body can be visualized, often in graphic detail. Although ionizing radiation still plays a major part other modalities especially electromagnetism and ultrasound are being increasingly used.

Ultrasonography

This investigation can be used to detect intramuscular cysts and other soft tissue swellings. However, it is particularly helpful in the early diagnosis of stress fractures in sportsmen and women. Such stress lesions become painful after therapeutic ultrasound whereas soft tissue lesions usually respond positively by re-mission. Negative reactions to ultrasound do occur if the fracture is healing, but in most cases of recent fracture the patient will complain of subsequent pain and discomfort (Moss & Mowat 1983).

Tears of the rotator cuff may be demonstrated by high definition ultrasound (Middleton et al 1985) and if due to an impingement syndrome may be accompanied by radiological changes such as a subacromial spur. Ultrasound is more widely available than MRI but the quality and interpretation of the films depends on an ex-perienced radiologist.

Splenic and renal trauma may also be detected by combinations of ultrasound and CT scanning. In some patients with splenic trauma combined ultrasound and contrast enhanced images pro-duced by CT scanning have facilitated non-operative management (Buntain et al 1988).

Scintigraphy

In the investigation of stress fractures scintigraphy gives a high positive response of almost 100%. It also gives a positive response within 24 hours of injury, compared to radiography which may not be positive until 14–21 days after the initial symptoms present. Bone scintigraphy is therefore an early and accurate means of detecting stress fractures even in the absence of positive radio-graphic findings, especially when coupled with the clinical his-tory of increased or unusual exercise and pain in an extremity (Greaney et al 1983).

Computerized tomography (CT)

Though occasionally plain X-rays may give rise to a suspicion of intracranial bleeding (indicated by lateral shift of a calcified pineal) CT scanning remains the investigation of choice and should be undertaken quickly when this is suspected (Gentry et al 1988). Even in sport around 6000 people die worldwide from the effects of head injuries sustained in their activity (Wallace 1988). It is also of use in detecting cortical atrophy or tears in the septum pellucidum in patients who have sustained progressive post-traumatic encephalopathy (Corsellis et al 1983).

Other uses include the detection of orbital floor fractures, spinal injuries and abdominal trauma.

Magnetic resonance imaging (MRI)

MRI is of particular value, in association with plain films, in evaluating damage to the intervertebral discs and ligaments. It can also demonstrate paraspinal haematomas and injuries to the cord.

Its general indications are wide but its availability limited. However imaging of shoulder problems such as tendonitis and sub-acromial bursitis, knee and hamstring injuries has been particularly encouraging. In tendo-achilles lesions MRI has been used to demonstrate the lesion precisely before surgery.

Peroneal tenography

This may be used in conjunction with inversion and anterior stress tests for the investigation of ankle injuries and the integrity of the calcaneal tibial and talo-tibial ligaments.

Arthrography

This is being used less now but may be useful in detecting abnormalities in the rotator cuff of the shoulder joint or investigating the integrity of the articular cartilages of a joint (e.g. knee).

Radiological techniques can therefore be seen to be of value in complementing the clinical picture. They can allow the clinician to exclude areas in his differential diagnosis and it is especially important in sport, as in all branches of medicine, to exclude serious or malignant disease which may masquerade as soft tissue or bone injury. The areas of particular concern are the differences between myositis ossificans in young patients and osteoblastic sarcoma, for the two may be similar in the early stages. Patients who present with a history of breast trauma may report that they felt the lump in the breast only after the injury occurred. Clinically there may be a lump with surrounding bruising. If there are any grounds for suspicion of such lumps they must be excised and examined microscopically and appropriate referral should be made. Although testicular cancer may not require radiological investigation except in the form of lymphangiography or computerized axial tomography, clinicians should bear in mind that a scrotal lump with a history of trauma in a young man must be thoroughly investigated.

REFERENCES

Buntain W L, Gould H R, Maull K I 1988 Predictability of splenic salvage by computed tomography. Journal of Trauma 28: 24–34

Corsellis J, Bruton C, Freeman-Browne D 1983 The aftermath of boxing. Psychological Medicine 3: 270

Gentry L R, Godersky J C, Thompson B 1988 Prospective comparative study of intermediate field MT and CT in the evaluation of closed head trauma. American Journal of Traumatology 150: 673–682

Greaney R B et al 1983 Distribution and natural history of stress fractures in US Marine recruits. Radiology 146: 339–346

Middleton W D, Edelstein, G, Reimus W R 1985 Serographic detection of rotator cuff tear. American Journal of Radiology 144: 349

Morgan W J, Ogden E G, Martin A, Singh L 1980 Correlation between clinical and radiological diagnosis for fractures and dislocations in an accident department. Injury 11: 225–227

Moss A, Mowat A G 1983 Ultrasonic assessment of stress fractures. British Medical Journal 286: 1479–1480

Wallace R B 1988 Application of epidemiologic principles to sports injury research. American Journal of Sports Medicine 16 (Suppl) 522–524

17. Injuries to the face, teeth and jaws

Traditionally injuries to the face in sport are accepted as unavoidable, which reflects prevailing attitudes towards dental health and the machismo element present in many sports. The smiling prop forward with his absent maxillary teeth is a common but unnecessary sight.

Orofacial injuries account for up to 50% of injuries in some contact sports (Turner 1977, Davies et al 1977). This is a particularly sad indictment of attitudes towards prevention of such injuries, for simply wearing a gumshield can reduce the number considerably. Almost all dental injuries in children occur during sport or games. Irreversible functional and cosmetic disturbances result which can become an expensive and recurring problem in later life.

ANATOMICAL CONSIDERATIONS IN FACIAL INJURY

The primary function of the facial bones are:

1. To support the teeth in their masticatory role
2. To maintain a nasal airway
3. To form the margins of the orbit.

These developmental features make the facial bones unsuited to withstand lateral force.

The maxilla

The maxillary sinuses and nasal passages are structured to transfer load from the teeth to the base of the skull. They are therefore well suited to accept a blow directed along the long axis of the maxillary teeth, but not from other directions. The malar complex is attached to the facial skeleton at the zygomatic arch, zygomatico-frontal suture and the lateral antral wall. Lateral pressure on the malar can fracture the arch and antral wall and rotate the malar bone medially, sometimes producing distraction at the zygomatico-frontal suture.

Le Fort II and III fractures are unusual sports injuries because considerable force is required to detach the facial bones from the cranial base, but Le Fort I injuries and dento-alveolar fractures (fractures of a segment of bone carrying two or more teeth) do arise.

The mandible

The mandibular condylar neck is a weak point but acts as a protective device in as much as it will normally fracture, therefore dissipating energy, rather than being forced intact through the glenoid fossa into the middle cranial cavity. Unerupted teeth and teeth with large roots, by virtue of reducing the bulk of bone, are also potential sites of weakness and are normally located at the third molar and canine regions.

The teeth

Erupted teeth are maintained in their bony sockets by elastic tissue, the periodontal membrane, which permits some movement after a blow; but the blow may disrupt the neurovascular supply rendering the tooth non-vital. For this reason apparently sound teeth which have been traumatized, commonly the upper anterior teeth, should be kept under observation as they may abscess later.

Dental injury can be caused by direct trauma or by the mandibular teeth being forced against their maxillary counterparts. There may be temporary discomfort with no physical damage to the teeth or a range of horizontal or vertical crown and root fractures extending to subluxation or avulsion of the tooth. If the upper anterior teeth are prominent they are more liable to injury.

Most lip and cheek lacerations are self-inflicted bites. Irregularities in the dental arch increase the likelihood of soft tissue injury.

CLINICAL EXAMINATION

In the normal course of events, the dentist sees the athlete, by now a patient, in the familiar surroundings of his own surgery or practice in optimum conditions. If the examination has to be made at the source of the injury the facilities may be far from ideal, but the examination should follow the same pattern.

Patients will usually give an accurate history. Close scrutiny of the face and mouth during this verbal exchange will pick up the presence of restricted or guarded movements suggestive of underlying bony injury. Ask specifically about areas of anaesthesia over the distribution of the infra-orbital and mandibular nerves and check for diplopia.

The examination is conducted with the patient sitting and the clinician behind him. This permits bimanual examination of the facial bones for areas of tenderness, anaesthesia and asymmetry. The examination should begin with gentle but firm palpatation of the frontal bones and supra-orbital rims and extend laterally and inferiorly round the orbital rim to the lower orbital margins. Fractures of the malar bone will commonly cause step deformities of the lateral and inferior orbital margins. From a position above and behind the patient, depression of the malar bone is readily seen or palpatated provided there is no gross oedema. Gentle inward pressure on the malar eminence will be painful if there is a malar fracture. Following examination of the globe for restriction of movement and sub-conjunctival ecchymosis, both of which suggest malar fractures, the malar bones are palpated for abnormalities of contour and mobility.

The examiner's fingers should then trace the malar bones and zygomatic arches backwards to come to rest over the mandibular condyles. The external auditory meatus should be examined for signs of haemorrhage and, in severe injury, cerebrospinal fluid. The former suggests fracture of the mandibular condyle, the latter middle cranial fossa injury.

Bimanual examination then proceeds along the lower border of the mandible towards the mandibular symphysis, again principally looking for bony irregularities but also for areas of tenderness and swelling. The presence of dental anaesthesia is strongly suggestive of mandibular fracture.

At this point check for occlusal irregularities and loss of mandibular function. This is done with three simple questions, 'Do your teeth meet together properly?', 'Can you open your mouth wide?' and 'Can you move your jaw from side to side?' If the patient can perform these functions without pain and his teeth meet together as they should do, it is unlikely that he has a mandibular fracture. A further check for mandibular fracture is to apply gentle inward pressure bilaterally over the mandibular angles. Pain accompanying this manoeuvre is again strongly suggestive of mandibular fracture.

The oral cavity is then examined under a strong light source; a pen torch is scarcely adequate. Blood and debris should be aspirated. Disposable portable aspirators are a sensible acquisition for those likely to be dealing with injuries 'on the spot'.

Salient points for intra-oral examination

1. The lower anterior teeth should normally meet the palatal surfaces of the upper anterior teeth
2. When the upper and lower anterior teeth are in contact the posterior teeth should also meet together
3. Look for 'steps' in the dental arches (Fig. 17.1)
4. Check for sub-lingual bruising. This is often associated with mandibular fractures

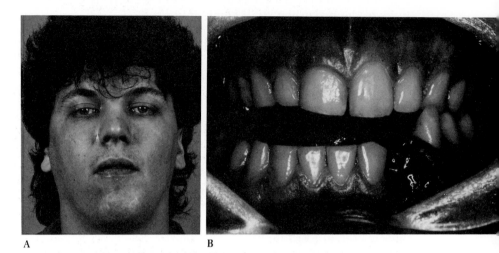

A   B

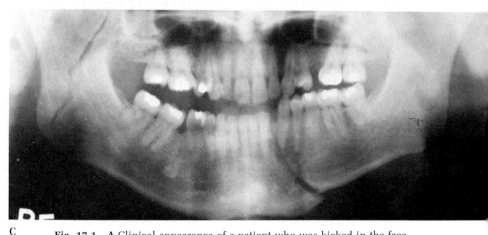

C

Fig. 17.1 A Clinical appearance of a patient who was kicked in the face
playing rugby **B** Irregularities of the dental arch imply fractures of the mandible
C Radiological appearance: there is a fracture of the left body of the mandible
and right ascending ramus

5. Check teeth for mobility either individually or in groups by
   grasping them between thumb and index finger and applying
   lateral pressure
6. Check for missing teeth or tooth fragments, especially if the
   patient has been unconscious. Where are they? Inhaled?
   Impacted in soft tissue? (Fig. 17.2)
7. Check for mobility of the hard palate by upwards and forwards
   pressure with the thumb in the vault of the palate.

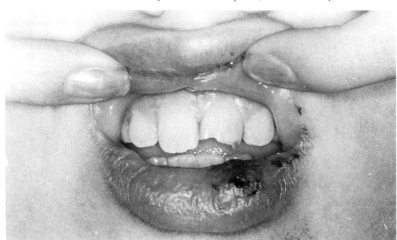

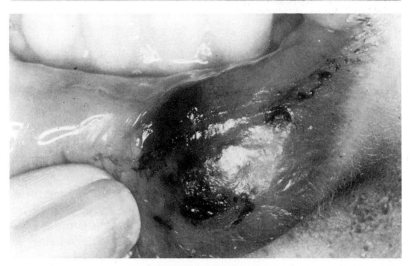

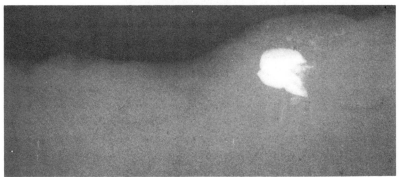

Fig. 17.2 When dental injury is associated with labial lacerations it is necessary to ensure that there are no retained fragments. This patient presented with a labial abscess 6 weeks after being assessed for a minor dental injury

If radiography is available, the X-rays of choice are:

Mandible—Orthopantomograph or lateral oblique mandible
           PA mandible
Maxilla —PA sinuses (15° occipitomental)
           30° occipitomental
           Lateral facial bones

AP radiographs are of little diagnostic aid.

TREATMENT OF SOFT TISSUE INJURY
Initial phase

      Aims: prevention of further injury
               prevention of haemorrhage
               prevention of contamination

These can be achieved by covering the wound with a clean dry dressing and applying pressure. Although facial wounds bleed freely direct local pressure is usually adequate to ensure haemostasis. Pressure on the superficial temporal vessels and the facial artery, where it crosses the lower border of the mandible anterior to masseter, can also be successful. It is unnecessary to clamp bleeders in the depth of a facial wound as a primary measure.

Elective phase

Treatment should be carried out under optimal conditions. Careful repositioning of soft tissue reduces scarring. Closure of facial wounds can be delayed for 6–8 hours, but contaminated wounds should be treated as soon as possible. When closure is to be delayed, cover the wound with a saline-soaked dressing.

Once the full extent of the wound and involvement of surrounding structures have been established the wound can be closed. Local infiltration with Xylocaine® (1% with 1/80 000 adrenaline) is used. The surrounding skin is cleaned with Betadine® or Phisohex® and a soft nylon nail brush is used to get rid of soil or grit, which can cause traumatic tattooing.

The wound should be closed from the inside out, in layers: i.e. oral mucosa, muscle then skin. It is unusual even in major lacerations to be forced to excise soft tissue.

Mucosa is sutured with 3/0 black silk on a cutting needle, muscle with 3/0 plain gut or dexon and skin with 5/0 monofilament nylon. The skin sutures may be removed in 4–6 days. The wound is best left uncovered and dry.

Intra-oral wounds inevitably develop infection and patients

should be instructed to wash out their mouths with warm hypertonic saline, in the morning, in the evening and after meals.

Grossly contaminated wounds, especially where closure has been unavoidably delayed should not be closed. They should be left to granulate and can be revised at a later date. Prophylactic antibiotics and tetanus prophylaxis should be given if indicated.

AVULSED OR DISLOCATED TEETH

During sport teeth are often avulsed or dislocated. Avulsed teeth should be replaced in their socket immediately. If this is not possible the tooth should be placed inside the player's mouth between the lip and gum margin and immediate dental treatment should be sought. When there is dislocation the doctor or team official should gently relocate the tooth in its socket. If both of these measures are initiated within the first hour of injury the tooth may survive.

FACIAL INJURY IN CHILDREN

The upper incisor teeth are those most commonly injured in children and, as parents will testify, such injuries are sustained under apparently innocuous circumstances. Lack of skill, co-ordination and common sense (on the part of supervisors) are the main factors.

Child patients are uncooperative and are therefore difficult to treat. Almost all injuries in children's sport can be avoided by wearing mouth guards.

Prevention of injury

Since protective equipment is accepted in most sports, mouth protectors must be used, but children and adults alike should also be forewarned of the risks. The onus is on the professions, dental and medical, to get the message home. If the Health Service adopted a preventive rather than a restorative attitude, mouth protectors could become available free of charge, to minors at least. It is therefore in the interest of dentally conscious parents to ensure mouth protection for their children. The dental arches change substantially between the ages of 6 and 14 so mouth protectors should be examined at regular 6–monthly intervals to ensure their continued suitability.

Mouth protectors

FUNCTIONS

1. Prevention of self-inflicted soft tissue injury
2. Prevention of dental injury
3. Reduction in the incidence and severity of mandibular fractures
4. Reduction in the incidence of concussion and intracranial injury

TYPES OF MOUTH PROTECTORS

1. *Professionally supplied protectors* constructed on a model made from an impression of the patient's teeth. This is normally a vacuum-formed silicone rubber appliance and is the best option (Fig. 17.3).
2. *Thermoplastic protectors.* These standard blanks are available at most sports shops. The protector is softened in boiling water, then chilled and adapted by the individual to fit the upper dental arch. It is a good second alternative.
3. *Standard rubber 'gumshields'* do not fit well and should not be used.

REQUIREMENTS FOR MOUTH PROTECTORS

1. *Comfort*—The protector should be as unobtrusive as possible and should not irritate the gingivae or buccal mucosa.
2. *Retention*—The appliance should be self-retentive to minimize interference with speech and breathing.
3. *Resilience*—The material should maintain its flexibility in use for a period of at least 2 years.
4. *Hygiene*—The protector should be easily cleaned and remain fresh in use.

DESIGN

The protector should be constructed for the jaw with the most prominent anterior teeth—normally the upper arch (Fig. 17.3). The biting surface should be thick enough to prevent its perforation in use and should allow the jaws to close comfortably. The design can be varied depending on the sport involved and therefore the degree of force to which it is likely to be subjected. In squash for example, where injuries are likely to be caused by the opponent's backswing, the potential site of damage is the upper teeth and lip. These injuries can be minimized by wearing a small flexible mouthguard covering the anterior teeth and buccal sulcus and extending back only as far as the first molar tooth. In rugby, a more substantial protector with full occlusal coverage is advised

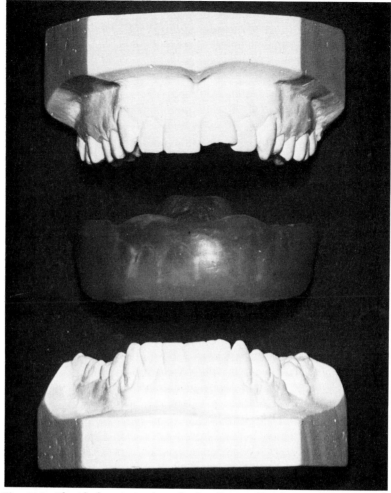

Fig. 17.3 The ideal protector is professionally supplied from an impression of the patient's teeth

because the potential loading is more substantial (Going et al 1974, Clegg 1977).

REFERENCES

Clegg J 1977 Mouthguards for rugby football players. British Journal of Sports Medicine 11: 191–193

Davies R M, Bradley D, Hale R W, Laird W R E, Thomas P D 1977 The prevalence of dental injuries in rugby players and their attitude to mouth guards. British Journal of Sports Medicine 11: 72–74

Going R E, Loehman R E, Chan M S 1974 Mouthguard materials, their physical and mechanical properties. Journal of the American Dental Association 89: 132–138

Turner C H 1977 Mouth protectors. British Dental Journal 143:81

18. Injuries to the eye and orbit

EPIDEMIOLOGY OF SPORTS ASSOCIATED EYE INJURIES

Eye injuries in sport are a major cause of serious eye trauma in this country. They have become relatively more common as occupational and road traffic associated ocular injuries have declined. Sport and all domestic and recreational activities taken together currently account for 75% of eye injuries requiring hospital admission (MacEwen 1989).

Although the majority of sports associated eye injuries are superficial and can be dealt with on an out-patient basis, approximately 30% are of a more serious nature, requiring hospital admission for treatment (Jones 1987, MacEwen 1989). There is a significant chance that surgical intervention will be required in such cases and permanent loss of visual acuity or field of vision occurs in almost 50% of those suffering from this type of severe sporting eye injury (Jones 1988). The majority of injuries occur in males under the age of 25, with children being commonly affected.

Risk of injury

There are quite clear regional differences in the types of sports which cause sporting eye injuries, reflecting varying popularity of sports in different areas, but in general the risk depends on the nature of the sport being played. Low risk sports such as walking, aerobics and jogging or other activities played on an individual basis without the use of implements or balls are unlikely to result in ocular injury. Sports which are played at high speed, in close proximity to other players, involve the use of missiles (balls, pucks) and rackets or sticks are of higher risk. The racket sports fulfil these criteria and therefore have been pinpointed as high risk sports and are a particular area of concern. In addition soccer and rugby are also implicated because of the high degree of physical contact involved in playing these sports. The very high risk sports are, of course, the combat sports, karate, judo and boxing, because they involve direct blows to the opposition.

THE NATURE AND MECHANISMS OF INJURY

There are five basic mechanisms of the eye injury, which can be classified as follows:

1. Blunt injuries
2. Injuries caused by large, sharp objects
3. Injuries caused by small flying particles
4. Chemical burns
5. Physical burns

Each of these causes a different spectrum of injury to the eye and surrounding adnexa and therefore will be described separately.

Blunt trauma

Blunt injuries are caused by a direct blow to the eye and/or surrounding tissues by an object such as a fist or a ball. No skin or ocular penetration takes place, although in severe cases rupture of the peri-orbital skin or eyeball may occur due to excessive force. Blunt trauma is the most common type of injury occurring in sport because the majority of sporting eye injuries are caused by the ball and most of the remainder by body contact.

The most frequent injury seen is the 'black eye' or peri-orbital haematoma. The tissues around the eye are very lax and have an excellent blood supply. Therefore extensive bruising occurs easily. This may prevent satisfactory examination of the underlying globe due to tense swelling of the eyelids. Otherwise peri-orbital haematoma is not a serious problem and spontaneous resolution occurs in a few days.

A direct blow to the eye results in well-documented changes in forces within the orbital and globe (Fig. 18.1). The eye is compressed antero-posteriorly and expands correspondingly in the equatorial plane.

There is an associated acute rise in intra-orbital pressure which may result in a blowout fracture as the weakest wall of the orbit fractures. This usually affects the floor or medial wall of the orbit with expansion of the contents into the maxillary or ethmoid sinus respectively. The rim of the orbit classically remains intact and no fracture is therefore palpable. The clinical features are enophthalmos (due to the expanded orbit), diplopia (due to the entrapped orbital contents preventing full range of movements (Fig. 18.2)), infra-orbital anaesthesia (due to the contused or severed infra-orbital nerve as it runs across the floor of the orbit) and in some cases surgical emphysema (due to the subcutaneous air from the sinus).

Other fractures of the malar complex surrounding the eye may occur, these are usually easily felt as palpable steps in the facial bones and are often associated with more extensive trauma to the head and neck.

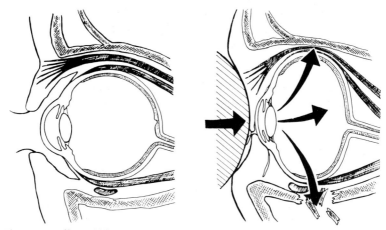

Fig. 18.1   Effect of blunt injury to the eye. The eye is flattened antero-posteriorly and stretched equastorially, causing a blowout fracture and damage to the intra-ocular contents

The flattening forces, as the eye is compressed, are responsible for direct damage to the structures in the anterior segment and contre-coup injury to the posterior segment. The corneal

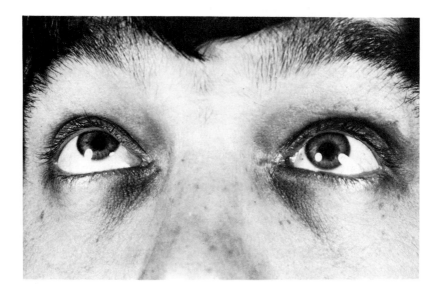

Fig. 18.2   Clinical appearance of a blowout fracture affecting the left eye. In attempted elevation the eye is tethered by the inferior orbital contents in the fracture site

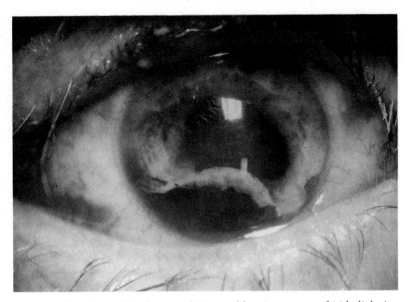

Fig. 18.3   The iris root has become disinserted leaving an area of iridodialysis

epithelium is frequently damaged by the blow, which causes a painful corneal abrasion. This heals without scarring in a few days. The iris comes into contact with the lens causing iris sphincter tears which result in a fixed dilated pupil. Early cataract formation is due to the traumatic interruption of lens metabolism which may cause a rapid reduction in vision. Retinal haemorrhages and oedema may reduce the vision if the macular region is affected. The optic nerve can be damaged by indirect shearing forces causing a reduction in visual acuity or visual field defects (see Fig. 18.9).

As the eye itself expands when struck (see Fig. 18.1) many structures are stretched from their origins and may become partially or completely disinserted. The iris is torn from the ciliary body, causing an iridodialysis (Fig. 18.3) or leading to drainage angle recession which predisposes to glaucoma. The supporting zonules of the lens become damaged, causing a total or partial lens dislocation. In the posterior segment the peripheral retina may be torn, predisposing to a retinal detachment and this may be associated with a vitreous haemorrhage. The choroid in the macular region may rupture (Fig. 18.4) causing a considerable reduction in the central vision.

Bleeding into the anterior chamber—hyphaema—indicates that the eye has received a significant blunt injury. This may be evident

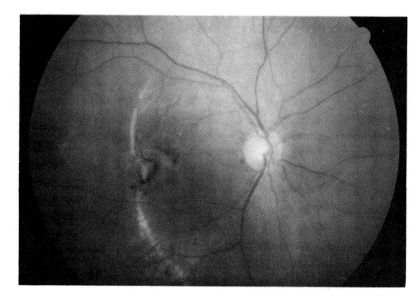

Fig. 18.4   The macular area has a large cresentic shaped choroidal tear running through it. This reduces the central vision

as a level of blood inside the eye (Fig. 18.5) or may be seen as a hazy looking anterior chamber with a poor view of the iris details. The site of bleeding is usually a tear in the highly vascular iris or ciliary body. The patient may be systematically upset with nausea and severe pain in the eye, which usually suggests that the intra-ocular pressure has become acutely elevated. This must be urgently assessed as secondary intra-ocular damage may be caused by this increased pressure. The main concern in the immediate period with hyphaema is that a secondary bleed will occur and rest and hospital assessment are mandatory to prevent this. The presence of hyphaema indicates that damage sufficient to predispose to future retinal detachment, glaucoma or cataract formation has occurred (Kaufman & Tolpin 1974). Full oph-thalmological examination is therefore essential in all patients within a few days of injury as any predisposing damage can be treated if indicated.

In very extensive blunt trauma the eye itself may rupture. This usually occurs at the corneo-scleral limbus or along the insertion of one of the extra-ocular muscles. The contents of the eye may prolapse through the rupture site, but this is not always evident. The vision is always significantly affected in such cases and sub-

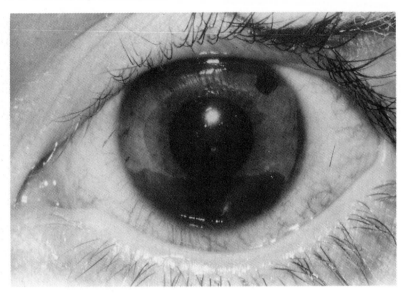

Fig. 18.5 A level of blood is seen in the anterior chamber (hyphaema)

conjunctival oedema and haemorrhages should create a high index
of suspicion.

Large sharp objects—sticks and rackets

Fortunately, penetrating injuries are rare in sport. Less than 5% of
sports eye injuries are caused by a stick, racquet or any potentially
penetrating object (MacEwen 1986). Superficial damage to the eye
in the form of corneal abrasions or lid lacerations are much more
common. Lid lacerations, like any facial injury, require careful
skin closure. However in addition it must be remembered that the
lacrimal drainage apparatus is situated at the medial aspect of the
lid and any injury in this area should be referred for specialist
evaluation and treatment.

Full ocular penetration which carries a very poor prognosis is
fortunately a rare sporting injury. This should be suspected if the
anterior chamber appears shallower than that in the other eye. In
small penetrations an irregular pupil may be present as the iris
plugs the wound to prevent loss of aqueous or the intra-ocular
contents. Larger wounds are usually associated with more extensive intra-ocular damage to the iris, lens and retina (Fig. 18.6).
Lacerations through the sclera involve the retina directly and these
often take place through closed lids. Therefore, any patient with a

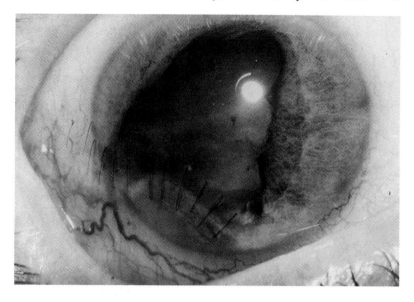

Fig. 18.6 The appearance of a corneo-scleral laceration after repair has been performed. Part of the iris has been removed.

full thickness lid laceration should be suspected as having an associated ocular laceration until proved otherwise. Multiple surgical procedures may be required in order to repair such damaged globes.

Small flying particles

A small piece of foreign material, such as grit or dust may be blown or thrown into the eye. This causes a corneal foreign body which is a superficial but acutely painful injury (Fig. 18.7). These foreign particles remain on the surface of the eye or may settle under the upper lid as sub-tarsal foreign bodies which rub up and down on the cornea each time the eye opens and closes causing a corneal abrasion. Removal of the foreign body results in immediate relief.

Fortunately, small particles rarely travel with sufficient momentum to penetrate the sclera to become intra-ocular foreign bodies in sport.

Chemical burns

Swimmers may suffer corneal burns from excessive chlorination of swimming pools. These are superficial but extremely painful,

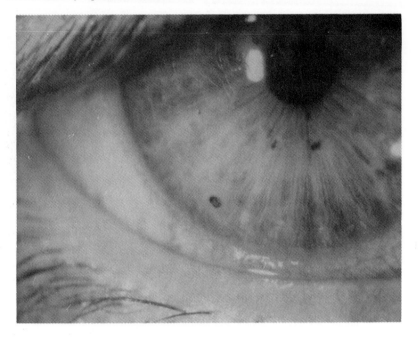

Fig. 18.7 A corneal foreign body

and can be prevented by the use of goggles. Strong acids or alkalis
are not in common use in sports, but the use of lime to mark lines
on football and rugby pitches has resulted in corneal and conjunctival burns from particles being kicked up into the conjunctival sac. The resultant burns may be extensive and cause
reduction in vision.

Physical burns

A more recently recognized type of burn is the physical burn
which is common in mountaineers, skiers and sailors. 'Snow
blindness' is due to the absorption of ultra-violet radiation by the
DNA in the superficial corneal epithelium. This prevents normal
turnover of the affected epithelial cells and 4–6 hours after exposure the epithelium sloughs off leaving a painful raw surface.
The dangers of the blue end of the visible spectrum have also become recognized and chronic over-exposure to bright light in outdoor activities may predispose to early cataract formation and
macular degeneration.

ASSESSMENT OF EYE INJURIES

Touch line assessment and examination of eye injuries

Early assessment of eye injuries is very important as appropriate, immediate management can reduce further damage and therefore prevent any unnecessary visual loss.

Injuries tend to occur in situations which make detailed examination of the eye virtually impossible. The role of the attending doctor in these adverse circumstances, without any specialized equipment or effective treatment, is simply to exclude or confirm serious eye injury and to transfer the patient to the local hospital as safely and as soon as possible, if required.

Any evaluation should always be carried out bearing in mind the nature (blunt, sharp, etc.) of the injury to ensure appropriate examination. If the incident was not directly observed then a good and accurate history must be elicited. An attempt to use good illumination should be made as this assists in the examination. The lids should not be forced apart, they should be allowed to open spontaneously or be gently parted as the underlying globe may be damaged. The visual acuity should be roughly assessed, evaluating each eye in turn, first by asking about any subjective alteration in vision and then asking the patient to count fingers or identify facial features. The size and shape of the pupils should be assessed and compared to the opposite side; the direct and consensual pupillary reactions to light tested. The anterior chamber depth and presence or absence of hyphaema should be noted.

Immediate referral to hospital should be arranged if there is any doubt about the severity or nature of the injury or if there is any difficulty in making an informative assessment. Other features of eye injury which should alert attention to early and careful hospital transfer are: significant pain, reduction in vision, double vision, marked conjunctival swelling or sub-conjunctival haemorrhage, presence of hyphaema or an irregular pupil.

Casualty assessment

Once transferred to hospital, a better evaluation of the injuries sustained should be possible in the casualty department as better lighting and equipment are available. The examination should take place in a systematic fashion, assessing the visual function first followed by examination of the eyes themselves. Each eye should be examined in turn, but it is helpful if both eyes remain open at the same time (cover one eye when assessing the visual acuity).

The visual acuity should be evaluated using a standard Snellen

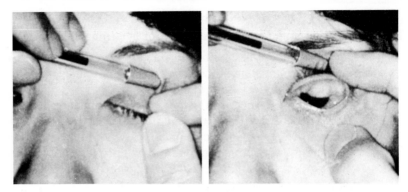

Fig. 18.8   Eversion of the upper lid is essential in the evaluation of the patient with a sub-tarsal foreign body

chart, and if this is not available then reading newsprint is an alternative method of assessment. The field of vision can be assessed using the confrontation method. The range of eye movements is tested using a fixation target and the presence or absence of diplopia assessed in all positions of gaze.

The examination should be carried out systematically, the lids first, followed by the conjunctiva and cornea, and moving on to examine the anterior chamber and posterior chamber in turn.

Superficial corneal abrasions and foreign bodies can be identified with the assistance of one drop of fluorescein 2% which stains the affected area. They may be too painful to allow examination of the eye due to blepharospasm, and a drop of topical anaesthetic, such as amethocaine or benoxinate drops, may provide sufficient relief to allow the eye to open. This must not be used routinely as the drops inhibit epithelial healing. A sub-tarsal foreign body may be identified by everting the upper lid and examining the under-surface of the tarsus (Fig. 18.8). The conjunctival sac should be examined for lacerations, haemorrhages or the presence of foreign materials. The anterior chamber depth must be assessed and the presence of any hyphaema noted. The pupil reactions are tested to a light and the size and shape documented. The lens is usually clear in the early stages but may have become dislocated, this is usually seen as a shimmering movement behind the iris. It is acceptable to carry out this examination using a direct light source, but examination with a slit lamp provides better magnification.

The fundus should be examined with a direct ophthalmoscope to evaluate the clarity of the ocular media and fundal appearances.

This should be done in all cases as soon as possible since after even a short period the view of the posterior pole may be impossible due to rapidly developing lens opacities or vitreous haemorrhage. The pupil should be dilated using a short acting cycloplegic, such as tropicamide 0.5% drops to obtain a good view of the fundus, although this should not be done in cases of hyphaema, nor in those with associated head injuries.

Specialist referral

Patients in whom there is difficulty in making a full evaluation or in those where there is evidence of significant intra-ocular damage or ocular penetration must be referred to an ophthalmologist for specialist examination and treatment.

TREATMENT OF EYE INJURIES

The majority of sports associated eye injuries can be treated on an out-patient basis. The closure of lid lacerations, as long as they do not involve the lid margin, does not differ from the closure of other facial wounds. The lid should be repaired using an interrupted fine monofilament suture (6.0 or 7.0 nylon or prolene). If the lid margin is involved the patient should be referred for specialist repair as improper closure may result in permanent lid notching with associated functional and cosmetic implications. Similarly, lacerations which involve the medial aspect of the lid require specialist evaluation because of the proximity of the lacrimal drainage apparatus. The tetanus status of such patients should be ascertained as a further booster or complete new course of toxoid may be required.

Superficial corneal abrasions heal rapidly. However, they are extremely painful and treatment is aimed at reducing the discomfort and preventing any secondary infection. A firm pad and bandage will reduce the pain (ensuring that the eye is closed under the pad) and broad spectrum antibiotic ointment should be applied four times a day. Chemical abrasions (swimming pool chemical burns) and snow blindness require the same treatment.

The ability to remove a corneal or sub-tarsal foreign body is essential for any casualty officer, although great care must be taken and good illumination is essential. Lid eversion (Fig. 18.8) may reveal a foreign body which can be swept away from the under surface of the lid using a cotton bud. Corneal foreign bodies are removed from the surface of the eye first by irrigation with saline after the instillation of topical anaesthetic. If this is unsuccessful, a sterile needle may be used to remove the material.

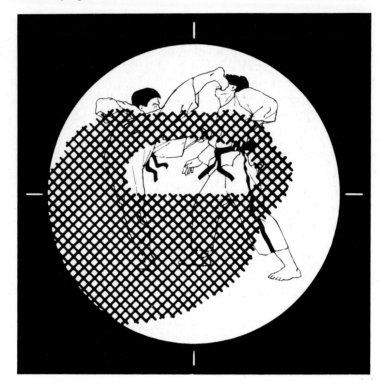

Fig. 18.9 Visual field defect in a patient who sustained a blowout fracture while taking part in karate

Any chemical materials require urgent irrigation and this is done most easily using a drip set and directing the normal saline into the lower conjunctival sac. Any particular material should be removed using a pair of fine forceps.

A blow out fracture should be suspected in all patients who have sustained a significant blunt injury (usually with peri-orbital bruising) and have infra-orbital anaesthesia, enophthalmos and limitation of vertical eye movements (Figs 18.2, 18.9). X-ray examination is unlikely to demonstrate the presence of the fracture, without tomography or CT, but opacity of the maxillary antrum (Fig. 18.10) due to blood in the sinus provides a clue to an underlying fracture. The diagnosis is however primarily based on the clinical evidence. The treatment is usually conservative, observing gradual improvement of the signs and symptoms. However if the patient continues to suffer from diplopia in the primary position or has significant enophthalmos then surgical repair of the

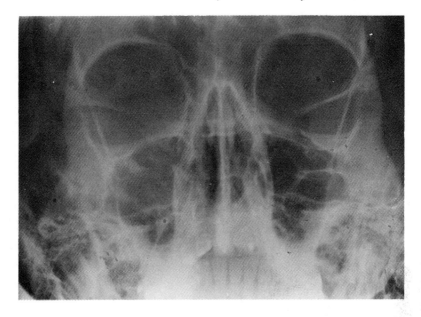

Fig. 18.10 X-ray demonstrating reduced clarity of the right maxillary antrum in a patient with a blowout fracture

orbital fracture should be undertaken, usually between 10 and 14 days from the injury.

Certain injuries require more specialist attention. Intra-ocular bleeding, full thickness penetrations and ruptures or retained intra-ocular foreign bodies must be referred to an ophthalmologist. Any patient who has had an injury consistent with the presence of an intra-ocular foreign body should have a X-ray performed. Further examination and treatment of these patients may be impossible without the use of specialized instruments.

The current treatment of hyphaema is to encourage rest to prevent the development of a secondary haemorrhage. This may involve hospital admission, depending on the severity of the bleed and of the associated symptoms (raised intra-ocular pressure, general systemic upset). The requirement for follow-up to identify the possible complications such as retinal detachment, glaucoma or cataract formation, varies depending on the extent and severity of the injury. Corneal and scleral lacerations are closed microsurgically with 10.0 monofilament sutures after careful examination of the other potentially damaged intra-ocular contents. Retinal detachments are replaced using cryotherapy and internal or external tamponade.

REHABILITATION AFTER INJURY

Players who have suffered superficial injuries (e.g. foreign bodies or corneal abrasions) may return to work and sport as soon as they feel fit to do so. Patients who have suffered from hyphaemas require a period of rest to allow the blood to resorb. Follow-up at the eye clinic is usually 2–3 weeks after the injury and if all the potential complications of blunt injury are excluded, return to training and sports is permitted at this point. If there are any associated problems (e.g. cataract, glaucoma or retinal detachment) they must be treated and fitness to return to sport reconsidered after convalescence. Retinal detachment surgery, if successful, should not leave any areas of weakness in the operated eye. However, this may demonstrate a predisposition to the development of this potentially blinding condition.

All cases of penetrating injury leave an area of ocular weakness and such eyes should be protected during sports at all times. If the vision is significantly reduced after such an injury, consideration should be given to the continued participation in dangerous sports.

Following injury, players are frequently stimulated into the use of eye protection to prevent further damage.

PREVENTION OF EYE INJURIES

It has been estimated that the majority of sports associated eye trauma is preventable (Vinger 1981). It is essential that all steps are taken to protect the eye against these potentially blinding injuries. In view of the amount of time and expense involved in treating eye injuries and the poor visual outcome in cases of serious injury the emphasis has shifted from treatment to prevention.

In general prevention of eye injuries can be achieved by four main methods:

1. Protection of the eyes using goggles, plastic glasses or face masks
2. The rules of certain sports may be changed to make them safer
3. Greater emphasis should be placed on the training and tuition of players to promote safer play
4. The prevention of certain 'at risk' players (such as those with only one useful eye or those at increased risk of certain eye conditions) from participating in the more dangerous sports.

The use of eye protectors has been resisted by many sporting authorities and players as they feel that such devices may reduce both visual acuity and field of vision which will reduce performance. Recently designed goggles and other eye protectors, made of the strong polymer, polycarbonate, have reduced these potential problems. This material, which has been used for many years as an industrial eye protector will permanently deform before it fractures. It is light and easy to wear and if treated appropriately it can be made fog and scratch resistant. The visual acuity is unaffected (and contact lenses or glasses can be safely worn under such devices) and the field of vision unimpeded. Prescription lenses can be incorporated into these protectors. The device of choice is the one-piece polycarbonate goggle which has no hinges, as these are areas of potential weakness. Open eye guards, or those without complete protection of the eyes are potentially harmful as they can funnel the softer balls in to the eye and therefore increase the amount of damage. Prescription lenses made of glass provide no protection because particles of glass from broken spectacles may convert a blunt injury into a penetrating injury. Contact lenses also fail to provide any protection.

All sports must be made as safe as possible and, if necessary the rules must be altered to make them safer. In ice hockey the sticks rule was altered in the Canadian game to prevent raising the stick above the shoulder. This had a beneficial effect on the numbers of eye injuries incurred in this sport (Pashby 1985) (although the opposite effect was seen in this country in field hockey when the sticks rule was altered to allow high sticks). In the racket sports there should be no crowding at the net as this has been identified as a cause of injury. To this end, the observance of the rules of play must be encouraged to improve safety standards. It is important that dangerous or irresponsible play is discouraged as this is often a factor in the development of injuries. The idea that an experienced sportsperson is at less risk than a novice has been shown to be erroneous and level of skill is not a factor.

There are some people who are at very high risk of developing a more serious injury (e.g. high myopes, those with previous penetrating injury) and people in whom an injury would have more devastating effects than others (those with only one useful eye) and they should be discouraged from participating in dangerous sports, and any other sports without the use of eye protection.

The risk of eye injury in each sport must be weighed up against the possible advantages of using protectors or other methods of reducing the injury. The low risk sports such as jogging or aerobics do not require any form of protection, as injury is unlikely. The racket sports are an area most amenable to wearing eye protection (Easterbrook 1978). There is little in the way of physical contact and therefore the goggles would be unlikely to cause injury to other players. Injury in these sports, caused by the fast-moving balls or shuttlecocks, is easily preventable. As the evidence has accumulated for the use of sports eye protection in the games of squash and badminton these have become compulsory in some states in the USA. In this country the sporting authorities and players remain to be convinced that the use of these devices is desirable. There is still a need for a British Standard so that protectors can be made widely available.

The combat sports such as boxing confer such a high risk of eye injury that appropriate protectors must be worn at all times to prevent injuries to the head as well as the eyes. Furthermore, individuals at particularly high risk of injury should be prevented from participating. Examinations for the fitness to continue to participate are compulsory at regular intervals. Any player with a significant degree of myopia or a visual acuity below a certain standard in either eyes is prevented from participating.

As the majority of sports associated eye injuries can be predicted and therefore prevented, (National Society for the Prevention of Blindness 1978) the emphasis must continue to be in the field of protection and safe play.

Acknowledgments

I would like to thank Mrs Angela Ellingford for the illustrations.

REFERENCES

Easterbrook M 1978 Eye injuries in squash, a preventible disease. Canadian Medical Association Journal 118: 298–305

Jones N P 1987 Eye injuries in sport: an increasing problem. British Journal of Sports Medicine 71: 701–705

Jones N P 1988 One year of severe eye injuries in sport. Eye 2: 484–487

Kaufman J H, Tolpin D W 1974 Glaucoma after traumatic angle recession. A ten year prospective study. American Journal of Ophthalmology 78: 648–654

MacEwen C J 1986 Sport associated eye injuries: a casualty department survey. British Journal of Ophthalmology 771: 701–705

MacEwen C J 1989 Eye injuries: a prospective survey of 5671 cases. British Journal of Ophthalmology 73: 888–894

National Society for the Prevention of Blindness 1980 Fact sheet. New York, National Society to Prevent Blindness

Pashby T 1985 Eye injuries in Canadian amateur hockey. Canadian Journal of Ophthalmology 20: 2–4

Vinger P F 1981 Sports eye injuries; a preventable disease. Ophthalmology 88: 108–112

19. Head injuries

Of all patients with head injuries attending Accident and Emergency Departments, 10% sustained their injury in sport. One-quarter will need to be admitted for primary care or observation in a surgical or casualty ward, but less than 1% require admission for neurosurgical care (Strang et al 1978). Another study of head-injured patients admitted to a neurosurgical department showed that sport was responsible for 2.7% of the injuries. Thus serious head injury is uncommon in sport (Lindsay et al 1980).

Since the ethos of sport dictates that players should ignore their injuries and carry on, most figures are likely to be an underestimate, particularly of the more minor injuries. Yet it is these which may present most problems for, although the management of a seriously head-injured patient is obvious, considerable doubt may arise when a player is knocked out for several seconds or simply appears confused after a bump on the head. How safe is it for these players to continue? If they are taken off the park how soon can they return?

THE PATHOLOGY OF BRAIN DAMAGE

Following head injury it is damage to the brain that matters. Skull fractures or lacerations provide clues to possible brain damage or indicate future problems. Diffuse brain damage is produced by acceleration/deceleration forces acting on the brain as a whole. Lesions are widespread and consist of varying amounts of neuronal damage with shearing lesions of nerve fibres in the subcortical region and in the brain stem. There are also superficial contusions and lacerations of the cerebral cortex. The extent of such diffuse injury depends on the severity of the trauma. However, even after injuries associated with the briefest period of unconsciousness, structural brain damage is present, some of which is permanent (Oppenheimer 1968). Therefore the word 'concussion', used to imply transient dysfunction and exclude structural brain damage, should be abandoned. Repeated minor head injuries have a cumulative effect. This has been demonstrated in boxers and in steeplechase jockeys (Critchley 1957, & Foster Leiguarda 1976) and the clinical findings in such people are corroborated by postmortem examinations in persons dying after single or repeated brain injuries (Hume Adams et al 1981).

The best clinical measure of the extent of diffuse brain damage is the duration of post-traumatic amnesia (PTA). This is the time from the moment of injury to the onset of continuous memory. It can last from minutes to months and may endure for some time after consciousness has been judged to return by observers who believe that this is gauged by the patient's ability to speak.

Focal brain damage generally results from depression or penetration of the skull. Although there may be no loss of consciousness there is often a neurological deficit such as hemiparesis.

It is also useful to distinguish between primary or impact damage and secondary damage. Primary damage occurs at the time of the inquiry, is irreversible and is unaffected by treatment. Prevention of such injury depends on changes in the philosophy of sport, for example removing the head as a target in boxing would prevent primary damage being sustained. Secondary brain damage is due to complications such as intracranial haematoma, infection, hypoxia and ischaemia. These things can convert a trivial injury into a life-threatening one. Their onset must be recognized, and their effects are preventable with treatment.

PRIMARY BRAIN DAMAGE

There are two lesions produced by impact injuries: cerebral contusions and diffuse axonal injury.

Cerebral contusions

These are haemorrhages on the surface of the cerebral cortex, frequently on the undersurfaces of the frontal lobes and on the temporal lobes irrespective of the site of initial impact on the head. They are usually bilateral.

Diffuse axonal injury

Loss of white matter has been demonstrated in patients who die some time after sustaining serious head injuries (Strich 1956). The changes are due to shearing stresses on the white matter at its interface with the grey and they are observed in primates which were unconscious for more than 2 hours after head injury but which recovered consciousness (Genarelli et al 1982). Naked-eye changes are seen in the region of the corpus callosum and hindbrain, but on histological study the sites of axonal shearing are seen throughout the brain. These are known as neuronal retraction balls.

SECONDARY BRAIN DAMAGE

This may arise even from injuries which initially appear to be mild. Extracranial factors such as hypoxia or hypotension from injury elsewhere may also be implicated.

Intracranial haematomas

These may be intra- or extradural. Intradural haematomas are three times more common than extradural ones and may be subdural, intracerebral or a mixture of the two. An extradural haematoma is classically, but not always, associated with a skull fracture that has torn the middle meningeal vessels. Whatever the type of haematoma, it will produce deterioration in level of consciousness and, unless removed, will lead to pathological changes associated with compression or distortion of the brain.

Infection

This may present as a cerebral abscess or meningitis some days after a head injury such as depressed skull fracture or fractures of the anterior or middle cranial fossae giving access to the nasal sinuses or external auditory meatus. Leakage of cerebrospinal fluid (CSF) in the form of rhinorrhoea or otorrhoea should arouse suspicion of the latter.

Brain swelling

This may be caused by obstruction to the flow of CSF or by increased cerebral blood flow. Intracranial pressure rises and there is deterioration of the conscious level.

Sequelae of brain damage

The long-term effects of severe brain damage, both physical and psychological, are well-known. It is not generally appreciated, however, that even minor head injuries with brief periods of PTA are associated with impairment of psychological function. The processing and recall of information is especially impaired (Fig. 19.1). The defect can persist for up to one month and although in many people no direct symptoms can be attributed to it, in others a 'post-traumatic syndrome' of headaches, irritability and difficulties with concentration and sleeping develops. Such symptoms may take months to resolve (Gronwall & Wrightson 1974).

In any sport where there is a risk of recurrent head injury there is

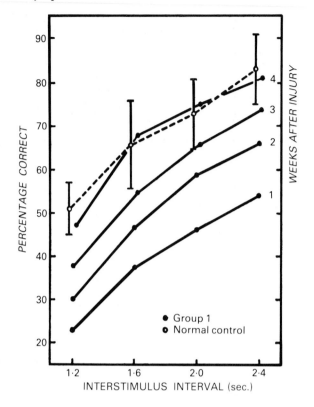

Fig. 19.1 Psychological and intellectual disruption after head injury (Gronwall & Wrightson 1974). Group 1 = head injured patients.

a risk of cumulative damage (Fig. 19.2). After apparent recovery from the initial injury, further trauma produces greater psychological impairment and is more likely to lead to the post-traumatic syndrome (Gronwall & Wrightson 1975). To date only two sports— boxing and steeplechase riding have been implicated in cases of

Table 19.1 Head injury in sport: lasting brain damage (Corsellis 1974) Questionnaire sent to 165 British neurologists: Have you ever seen a condition resembling the punch-drunk state in any sportsmen?

1. Professional soccer	5 cases
2. Rugby football	2 cases
3. Professional wrestling	2 cases
4. Parachute jumping	1 case
5. Steeplechase jockeys	12 cases
6. Boxing	290 cases

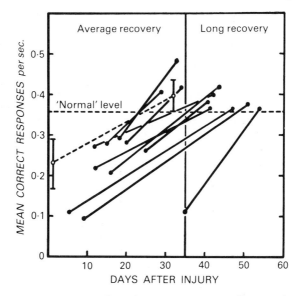

Fig. 19.2 The cumulative effect of concussion (Gronwall & Wrightson 1975)

cumulative brain damage, but there are anecdotal reports of cerebral damage in other sportsmen (Corsellis 1974) (Table 19.1). Certainly, the record of cumulative brain damage in sports such as rugby, soccer and American football might repay systematic investigation. Although both boxers and steeplechase jockeys suffer obvious recurrent minor head injuries in their sport, it is possible that a centre-half in football, who may head the ball up to 500 times each year, or a rugby prop forward sustains similar injuries.

MANAGEMENT OF SPORTSMEN AND WOMEN WITH ACUTE HEAD INJURIES

Everyone who is involved with athletes should be aware of the implications of head injuries. Their only clinical manifestation is alteration of the conscious level. This may take the form of a knockout, a period of post-traumatic amnesia with automatism, or profound coma. Although all these states represent diffuse brain damage in varying degrees the dilemma arises with regard to the person who has been briefly amnesic but, because he is able to talk, appears to be fully recovered. Frequently the duration of PTA includes such an apparently lucid interval. The story of the footballer who completes the game after a brief knockout but remembers nothing between the time of his injury and the shower is

Northern Region
GUIDELINES FOR HEAD INJURY

IN ALL CASES DIAGNOSIS AND INITIAL TREATMENT OF SERIOUS EXTRACRANIAL INJURIES TAKES PRIORITY OVER INVESTIGATION AND TRANSFER TO NEUROSURGERY.

INITIAL ASSESSMENT

AIRWAY: Clear and maintain a patient airway
Control cervical spine until injury excluded*

BREATHING: Oxygen 100% by mask (then blood gases)
Intubate if airway obstructed, threatened or post-aspiration
Exclude tension/open pneumothorax clinically and treat if present*
Indications for ventilation include:
  Cyanosis or Oxygen saturation $<$90%
  PaO2 $<$60mmHg ($<$8kPA)
  PaCO2 $>$45mmHg ($>$6kPA) Or $<$30 mmHG ($<$4kPA)
  Not obeying commands AND not localising to a painful stimulus

CIRCULATION: Commence IV infusion
Assess degree of shock and transfuse as appropriate for age/weight (shock in infants may follow intracranial blood loss)

Record pulse, BP, and respiratory rate
Control external haemorrhage by direct pressure and immobilise fractures
Exclude occult haemorrhage
  (chest/abdomen/pelvis/lower limbs)

DISABILITY: Record pupils, consciousness on Glasgow Coma Scale (appropriate for age) and limb motor responses

EXAMINATION: All clothing should be removed
Seek senior advice (children below five years are particularly difficult to assess and paediatric advice should be sought after initial assessment and resuscitation)

*Adequate lateral cervical spine and chest x-ray to be performed after resuscitation.

familiar to many people. Such patients should be encouraged to leave the field and indeed may now be sent off for their own safety in rugby football. They are more liable to sustain a second head injury or to develop secondary brain damage from an intra-cranial haematoma. Although the latter risk is small it is increased tenfold if there is a skull fracture (Galbraith & Smith 1976).

CRITERIA FOR SKULL X-RAY AFTER RECENT HEAD INJURY:

Skull x-ray not necessary if CT scan is to take place.

Clinical judgement is necessary but the following criteria are helpful:

1 Loss of consciousness or amnesia suspected at any time
2 Neurological symptoms or signs (including headache &/or vomiting)
3 Cerebrospinal fluid or blood from the nose or ear
4 Suspected penetrating injury
5 Scalp bruising or laceration (to bone or >5cm long)
6 Falls from height (>60cm) or onto a hard surface (<5 years)
7 Suspected Non-Accidental Injury
8 Tense fontanelle
9 Inadequate history

CRITERIA FOR ADMISSION TO HOSPITAL:

1 Confusion or any other depression of the level of consciousness at the time of examination (<5 years AT ANY TIME FOLLOWING THE INJURY)
2 Skull fracture
3 Neurological symptoms or signs even if minor, particularly in children (eg headache or vomiting)
4 Other medical conditions - eg coagulation disorders
5 Difficulty in assessing the patient (eg suspected drugs/glue/alcohol/non-accidental injury)

Patients sent home should be accompanied by a responsible adult who should receive written advice to return immediately if there is any deterioration.

CRITERIA FOR CONSULTATION WITH NEUROSURGICAL UNIT:

1 Deterioration in level of consciousness or other neurosurgical signs
2 Confusion or coma continuing after adequate resuscitation
3 Tense fontanelle
4 Skull fractures
5 Sutural diastasis
6 Compound depressed factures of the skull vault
7 Suspected fracture of skull base

TRANSFER TO NEUROSURGICAL UNIT:

1 Consultation process to be completed and recorded
2 Personnel able to insert or re-position endotracheal tube and to initiate or maintain ventilation should accompany the patient
3 Ensure adequate IV access and fluid to maintain systolic BP appropriate for age
4 Adequate notes, trauma charts and x rays to accompany patient. Observations should be continued during transfer.

Fig. 19.3 Example of guidelines card (both sides) for the management of patients with head injuries. By courtesy of the Northern Children's Head Injury Group, 1991. Northern RHA, Newcastle.

The crucial question is whether admission to hospital is required. If there is a scalp laceration, with the possibility of infection, or a depressed skull fracture careful attention and assess-

Table 19.2   The Glasgow Coma Scale

Function	Response	Scale
Eye opening	Spontaneous	3
	To speech	2
	To pain	1
	None	0
Best verbal response	Orientated	4
	Confused conversation	3
	Inappropriate words	2
	Incomprehensible sounds	1
	None	0
Best motor response	Obeys commands	5
	Localises	4
	Flexes {normal	3
	{abnormal	2
	Extends	1
	None	0

ment in an Accident and Emergency Department is necessary; if the patient experiences a period of altered conscious level, even if he is walking and talking, there is a need for a skull X-ray in order to identify (and detain under observation) the small number of such patients who have suffered a skull fracture (see Fig. 19.3).

The Glasgow Coma Scale (Table 19.2–Teasdale & Jennett 1974) permits a ready means of assessing, recording and displaying levels of consciousness. It records in a scaled form the functions of eye-opening, best verbal response and best motor response. Its simple terms have a low interobserver variability (Braakman et al 1974) and the state of responsiveness can be summarized.

If there is prolonged unconsciousness the patient should be placed in the coma position or nursed supine if aspiration equipment is available. The airway must be cleared and maintained during transport.

If a player sustains a head injury at an away match he must be assessed by the doctor present and referred to hospital if indicated. Following assessment, advice should also be given to relatives, friends or club officials about the journey home and what should happen after. No alcohol should be drunk. If focal neurological signs develop, or if there is vomiting or persistent headache, further medical aid should be sought. These instructions can be given on a printed card, as illustrated in Chapter 3.

RETURN TO SPORT

Any person who has sustained a head injury (no matter how trivial) should be discouraged from returning to any sport likely to cause another head injury for a period of 3 weeks–1 month. If there are symptoms of the 'post-traumatic syndrome' he should not return to sport until it has resolved completely. Further injuries will compound existing damage.

Anyone who has been in a coma or has had a neurosurgical procedure should be advised to give up combat or contact sports altogether. There is always underlying neuronal damage in such cases and further injury could be very serious.

PREVENTION OF HEAD INJURY

In non-combat sports most head injuries are accidental. In many, head injury can be anticipated and suitable protective equipment should be worn (Ch. 8). The age-range of patients with injuries caused by golf clubs suggests that young children should be supervised or forewarned of the need to stand well clear when others are swinging (Lindsay et al 1980). In combat sports such as boxing and karate sprung or padded flooring has reduced the incidence of second head injuries (McLatchie 1979) and the use of adequate headgear in boxing has reduced the number of knockouts in Czechoslovakia (Schmid et al 1968). Paradoxically, however, a knockout will stop the fight whereas wearing protective headgear may permit a fighter instead to sustain multiple PTAs with the attendant risk of cumulative damage. If a fighter sustains three knockouts, he cannot box again in that year. There is no such rule in relation to PTA.

The design of headgear is also important. The best model is the motor-cycling crash helmet. In high-risk sports such as horse riding similarly designed helmets should be available for social riding as well as for the professional sport.

Secondary and cumulative damage can only be prevented by making sports officials and participants aware of the risks of continuing to play with a head injury. The ethos of sport demands that the player should continue: we need a change of philosophy, which could be fostered by the governing bodies. If foul play were more strictly controlled and referees, trainers and players were more aware of the risks involved, the incidence of head injury in sport could be reduced.

REFERENCES

Braakman R, Avezaat C J J, Maas A T R, Roel M, Schouten H J A 1977 Inter-observer agreement in the assessment of the motor response of the Glasgow Coma Scale. Clinical Neurology and Neurosurgery 80: 100–106

Corsellis J A N 1974 Brain damage in sport. Lancet i: 401–402

Critchley M 1957 Medical aspects of boxing, particularly from a neurological standpoint. British Medical Journal i: 357–362

Foster J B, Leiguarda R 1976 Brain damage in National Hunt jockeys. Lancet i: 981

Galbraith S, Smith J 1976 Acute traumatic intracranial haematoma without skull fracture. Lancet ii: 501–503

Genarelli T A, Thibault L E, Hume Adams J 1982 Diffuse axonal injury and traumatic coma in the primate. Annals of Neurology 12: 564–574

Gronwall D, Wrightson P 1974 Delayed recovery of intellectual function after minor head injury. Lancet ii: 605–609

Gronwall D, Wrightson P 1975 Cumulative effect of concussion. Lancet ii: 995–997

Hume Adams J, Graham D I, Murray L S 1981 Diffuse axonal injury due to non missile head injury in humans: an analysis of 45 cases. Annals of Neurology 12: 557–563

Lindsay K W, McLatchie G R, Jennett B 1980 Serious head injury in sport. British Medical Journal 281: 789–791

McLatchie G R 1979 Surgical and orthopaedic problems of sport karate. Medisport 1: 40–44

Oppenheimer D R 1968 Microscopic lesions in the brain following head injury. Journal of Neurology, Neurosurgery and Psychiatry 31: 299–306

Schmid L, Hajiik E, Votipka F, Teprik O, Blonstein J L 1968 Experience with headgear in boxing. Journal of Sports Medicine and Physical Fitness 8: 171–173

Strich S J 1956 Diffuse degeneration of the cerebral white matter in severe dementia following head injury. Journal of Neurology, Neurosurgery and Psychiatry 19: 163–185

Strang I, McMillan R, Jennett B 1978 Head injuries in accident and emergency departments at Scottish hospitals. Head Injury 10: 154–158

Teasdale G, Jennett B 1974 Assessment of coma and impaired consciousness. Lancet ii: 81–84

20. Injuries to the neck and spine

The incidence of spinal injuries due to sport varies between communities and in different countries depending on the particular sports and leisure activities enjoyed by each. However, after road traffic accidents sport remains the commonest cause of tetraplegia but a relatively uncommon cause of paraplegia (Table 20.1). The sports most often implicated are casual diving into water that is too shallow, rugby, American football and gymnastics. Mountaineering figures may be falsely low because the violence involved in a fall usually kills rather than paralyses.

MECHANISM OF CERVICAL INJURY

Determination of the mechanism of injury is of more than academic interest in cases of spinal injury. Prevention depends on accurate knowledge of risks. The use of protective equipment, if appropriate, can then be encouraged, or alternatively the philosophy or regulations of certain aspects of the sport can be changed.

Hyperflexion

This cervical posture results when an individual dives into water that is too shallow or is involved in a collapsing scrum (Fig. 20.1).

In American football only 10% of injuries are caused by hyperflexion (Torg et al 1979) but collapse of the scrum with hyperflexion and rotation accounts for one-third of tetraplegias in rugby both in South Africa and New Zealand (Scher 1977, Burry & Gowland 1981). Forced cervical flexion associated with rotation can produce either a fracture or fracture dislocation (Fig. 20.2).

Table 20.1 Causes of spinal cord injuries—2296 cases (From the National Spinal Cord Injuries Research Centre 1979). Percentages are approximate

Lesion	Road traffic accidents (%)	Penetrating wounds (%)	Sport (%)	Falls (%)	Other (%)
Paraplegia (47%)	47	19	2	19	13
Tetraplegia (53%)	46	6	28	14	11

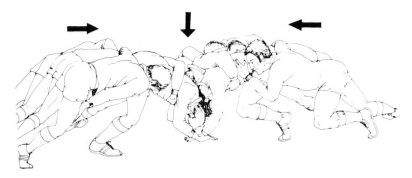

Fig. 20.1   Hyperflexion and rotation of the neck can produce fracture or fracture dislocation

Hyperextension

This too is an uncommon mechanism of tetraplegia (Carter & Frankel 1980), being responsible for only 3% of all American football tetraplegias. However, it has been a frequent cause of fatal cervical dislocation in Soviet wrestlers sustaining cervical dislocation during bridging because of downward pressure by their opponent (Gabashvili 1971). The risk of cervical injury in the bridge is obvious and it should only be broken by flexion of the neck (Ch. 13; Fig. 13.9). This is now the standard method.

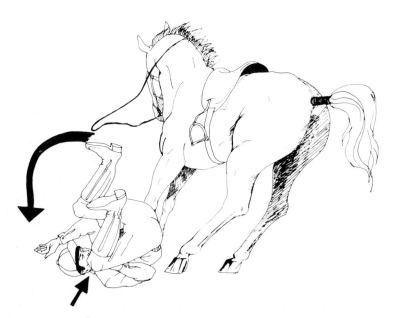

Fig. 20.2   Hyperflexion injury of the neck

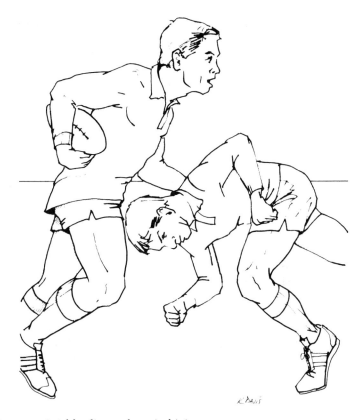

Fig. 20.3   Axial loading and cervical injury

Axial loading

In Torg's (1978) study, 52% of all tetraplegias in American football were neither accidental nor due to either hyperflexion or hyperextension. In most cases the injured player was executing a tackle voluntarily using his head as a battering ram (Fig. 20.3). The initial contact in these injuries was made with the top of the helmet at speed—a technique known as 'spearing'. In the studies of rugby football tacklers were injured most often during 'head-on' attempts to stop an opponent. High tackles, usually executed by more than one opponent, accounted for most injuries to tackled players. Spearing is also a cause of neck injury, in rugby involving two players driving another head first to the ground.

In other sports, such as gymnastics, judo, horse-riding and diving, a combination of axial loading with hyperflexion and rotation would seem to be responsible for most cases of tetraplegia (Fig. 20.4). Biomechanically, compression on the neck will ulti-

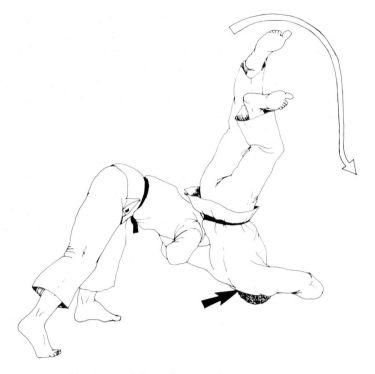

Fig. 20.4   Axial loading with hyperflexion and rotation

mately produce 'buckling' of the cervical vertebrae. This in turn will lead to cervical flexion or rotation with fracture, subluxation or facetal dislocation.

It is now believed that compression of the flexed neck (i.e. straight cervical spine) is the first stage of serious neck injury. As the compressive force increases, buckling with angulation occurs because this is the only way that the spinal column can cope with the increasing compressive energy. Such mechanical loading is a low-velocity phenomenon compared to the high-speed road-traffic accident.

RISK SPORTS

Rugby and American football are the sports most commonly associated with serious cervical injury. In American football much has been done to prevent this problem, with the result that serious cervical injury is becoming increasingly rare. In rugby football also, positive moves have been made. Collapsing the scrum has been made illegal, and dangerous play in the form of high tackles has been more heavily penalized. There still remains, nevertheless, a degree of risk which has not reached the ideal acceptable level: one-third of neck injuries still occur in the 'ruck and maul' phase of the game when a player at the bottom is 'rolled over' with his head trapped on the ground.

Other organized activities, such as gymnastics and wrestling in Eastern Europe, have benefited from changes in the rules. Even in sports parachuting, cervical dislocation in the past has been associated with excessively weighty helmets, which have now been modified.

So far mention has been made of organized sport, but possibly the commonest leisure activity associated with serious cervical injury is diving into water that is too shallow. This is to be distinguished from sports diving: most of the injuries have occurred in people on holiday. Alcohol intoxication is frequently associated with such injuries, but holiday-makers could be forewarned of the problem if shallow water areas were to be identified by local government or local sports authorities. This would be especially useful if a tetraplegia or drowning had previously occurred in that spot. Perhaps even the use of a gimmick slogan such as 'Don't drink and swim or dive' might be more effective than a more formal warning.

CLINICAL PRESENTATION

Two clinical situations present after a neck injury—the patient may be conscious or unconscious. Although management of the neck injury remains essentially the same, the unconscious player's life may be threatened by airway obstruction.

The conscious patient

The injured player will complain of neck pain and perhaps of breathing difficulties. The attendant should confirm that a cervical injury has indeed occurred by simple questions such as 'Can you move your arms or legs? Do you have any pain, or tingling?' Depending on these answers and the posture of the patient a decision can be made that cervical damage exists. It is safer to assume the worst than to move the injured player quickly.

Provided there are no airway problems the player should remain where he lies. Movement, by the log-rolling method, should only be made when rigid stretchers and appropriate transport facilities are available. Log-rolling is a complex manoeuvre which must be rehearsed in mock injury situations, for there is no place for attempting it haphazardly on the field of play.

The unconscious patient

It should be assumed that a potential cervical injury is present when a player is unconscious. In this case the airway is of vital importance and must be given priority. If spontaneous breathing is present the injured person should lie in the coma position until transport is available. If the patient is not breathing then mouth-to-mouth resuscitation, with the spinal column straight and the head held in neutral, is indicated.

An unconscious player lying on his back may have to be log-rolled into the coma position. This must be done in such a way as to ensure a straight spinal column. Such a manoeuvre is necessary because of the risk of aspiration of vomitus. (See Ch. 15)

Posture and cervical injury

Since there is segmental representation of sensation and muscle supply throughout the grey substance of the cord, muscle paralysis and dermatomal sensation losses have value in localizing the site of the injury.

1. C6/C7 FRACTION/DISLOCATION

In this lesion the upper limbs lie parallel to the trunk with the elbows flexed to 90° and the forearms across the chest, a posture due to the unopposed contraction of the forearm flexors.

2. C5/C6

At this level the unopposed action of the deltoids and supraspinatus muscles causes the upper limbs to lie abducted with the elbows flexed and the forearms alongside the player's head.

3. C4/C5

All the roots of the brachial plexus are at or below the level of the lesion. The arms lie flail and at the sides in no ordered position.

4. C3/C4

Since the phrenic nerve roots are at this level respiratory paralysis exists with flail arms.

TECHNIQUE OF THE LOG-ROLL (Fig. 20.5)

Proper training for this manoeuvre is essential. At the time of injury it is inefficient and dangerous to attempt it without previous

Fig. 20.5 Technique of the log roll. The head is first gently controlled then held in the neutral position (**A**). Under instruction from the person controlling the head, the injured player is log-rolled into the supine position (**B–D**)

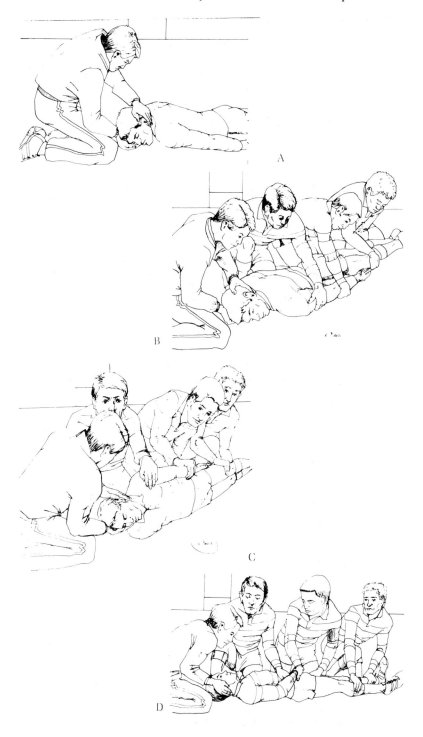

A

B

C

D

practice: everyone should already know what to do. The governing bodies of high-risk sports should therefore ensure that such instruction is freely available to participants and officials.

A rigid spine board and stretchers should be available. The aim is first to PREVENT FURTHER INJURY. The neck is manually immobilized in the neutral position by holding the head. This places considerable responsibility on the person controlling the head, who must both maintain the neutral position and also give all commands. If the athlete is conscious and breathing, this position should be maintained with light traction until transport arrives. The ambulance should be brought on to the field.

In the ideal log-roll five people are involved: the leader who controls the head and gives commands, three who roll the athlete and the fifth who helps to lift when it becomes necessary. The position to be taken up are one person at the shoulders, one at the hips and one at the knees. The body must be maintained in line with the head and spine throughout the roll. Immobilization of the head is maintained by slight traction with the hands.

PROGNOSIS OF 'ON-FIELD' INJURIES

The outlook for patients with immediate tetraplegia is uniformly poor. In most instances there is no doctor and the patient is first seen by medical staff in an accident and emergency department, when the head and neck are invariably immobilized and traction applied. There is some evidence, although tenuous, that skilled reduction of the dislocation coupled with transport in traction reduces the risk of permanent tetraplegia and that the correct transport position is with the patient supine (Piggott & Gordon 1979). In this posture the lumen of the spinal canal is at its widest (Edmond 1984).

RECOMMENDATIONS FOR THE MANAGEMENT OF IMMEDIATE INJURY

Since casual water sports, especially diving, are the commonest cause of tetraplegia, training in life-saving techniques which protect the head and neck at the same time would be extremely valuable. Once on dry land the principles of prevention of secondary damage will apply. Further research and assessment in this whole area is vital.

In sports where the organizers cannot always rely on the services of a Flying Squad or even await an ambulance, the early application of skilful First Aid significantly influences the degree of morbidity and mortality following cervical spine or cord injury.

PREVENTION OF TETRAPLEGIA IN SPORT

Alcohol intoxication is responsible for 30% of all cases of tetraplegia in casual sports activities and the public should be aware of the implications of mixing whisky with water! The identification of danger areas is important, for it is now clear that few accidents happen in public pools. Most occur at private swimming parties or in open water.

In organized collision sports speed and skills have increased. There are two reasons for this. Firstly, the rules of many games have been changed to allow more fluid movement of the ball, and secondly most ball players now demonstrate superior fitness to their predecessors. Perhaps also there has been a proportional increase in 'non-accidental injury', i.e. deliberate attempts to take a good player out of the game.

Coaching and neck-strengthening exercises are two further methods of reducing risks. It is also vital that the laws of the game involved be enforced, ensuring adequate respect for the referee and, where necessary, that the laws of the game should be changed if appropriate investigation shows them to be deficient.

The identification of high-risk sports and of increasing injury trends can only be made by collecting accurate standardized and relevant data. This could be best achieved by ensuring that tetraplegia becomes a notifiable condition. Such a step is essential because many of the accidents are preventable and costly to both the individual and the community. From such centralization of information high-risk leisure and organized sports could be identified, preventive measures instituted and organized immediate care established in these sports. The example of such a register in American football has acted as a precedent where spinal injuries have been markedly reduced (Torg et al 1979). Such a successful outcome is also feasible in other sports.

LESS SERIOUS INJURIES
Acute cervical sprain

This injury occurs frequently in contact and high-velocity activities including motor sport and parachuting. After a twisting movement there is localized neck pain with limitation of movement and/or radiating pain and paraesthesia. Radiological changes are absent. Such injuries probably relate to intravertebral structures or supporting ligaments and joints. Repeated injuries such as result from heading a football may be responsible for chronic changes.

TREATMENT

After facetal dislocation or other bone or soft tissue injury has been excluded the neck should be immobilized in a soft collar. Anti-inflammatory drugs are effective if given within 6 hours and should be taken for at least 7 days or until there is an increased range of neck movement. If pain persists this should be regarded as an indication for further hospital investigation with appropriate physiotherapy and possible traction.

Disc injuries

Acute herniation of the nucleus pulposus resulting from sport is rare. In such cases absolute rest and/or hospital admission is necessary with myelography being required in some cases.

Low back pain

In common with the general population low back pain is a frequently encountered complaint in athletes. In most cases there is no radiological abnormality but conditions such as osteochondritis of the thoraco-lumbar spine and 'juvenile disc' must be excluded in children and adolescents. Other causes of low back pain with or without radiation to the limbs include spondylolysis, spondylolisthesis, lumbo-sacral strain, stress fracture, prolapsed intervertebral disc, ankylosing spondylitis, osteoarthrosis and also neoplasia.

TREATMENT

Vague symptoms are difficult to treat successfully. However, after specific lesions have been excluded analgesic and anti-inflammatory agents may be used during the acute stage. Once pain is relieved strengthening exercises, usually in the form of sit-ups, should be prescribed. In both acute and chronic backache physical therapies such as short-wave diathermy or even local anaesthetic injection can be of considerable value.

The prognosis is good. Most well-motivated sports participants will successfully return to full activity.

REFERENCES

Burry H C, Gowland H 1981 Cervical injury in rugby football—a New Zealand survey. British Journal of Sports Medicine 15 1: 56–59
Carter D C, Frankel V H 1980 Biomechanics of hyperextension injuries to the cervical spine in football. American Journal of Sports Medicine 8: 302

Edmond P 1984 Consultant in charge of spinal injuries centre, Edinburgh, Scotland. Personal communication

Gabashvili I 1971 Death of sportsmen in the Georgian SSR 1955–1970. In: Abstracts of XVIIIth World Congress of Sports Medicine. British Association of Sports Medicine, London, p 57

Piggott J, Gordon D S 1979 Letter. British Medical Journal ii: 193

Scher A T 1977 Rugby injuries to the cervical spinal cord. South African Medical Journal 51: 473–475

Torg J S et al 1979 The national football head and neck injury registry. Report and conclusions 1978. Journal of the American Medical Association 241: 1477

21. Injuries to the thorax and abdomen

This region accounts for just over 6% of all sport-related injuries (McGregor & McLatchie 1984). The incidence of abdominal trauma in sport is rising (Bergqvist et al 1982) and major intrathoracic or intraabdominal organic rupture remains the commonest cause of death in young people (National Safety Council 1978). The recognition of such injuries is often delayed in sporting activity due to a low index of suspicion, and a thorough knowledge of the evaluation and management of these problems is essential to every doctor who sees injured patients.

MECHANISM OF INJURY

Three mechanisms are possible.

1. Penetrating injury

This is not a common type of injury in sport. Most are due to freak accidents in fencing, javelin and rock-climbing. Shooting accidents may be associated with excessive alcohol intake (grouse shooting, etc.) or careless handling of firearms. These take the form of high- (rifle) or low- (shotgun) velocity missile injuries.

2. Blunt injury

Falls during horse-riding or mountain-climbing are frequent causes of blunt injury to the thorax and abdomen but motor sports are not common causes. However, jogging can be extremely risky in the United States. In one year 8300 joggers were killed and more than 100000 were injured by motor vehicles. In contact sports most injuries are due to kicks, falls or being fallen upon.

3. Deceleration injuries

These are seen in motor sports, combat sports, parachuting and hang-gliding. Classically there is duodenal–jejunal disruption. The junction of the duodenum with the jejunum is at risk because of the retroperitoneal position of the duodenum. Other sites of avulsion are at the junction of the great vessels with the heart and the renal vessels with the kidneys.

THORACIC INJURIES
Superficial

CONTUSIONS AND HAEMATOMA

These are common in all contact and combat sports. Treatment involves the relief of pain with analgesics, aspiration of large haematomas and the application of cooling with a compressive dressing for a variable period. It is quite possible to return to sport within minutes of the injury.

STRAIN-INJURIES TO THE MUSCLE TENDON UNIT

Depending on the severity of the injury return to sport can again be rapid and the treatment methods mentioned above are usually satisfactory.

SPRAINS/SUBLUXATIONS/DISLOCATIONS

The tendo–periosteal junction may be injured in most activities. The principles of immediate care can be effectively applied but when subluxation or dislocation is suspected, transfer to hospital for radiological confirmation is necessary. Common sites are at the costo–chondral or even the costo–vertebral junctions. Discomfort can persist for several weeks afterwards, so return to training needs to be carefully graded.

RIB FRACTURES

Pain and splinting of respiration are the main symptoms after rib fracture. Those most frequently fractured are the fourth to the ninth. They can be complicated by pneumothorax, haemothorax or pulmonary contusion. Therefore, early attendance at an accident and emergency department is advisable if such an injury is suspected.

Treatment is directed towards the effective relief of pain which may require narcotic analgesia or intercostal nerve blocking techniques. Although associated with a 20% mortality rate in the elderly (Conn et al 1963), recovery in the young is usually uncomplicated.

STERNAL AND SCAPULAR FRACTURES

Both are uncommon but important because they imply severe trauma. Sternal fractures are seen in motor-sport accidents and parachuting. Cardiac contusion or rupture is the most serious associated injury. The site of fracture may be felt when there is overlapping of the fragments. In such instances, operation with realignment and sternal wiring is indicated, otherwise a pseudo-arthrosis with persistent sternal pain may result.

Scapular fractures occur in motor-sport and climbing accidents and have a high incidence of associated injuries—almost 50% of patients also have head injuries. The remainder sustain renal, pulmonary, cardiac and brachial plexus lesions (Imatani 1975). These associated injuries must be looked for if a scapular fracture is confirmed or suspected.

Local pain and tenderness are the main symptoms and im-mobilization of the arm in a sling until the pain settles is all that is required. Good healing is inevitable because of the excellent blood supply. The importance of the injury lies not in the fracture itself but in its more sinister associations.

BREAST INJURIES

The female breast is liable to injury in many activities. Nipple contusion and bleeding is common in joggers and marathon runners. The use of Vaseline or oil is an effective means of preven-tion but if symptoms persist, or the nipple bleeds or scabs when not training, further investigation is necessary.

A woman will often present to the surgery to report a lump in the breast which first came to her notice after a knock or bump. While haematoma or fat necrosis are both frequent sequelae of trauma it is important to realize that breast cancer may first present in this manner. Any lump, therefore, which does not resolve within a few days or which does not appear to be related to significant trauma should be treated with suspicion and excision biopsy performed.

Prevention of traumatic breast injuries is possible through the use of protective brassieres or tight-fitting tops. However, there is considerable variation among women as to how effective such measures are.

Deep injuries

The heart, lungs, major vessels, oesophagus and diaphragm may be injured in major trauma. Although life-threatening, their early recognition can considerably reduce the high mortality rate.

BLUNT CARDIAC TRAUMA

This can produce two problems

1. Cardiac rupture
2. Cardiac contusion.

Cardiac rupture has been reported in sports parachutists (Simson 1971) and other aerial activities. In 80% of cases death will occur at the site of the injury before transport can be arranged, usually due to cardiac tamponade in association with an atrial tear (Smith et al 1976). Successful treatment will increasingly depend on rapid and effective transport from the accident site.

Cardiac contusion is difficult to diagnose but should be suspected when the history is of trauma to the chest wall and there is evidence of chest or sternal bruising or fracture. Arrhythmia is another presenting feature. The danger run by such patients is of cardiac failure, which is of a type similar to that seen in myocardial infarction (as are the ECG changes). Admission to hospital is therefore indicated. Exercise should be restricted for at least 6 weeks after the injury. Return to full training is dependent upon a normal exercise ECG.

PENETRATING CARDIAC TRAUMA

Fortunately, this is rare in sport. Most cases arise during shooting events or freak missile injuries. Tamponade or haemorrhagic shock are the causes of death. Only 15–20% of all such patients reach hospital alive.

PULMONARY INJURIES

Pneumothorax and haemothorax can complicate both blunt and penetrating thoracic injuries. If there is an open wound connecting the pleural cavity with the environment the risk of a tension pneumothorax exists. This can be effectively decompressed by inserting a syringe (large-bore) needle intercostally. The wound should be covered with a sterile dressing.

Closed injuries can produce local contusion and may also be associated with haemothorax or pneumothorax. There is a degree of pulmonary oedema underlying the contusion with disruption of alveoli and rupture into the large air spaces. If the injury is extensive, considerable pathological shunting of blood can occur, with resultant hypoxia. When multiple rib fractures exist the so-called flail chest with paradoxical respiration may result.

Clinically, there may be some delay between the incident and the onset of respiratory distress. The suspicion of multiple fractures, the presence of surgical emphysema or of reduced breath sounds with or without hyperinflation and resonance should therefore alert the doctor at sporting events to the possibility of significant lung injury.

MANAGEMENT OF THORACIC INJURY

In all cases the priority is to ensure airway patency and maintain respiration, artificially if necessary. Circulation should also be assessed and maintained. Sucking wounds of the chest wall should be covered with an occlusive dressing and suspected tension pneumothorax should be decompressed. Control of pain can be successfully effected by intercostal nerve block. The injured party can then be transported by ambulance to hospital for radiological assessment and blood gas analysis. Oxygen therapy, mechanical drainage of pneumothorax and colloid replacement of blood volume, with diuretic cover if indicated, can then be logically carried out.

RUPTURE OF MAJOR VESSELS, OESOPHAGUS AND DIAPHRAGM

Major vessel and oesophageal disruption are exceedingly rare in sport. In major vessel injury abnormal pulses may be felt with audible bruits in a shocked patient. Oesophageal rupture from trauma is often rapidly fatal. It requires urgent operative treatment.

Acute diaphragmatic rupture presents initially with symptoms and signs related to damage of intraabdominal or intrathoracic structures. Radiology may reveal a viscus in the chest. Late symptoms present weeks to years after the injury as progressive recurrent intestinal obstruction and gangrene or as a progressive respiratory or cardiac problem. If the complication is considered early, operative repair will prevent late complications.

ABDOMINAL TRAUMA

The liver is the most commonly injured intraabdominal organ, with the spleen second (Bolton et al 1973). Pancreas, kidney and intestine may all be damaged. Clinically, signs vary from discomfort to abdominal rigidity and shock but are often undramatic.

Diagnosis

If the medical officer has not witnessed the injury a history confirming direct trauma should be elicited either from the patient or from witnesses. Special note should also be taken of symptoms, such as shoulder-tip pain, which may indicate subdiaphragmatic irritation due to blood or leaking intestinal content.

Clinical examination may reveal specific abdominal tenderness, guarding or rigidity. If patterned abrasions exist on the abdominal wall, e.g. marks made by a belt, buttons or clothing, it can be assumed that significant intraabdominal injury has occurred. Remember too, that pelvic, back and thoracic injuries may all be associated with intraabdominal catastrophe. A shocked, clammy patient with a rapid pulse and respiratory rate is a frequent presentation.

Management

All patients who show signs of shock with increasing pain and distress, or who have patterned abrasions, must be transferred to hospital. In all other cases a careful history and clinical assessment of the injured person will allow a reasonable decision to be made. We believe that all patients with significant blunt trauma should be assessed clinically at 15-minute intervals. Parameters include pulse, blood pressure and abdominal examination. If there is evidence of clinical deterioration, transfer must be effected. To facilitate fluid and drug therapy, an intravenous infusion of sodium chloride should be established before transport.

Delayed rupture?

The spleen is notorious for bleeding torrentially several days after sustaining injury. Usually, there is a history of significant trauma to the splenic area, with associated rib fractures on occasions. However, the patient settles and may be allowed home only to collapse from late haemorrhage when straining (usually at stool) some 10 days later. The liver can also be involved in this process.

It is believed that an initial clot seals a tear in the organ but this becomes dislodged when intraabdominal pressure increases. Only awareness on the part of the attending physician can avert such disasters, and patients with multiple rib fractures should be carefully monitored. Unfortunately, procedures such as peritoneal lavage and four quadrant tap can give equivocal or false positive results. If suspicion of major organic damage exists, however, 'it is better to look and see, then wait and see'—laparotomy is indicated.

PREVENTION OF THORACIC AND ABDOMINAL TRAUMA

This can be achieved by ensuring that the following guidelines are observed:

1. Safety barriers to protect spectators in motor sport
2. Improved safety standards on all race tracks if there appear to be danger areas
3. The attendance of a well-equipped medical team at high-risk events, i.e. motor sport, aerial sport, combat/contact sport and horse-riding events
4. Prevention of cheating in sport by foul play. This would apply

to all combat and contact sports and can only be effected by the governing bodies of individual sports.

REFERENCES

Bergqvist D, Hedelin H, Karlsson G, Lindbald B, Matzsch T 1982 Abdominal injury from sporting activities. British Journal of Sports Medicine 16(2): 76–79

Bolton P M, Wood C B, Quantay J B, Blumgart L H 1973 Blunt abdominal injury. British Journal of Surgery 60: 657–663

Conn H J, Hardy J D, Fain W R, Natterville R E 1963 Thoracic trauma: analysis of 1022 cases. Journal of Trauma 3: 22–40

Imatani R 1975 Fractures of the scapula: a review of 53 fractures. Journal of Trauma 15: 473–478

McGregor H, McLatchie G R 1984 The frequency and nature of sport related injuries attending a city accident and emergency department. Unpublished.

National Safety Council 1978 Accident Facts. London, NSC, pp 96–100

Simson L R 1971 Chin–sternum–heart syndrome—cardiac injury associated with parachuting mishaps. Aerospace Medicine 42: 1214

Smith J M, Grover F L, Marcos J J, Arom F V, Trinkle J K 1976 Blunt traumatic rupture of the atria. Journal of Thoracic and Cardiovascular Surgery 71: 617–620

22. The assessment of the acutely injured joint

Note: This chapter should be read in conjunction with the appropriate chapter on the detailed injuries.

The acutely injured joint can present a major diagnostic problem whether on the field of play, the sidelines or the GP/hospital surgery.

Some so-called acute injuries may be the exacerbation of an existing condition such as chondromalacia patellae, tennis elbow, shoulder cuff impingement or an early osteoarthritic joint.

Acute injuries of any joint may be classified as open or closed.

OPEN INJURY

A penetrating injury of the joint is an acute surgical emergency. It results from a sharp object being driven into the region of the joint, most commonly during a fall to the ground. Such wounds should be regarded as having penetrated the joint until proved otherwise. X-rays taken may show air in the joint but its absence must *NOT* be taken as excluding the possibility. These wounds must be adequately explored, usually following general or regional anaesthesia and under tourniquet. Only this will allow adequate exploration with wound debridement and joint lavage as necessary. Antibiotic treatment is mandatory. Failure to observe the above rules will lead to the development of septic arthritis and joint damage.

CLOSED INJURY

Such injuries result from a direct blow or a twisting force applied to the joint.

A direct blow may simply cause a contusion or haematoma formation around the joint without involving the intra-articular structures. More serious injuries result from a force applied to the joint greater than the structure can withstand and failure (of the soft tissues or bone) occurs. This may occur in the plane of normal movement but more frequently in a plane in which movement does not normally occur.

Joints in which there is a good bony stability (ankle, hip) tend to sustain fractures and joints in which stability is dependent on soft tissues (ligaments, fibrocartilage, muscle) tend to suffer sprains and tears of varing severity with or without dislocation (knee, shoulder, fingers). However even in these latter joints significant bony injury may result from avulsion by attached soft tissue or osteochondral fractures from the shearing force within the joint.

The correct diagnosis of any injury will depend on taking an adequate history followed by an appropriate physical examination. Omission of either will increase the chance of an inadequate assessment of the situation with its inherent dangers for advice and treatment.

HISTORY

No matter where the assessment of the injury is taking place it is essential that the mechanism of the injury be ascertained as accurately as possible. On occasions this may prove difficult because of the circumstance in which the injury occurred or from the lack of full co-operation from an excited player.

In the *immediate* assessment the following should be determined:

1. Where is the pain?
2. Did the injury result from a direct blow, a twist or an overstretch?
3. If a direct blow, from which direction did it come, or in which direction did it push the joint?

At a *later* assessment the following additional information should be obtained:

1. Did the joint swell?
2. If so, did the swelling occur immediately (haemarthrosis) or sometime later (effusion)?
3. Was it possible to move the joint through its full movement or was it 'locked'?
4. In the lower limb joint was it possible to take weight through the joint?

EXAMINATION

Proper examination can only be performed if the injured area is adequately exposed. This exposure is likely to be less adequate on the field of play or sidelines but should be complete in the first aid room or surgery, together with its supposed normal fellow on the opposite side.

The following are the essentials of the examination:

LOOK

1. Is there any visible deformity?
2. Is there discolouration?
3. Is there swelling?
4. If so is it local or general?

FEEL

1. Is there tenderness?
2. If so, where is the tenderness in relation to anatomical structures?
3. Is there an effusion?

MOVE

1. Is there a full range of movement in the normal directions?
2. Is this movement painful?
3. Is there pain or movement when the joint is stressed in a direction in which movement does not normally occur?
4. Is there normal circulation and sensation in the limb distal to the injured joint?

If the limited examination possible on the field of play leads to a confident diagnosis of an insignificant injury, a functional assessment should be carried out and if satisfactory then the player can continue participating.

If there is any doubt the player should be removed to the sidelines where there will be more time for a better assessment of the injury. This will also allow for the pressure to be taken out of the situation, allow for some recovery time and a more leisurely assessment of function before deciding if the player can continue.

If after such a process the injury is still deemed not to be serious and the player continues after appropriate treatment, the performance on the field of play should be watched closely and if the player is seen to be clearly labouring under some disability then it may be appropriate to recall him or her from the field to avoid risking deterioration of the present injury or the occurrence of another injury as a result of the incapacity.

Players with more serious injuries may require to be referred to hospital for further investigation and treatment.

When hospital referral is necessary fractures and dislocations will be conformed by X-ray.

The further assessment of soft tissue injury is less easy. In the acute situation when instability of the joint is suspected it is usually wise to assess the degree of ligament laxity by stress testing under anaesthesia. This may be possible after infiltration of local anaesthetic (e.g. ankle) but in other joints particularly if it is anticipated that surgical treatment will be necessary it is best achieved under general or regional anaesthesia. Often this instability can be confirmed and measured visibly on X-ray. Only when this is done can the degree of damage be known and appropriate treatment instituted.

The use of the arthroscope is mainly confined to the knee joint where it can be used to diagnose and treat injuries of the intra-articular soft tissues.

Imaging of injuries of the soft tissues around and within joints is becoming increasingly employed. Arthrography is used less frequently now than formerly. In recent years computerized tomography (CT) scanning has been employed by itself or in combination with arthrography but the greatest advance has been the development in the use of magnetic resonance imaging (MRI). This is safer than the above techniques, gives a much improved image but unfortunately is not yet freely available throughout the UK although will become more so over the next few years.

SHOULDER

In sport, the shoulder area is most commonly injured by falling on to the outstretched arm or directly on to the point of the shoulder. These are the mechanisms which lead to fracture or dislocation. Throwing activities, or possibly jerking the arm result in injuries of the soft tissues, usually the shoulder cuff.

Careful inspection of the shoulder region can differentiate between fractures of the clavicle, dislocation or springing of the acromioclavicular joint or anterior dislocation of the shoulder. Palpation will certainly confirm any of the above diagnoses and it is not necessary to move the arm.

Players with other than a minor injury of the acromioclavicular joint will require treatment at hospital with assessment by X-rays but even with the latter diagnosis it may be necessary to X-ray the region to exclude a very distal clavicular fracture if the tenderness is over this part of the bone rather than the joint itself.

When there is a dislocation of the glenohumeral joint it is important to exclude a traction injury of the brachial plexus or more likely the axillary nerve.

Injuries of the tendons of the shoulder cuff are usually in the nature of contusions or sprains. Ruptures of the should cuff tend to occur in older athletes or in younger athletes after the injudicious use of local steroid infiltration. The presence of a cuff rupture is usually not appreciated until some time after the acute injury when there is specific loss of active movement in a particular direction (most commonly abduction due to supraspinatus rupture). Such a diagnosis can be confirmed by an arthrogram often coupled with a CT scan or MRI.

ELBOW

Injuries of the elbow most commonly follow a fall on to the outstretched hand.

The common posterior dislocation can be easily diagnosed by observing the arm held at approximately 90° with the forearm pushed backwards making the olecranon unduly prominent. In children a similar deformity exists with the usual supracondylar fracture of the humerus. However, with this injury the limb is much more unstable. With both there is the risk of a median nerve palsy which results from entrapment of the nerve. Of more critical importance is injury or compression of the brachial artery which results in ischaemia of the limb distally. This is a surgical emergency and there should be no delay in transporting the patient to hospital with the limb duly splinted.

In the absence of deformity there may be tenderness over the head of the radius in the presence of a fracture in that area or a palpable gap may be appreciated when there is a fracture of the olecranon which the triceps has displaced by its contraction.

Contusion of the elbow is a fairly common injury and results in swelling or effusion with loss of full flexion and full extension. This diagnosis should only be made after the exclusion of a fracture of the upper radius or an osteochondral fracture by X-ray.

Although rare, the most common specific soft tissue injury is rupture or avulsion of the biceps tendon. This is most common in the older tendon when the elbow is flexed against resistance but has also been described in younger power weight lifters performing the snatch lift. There is pain in the ante cubital fossa and examination reveals swelling, bruising and tenderness in the same area with weakness of active flexion and a bunched up appearance of the biceps muscle proximally. Surgical repair is necessary.

WRIST

By far the most common injury of the wrist is a simple sprain of the soft tissues.

If there is a displaced Colles' fracture of the distal radius the dinner fork deformity will be visible. Undisplaced fractures can be suspected by careful palpation and confirmed on X-ray.

The biggest pitfall in the assessment of injuries of the wrist is the failure to diagnose a fracture of the scaphoid. Delay in this diagnosis might mean delayed union, necessary surgery and if unsuccessful the development of post traumatic osteoarthritis.

The symptoms and signs of a wrist sprain or a scaphoid fracture are dangerously similar. Fracture should be suspected and X-rays arranged if there is specific tenderness over the scaphoid in the anatomical snuffbox or the volar aspect of the wrist. These X-rays may have to be repeated one to two weeks later if symptoms persist in the presence of an original normal X-ray.

HIP

Most injuries of the hip region affect the soft tissues, either tendons or capsule. They result from either a twisting injury or an overstretch. Most of these groin injuries occur anteriorly and in the acute situation it is usually difficult to decide which structure is involved i.e. psoas tendon, adductor tendon, rectus femoris tendon, rectus abdominis. When such an injury occurs the player should be exhorted not to continue in view of the prolonged disability which may develop if the condition becomes chronic. Over the succeeding hours or days it is important to try to define the source of the symptoms by careful palpation and stretch tests, so that treatment can be directed to the appropriate anatomical structure.

In the young adolescent (especially boys) it is important not to make this diagnosis until the possibility of a minimal slipped upper femoral epiphysis has been excluded by antero-posterior *and lateral* X-rays of the hip.

If displaced an acute slip in the adolescent has the same particular appearance as a displaced femoral neck fracture, namely shortening of the leg which lies in the externally rotated position. Such a slip may result from a fairly minor injury, particularly in a child who has had chronic pain for some weeks or months before indicating the developing pathology.

Posterior dislocation of the hip is rare in sport unless there is a violent injury to the joint. The appearance of the limb is characteristic as it lies in flexion, adduction and internal rotation in which movements are grossly restricted and painful. The limb distally should be examined to look for the signs of a sciatic nerve palsy which may complicate this injury.

KNEE

Injuries of this joint above all others constantly present difficulties in diagnosis. Sports trauma may occasionally cause a fracture, most commonly to the patella or the tibial plateau. Diagnosis of these injuries may be fairly difficult unless there is localized tenderness and palpation which may also reveal a fracture gap. This associated with loss of normal movement will raise sufficient suspicion to refer the player to hospital for X-ray which will confirm the diagnosis.

An osteochondral fracture may result from a shearing force within the joint and will be discussed later.

Since bony stability of the knee joint is minimal, trauma results in injury of the supporting and stabilizing soft tissues—capsule, collateral and cruciate ligaments, menisci and tendons.

Although isolated structures can be injured the interrelationship between all the soft tissues in stabilizing the joint often results in injuries of a complex nature.

Some attempt should be made to ascertain the mechanism of injury, e.g. valgus or varus stress with or without rotation. Occasionally a force may produce hyperextension which will injure posterior capsule with other structures.

One of the signs to which some importance should be attached is the development of an effusion. If such occurs immediately or within a short time after an injury then this will be blood. Since the only structures within the joint which are significantly vascular are bone and synovium then a haemarthrosis is an indication of injury to one or other structure. Synovial injury results from rupture of the structure which the synovium is investing, usually capsule or cruciate ligament.

An effusion developing some hours after injury is likely to be reactive in nature.

If after injury there is no effusion, no localized tenderness a full range of active movement and no ligament laxity on stress then there is unlikely to be a significant soft injury.

If there is no effusion, some tenderness over the bone attachment of the collateral ligament (at the epicondyle), a full range of active movement and no ligament laxity but some pain on stretching the appropriate collateral ligament then a mild partial tear of that ligament is likely. Provided the competitor's ability is not greatly affected by the pain then he or she may continue participating. However, if there is a greater degree of pain, such that full extension of the knee is not possible, then the player should not continue and appropriate treatment of the soft tissue injury should be instituted.

If the latter conditions exist and in addition the maximal tenderness is elicited over the joint line then a meniscal tear is likely and the player referred to hospital for possible arthroscopy.

All of the above injuries may develop a reactive effusion of synovial fluid some hours after the incident.

If after injury there is immediate effusion (of blood) then there is a 60–70% chance that there is a rupture of the anterior cruciate ligament. This will always be accompanied by injury to other structures such as capsule, ligaments or menisci. Therefore ideally all such injuries should be seen and assessed by an experienced doctor in hospital.

If on careful stress testing the integrity of all ligaments is assured then the other diagnoses which must be considered are a peripheral tear of the meniscus or an osteochondral fracture resulting from a shearing force applied to the joint surface. Routine X-rays if carefully examined are likely to show the osteochondral fragment which will necessitate exploration of the joint with reattachment of the fragment if appropriate. One source of such a fragment is the lateral femoral condyle from which it has sheared off during lateral displacement of the patella which then reduced spontaneously. This diagnosis should be suspected in knees such as the above in which there is tenderness all along the medial parapatellar region where the medial retinaculum and vastus medialis must of necessity have been ruptured.

If X-rays are normal then there is a good argument to proceed to arthroscopy which might provide the definitive diagnosis. Small osteochondral fragments and their source may be identified but more important, peripheral tears of the meniscus can be seen and repair carried out with an excellent chance of success.

Arthroscopy in the presence of a haemarthrosis is not easy but if after a careful search no specific injury can be identified then it is unlikely that any important structure has been injured. However, such knees should be kept under review until normal function, including sporting function has been restored.

If on initial examination there is obvious laxity of the cruciate and collateral ligaments on stress testing or if there is any doubt about the integrity of these ligaments then such tests should be performed under anaesthesia to confirm the degree of laxity. If present, surgical repair can give the best chance of success and since the knee joint will be opened on doing so there is little point in arthroscopy in the difficult situation of a haemarthrosis.

If the laxity is confined to the collateral ligament and it is not marked, then since cast immobilization is likely to give a good result it is wise to proceed to arthroscopy to make sure that none of the other causes of haemarthrosis are present which would necessitate arthrotomy.

Beware of the paradox where from the history, a serious injury has occurred yet there is little pain or effusion; this may indicate gross disruption of the capsule and ligaments such that no tension is present in the tissues to give pain.

A forced flexion injury can produce rupture of the quadriceps or patellar tendon especially in the older athlete. Such injuries can be missed since some active extension of the joint is possible through the medial and lateral retinacula. However, the mechanism of injury should alert to the possibility of this diagnosis especially if the knee cannot be actively fully extended home and can be confirmed by the palpation of a gap in the appropriate tendon. If available, MRI can demonstrate these tears beautifully.

The single most important feature in the examination of an injured knee is the assessment of stability. Failure to appreciate this in time for primary repair of the soft tissues will reduce the chance of restoring satisfactory function since the result of surgical treatment of chronic instability is uncertain.

ANKLE

Numerically the ankle is the joint most susceptible to injury. Most injuries result from a combination of inversion or eversion with rotation and most frequently result in damage to the ligaments and capsule. Fractures are associated with some degree of soft tissue injury.

When assessing injuries to the ankle region it is most important to exclude fracture of the calcaneum and rupture of the Achilles tendon which occur by quite a different mechanism to the above and which have a completely different appearance on clinical examination.

If after an injury there is obvious deformity of the ankle with displacement of the foot in relation to the leg then there will be a fracture or fractures present and an immediate referral to hospital is necessary.

If there is swelling alone and this is associated with tenderness over the bone then a fracture should be suspected and X-ray is required.

If swelling and tenderness lie distal to the malleolus or over the anterior tibio fibular ligament then it is likely that the injury is to the ligaments alone.

The only remaining question is the degree of injury and as a result the stability of the joint. If swelling is severe and associated with bruising (usually on the lateral side) it is important to carry out stress testing with X-rays in both the antero-posterior and lateral planes to assess instability since complete tears of the 'collateral' ligaments require immobilization whereas the stable joint does not. Such tests need to be performed under infiltration of local anaesthetic.

More detailed discussion and treatment of specific injuries can be found in the corresponding chapters.

23. Injuries to the upper limbs

MOVEMENTS OF THE SHOULDER AND THE ROTATOR CUFF

The glenohumeral joint is inherently unstable because of the shape of its bony components. Although these permit a wide range of movement, stability depends on the rotator cuff group of muscles around the joint.

THE ROTATOR CUFF

Four muscles contribute to the so called rotator cuff. These are:

1. *Subscapularis*. This is a medial rotator of the shoulder. It arises from the medial border of the scapula, passes in front of the shoulder joint and inserts into the lesser tuberosity of the humerus.
2. *Supraspinatus* muscle initiates abduction. It arises above the scapular spine and is inserted into the greater tuberosity of the humerus.
3. *Infraspinatus* is a lateral rotator. It arises from the inferior two-thirds of the dorsal surface of the scapula and its tendon inserts into the greater tuberosity of the humerus below the supra-spinatus but above teres minor.
4. *Teres minor* is also a lateral rotator. It arises from the dorsum of the lateral border of the scapula and is inserted into the lowest facet of the greater tuberosity of the humerus.

Other muscles, namely pectoralis major, teres major and latissimus dorsi, give some support to the anterior and inferior aspects of the joints. They insert into the ridges and gutter of the bicipital groove. the deltoid muscle arises from the anterior border of the lateral third of the clavicle, acromion and the lower lip of the crest of the spine of the scapula. Its fibres converge to be inserted into the deltoid tuberosity on the lateral aspect of the upper humeral shaft. Due to their insertion at some distance from the shoulder joint these muscles are very efficient power procedures for shoulder movement.

LIGAMENT AND JOINT INJURIES
The acromioclavicular joint

The acromioclavicular ligaments may be torn as a result of a fall on to the shoulder. More severe trauma may tear the conoid and trapezoid ligaments as well leading to acromioclavicular dislocation. This injury is commonly seen in contact sports and results from a fall directly on to the point of the shoulder.

SIGNS AND SYMPTOMS

There is well localized pain at the acromioclavicular joint and tenderness on examination. Unless swelling is extensive a visible step may be apparent which is easily palpable when the joint is subluxed or dislocated. Confirmation of the diagnosis is by straight X-ray taken in the sitting or standing position preferably with some weight held in the dependent arm.

TREATMENT

The injured player should be treated in a broad arm sling. Closed methods of reduction are ineffective. When the pain subsides the arm and shoulder are exercised—pendular movements initially followed by active exercises. In most cases function is unaffected by non-reduction. If displacement is severe, screw fixation between the clavicle and coracoid will permit improved healing and function long term. The screw should be removed after 6 weeks, before active movement is started.

PROGNOSIS

Most players have no residual disability. If there is excessive deformity or persistent pain, the lateral 2 cm of the clavicle may be excised.

The glenohumeral joint

Displacement of the head of the humerus results in an anterior dislocation of the shoulder, a common injury often resulting from a fall on to the outstretched hand. It may also occur during water sports.

Posterior dislocation is rare in sporting injuries and is caused by forced internal rotation when the arm is abducted or from a fall on to the elbow with the shoulder flexed to 90°.

Anterior dislocation

SIGNS AND SYMPTOMS

The injured player supports his arm which is held in abduction. There is loss of normal curvature of the shoulder which assumes an angular appearance and there may be an obvious hollow below the deltoid muscle. The arm appears to be 'too long'. Confirmation of the diagnosis is by X-ray, the head of the humerus being seen to lie below and anterior to the glenoid margin. Even if dislocation is obvious, films should be taken to exclude any associated fractures.

TREATMENT

In some cases immediate reduction by Kocher's or Hippocrates manoeuvre is effective, but should still be radiologically confirmed. In Kocher's manoeuvre the elbow is flexed and traction is applied to the humerus while it is in lateral rotation. The arm is then adducted and rotated medially. Using the Hippocratic method one places one foot gently in the patient's axilla, pulls the arm and levers the head of humerus into position. More often a general anaesthetic is necessary to effect reduction.

After reduction the arm should be immobilized in a restrictive sling which prevents external rotation and abduction for a period of 2 to 3 weeks which allows the stretched and injured anterior soft tissues to heal in the shortest length thus reducing the risk of recurrent dislocation (see below). After 3 weeks increasingly intensive exercises are encouraged but return to full contact sport should be delayed for 2 to 3 months.

COMPLICATIONS

Fractures of the glenoid margin, the neck of the humerus and the greater tuberosity must be excluded radiologically. The recognition of these is important if recurrent dislocation, avascular necrosis and post traumatic stiffness are to be avoided.

Neuropraxia due to stretching of the axillary nerve or less commonly the brachial plexus usually recovers spontaneously.

PROGNOSIS

Active movements prevent post traumatic stiffness and should be started within the limitations of the restrictive sling as soon as the shoulder is pain free. Uncomplicated dislocations have a good prognosis.

RECURRENT DISLOCATION OF THE SHOULDER

If as the result of an anterior shoulder dislocation damage is confined to the capsule and anterior shoulder cuff spontaneous repair will occur. However if there has been damage to the glenoid labrum, the glenoid margin or to the humeral head recurrent dislocation may result. This can happen with the most trivial arm movements but especially with the arm raised, abducted and externally rotated. Glenoid labrum detachment is most often seen in young people. If there is a history of recurrent dislocation advice

must be given to the athlete of the future prospect in his chosen
sport. If he is a thrower, or a hooker in a rugby team, his prognosis
is poor.

Procedures for the repair of recurrent dislocation

Two lesions of the shoulder may be present when there is recurrent dislocation. The first is the Bankhart lesion which consists of
a detachment of the glenoid labrum. On occasion there may be a
secondary bone defect of the postero-lateral aspect of the humeral
head which also predisposes to dislocation (the hatchet head or
Hill-Sachs lesion).

Several operations have been described. All attempt to stabilize
the shoulder in abduction and lateral rotation. The Bankhart, Putti-
Platt and Bristow-Helfet procedures are the best known. Successful operations result in slight reduction of full external rotation.

Bankhart's operation stabilizes the joint by reattaching the
glenoid labrum and shortening the capsule and subscapularis
tendon. The Putti-Platt procedure does not attempt to reattach the
glenoid labrum. In both procedures the arm is held in internal
rotation at the side for 4–6 weeks after which movements can
begin. The Bristow-Helfet procedure detaches the coracoid process with its attached tendons (short head of biceps and cora-
cobrachialis) and transferring this to a roughened area on the neck
of the scapula where it is reattached to reinforce in a dynamic
fashion the anterior soft tissues of the shoulder.

RECURRENT SUBLUXATION OF THE GLENOHUMERAL JOINT (THE UNSTABLE SHOULDER)

This term is given to the subjective sensation of shoulder instability with certain movements. It occurs more often in the
younger age groups (16–20 years) than does recurrent dislocation.
The condition can produce marked limitation in athletic activity.

SIGNS AND SYMPTOMS

Insecurity of the shoulder is the common presenting symptom and
clinical examination may reveal apprehension on abduction with
external rotation. There may be pain or even crepitus on external
rotation or an increased range of movement. The instability may be
multidirectional.

INVESTIGATIONS

Infraglenoid changes may be apparent in the AP X-ray with the
shoulder in neutral position and on the lateral view there may be
irregularity of the glenoid labrum or a notch on the humeral head

(see above). Arthrography coupled with CT examination is important in the diagnosis of this condition and will define more clearly the abnormal anatomy of the joint and in particular details of the capsular defect.

TREATMENT

When positive clinical and radiological signs are present in patients with a clear history of disability reconstructive surgery similar to that for recurrent dislocation may be indicated. If the condition is multidirectional rather than unidirectional, treatment is more difficult and the prognosis less good.

ROTATION CUFF LESIONS

Overarm bowling, serving a tennis ball, swimming and other activities involving overhead movements of the arm can cause pain around the shoulder. More than 20% of lesions causing the painful shoulder are due to extra-capsular soft tissue lesions, (Binder et al 1983). The changes which are seen are a direct result of abnormal repetitive stresses. These lead to mechanical irritation of the structures below the acromial arch—the rotator cuff tendons and the subacromial bursa. An inflammatory response is thus stimulated producing pain when the infected structures impinge upon the increasingly limited subacromial space. There is a painful arc of movement—the painful arc syndrome or rotator cuff impingement syndrome.

CLASSIFICATION

Three groups of affected patients are described by Neer and Welsh (1977), the young athlete under 25 years of age, the weekend sportsman and the middle aged worker. The prognosis differs in each group. In the very young the onset is often insidious and symptoms are usually reversible. In weekend sportsmen chronic pain is characteristic and may remain unrelieved by treatment. In older patients symptoms begin acutely and are often intractable.

Acute tendonitis

SIGNS AND SYMPTOMS

The supraspinatus tendon close to its insertion into the humeral head is the most commonly affected of the tendons of the shoulder cuff although any may be affected. The pain may begin initially as a soreness but in most cases it is exquisite and of rapid onset. There is pain on active and also passive abduction. Infraspinatus tendonitis is associated with pain on resisted internal rotation and a similar lesion of subscapularis results in pain on resisted external rotation. Well localized tenderness over the insertion of the affected tendon can usually be elicited. X-rays are usually normal unless there is calcification present (acute calcific tendonitis).

TREATMENT

In mild cases a broad arm sling should be applied for several days and a course of anti-inflammatory drug may be effective if commenced within the first 24 hours after the onset of symptoms. When the pain is severe an injection of local anaesthetic with a depot corticosteroid can be very effective in relieving symptoms quickly. There is some debate as to whether the injection should be given into the subacromial bursa or into the tender area. If calcification is present this procedure can be preceded by aspiration of the calcification. Such treatment is followed by a course of anti-inflammatory drugs.

REHABILITATION

Isometric exercises should be undertaken at first. When the patient is pain free isotonic exercises with weights are recommended. Light weights are used and the shoulder is exercised in abduction to isolate the supraspinatus muscle and strengthen it (Figure 23.1).

Chronic tendonitis

This condition affects occasional sportsmen. Symptoms gradually develop over several weeks and they are associated with degeneration and/or a minor tear of the shoulder cuff. The shoulder looks normal and there may be little or no tenderness but a painful arc of movement is present.

TREATMENT

Conservative treatment with short wave diathermy and injection of local anaesthetic and cortico-steroid into the subacromial area is usually effective. Repeated injections at short intervals may lead to complete rupture of a degenerate shoulder cuff (see below). Chronic persistent pain may require surgical decompression of the shoulder cuff by excising the coraco-acromial ligament and removing some of the thickness of the bone of the acromial arch.

Rupture of the rotator cuff

Partial tears produce the painful arc syndrome. Complete tears which may occur spontaneously or from repeated steroid injection

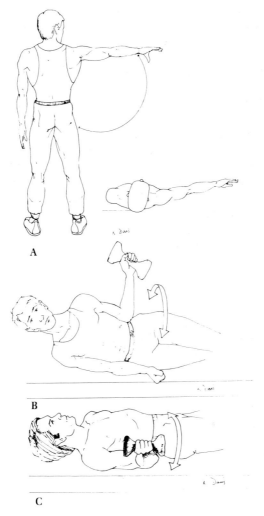

Fig. 23.1 Strengthening exercises for the rotator cuff **A** Supraspinatus **B** Infraspinatus **C** Subscapularis

are associated with weakness of the shoulder and inability to initiate abduction. The extent of the injury can be assessed by CT arthrography.

TREATMENT

Partial tears are treated in a similar manner to chronic tendonitis but with limited use of steroid injections. Complete tears require surgical repair.

Frozen shoulder (pericapsulitis)

The cause and pathology of this condition is not known. It leads to pain, often worst at night, and with restriction of all active and passive movements. Symptoms may last for 18 months or more but it is a self-limiting condition and eventually the shoulder will return completely to normal.

TREATMENT

It is most important to reassure the patient that recovery will take place albeit over a lengthy period of time. Exercises and steroid injections are of help and controlled manipulation under general anaesthetic may accelerate recovery.

Strengthening exercises for rotator cuff impingement lesions (Figure 23.1)

AIMS

Each muscle of the rotator cuff should be strengthened individually. Active exercises should start when the pain has diminished.

1. Supraspinatus can be exercised with weights with the arm in abduction.
2. Infraspinatus and teres minor can be exercised with the patient lying on the unaffected side and the affected arm at the side with the elbow flexed. The shoulder can then alternately be externally and internally rotated.
3. Subscapularis can be exercised in the supine position. The affected arm is held close to the side and the elbow flexed to 90°. The forearm is then turned into internal rotation then lowered again.

BICIPITAL SYNDROMES

Biceps tendonitis presents with pain and tenderness in the bicipital groove. Supination and flexion against resistance reproduce the pain. Rest and local heat are usually sufficient treatment with an early prescription of an anti-inflammatory drug.

Rupture of the tendon affects the long head of biceps and presents as a lump in the front of the arm due to the bunching of the contracted muscle belly. The condition is frequently preceded by the pain of biceps tendonitis which disappears suddenly when the rupture occurs. If this happens in a young athlete surgical repair can be carried out. Most frequently the diagnosis is delayed since the condition is painless and as a result repair is not possible.

However, even in this situation full activity can be reacquired and reassurance of the good prognosis should be given.

THE PAINFUL ELBOW
Tricipital tendonitis

Repeated forced extension produces pain over the triceps insertion. Rest, anti-inflammatory treatment and light exercises within the limits of pain permit resolution. If there is a suspected tear this should be repaired (McLatchie et al 1980).

Thrower's elbow

Javelin throwers who use an overarm action may develop avulsion fractures of the olecranon process. Medial symptoms may result from valgus stress. Forearm flexor strains, medial collateral ligament sprains and rupture, avulsion fractures and ulnar traction spurs are all variations found in throwers, bowlers and baseball pitchers. Loose bodies within the joint may cause locking and predispose to osteoarthrosis. They should be removed arthroscopically or at open operation. Such lesions are commonly seen in baseball pitchers and when distal humeral hypertrophy occurs. In children, partial avulsion of the medial epicondyle results from repetitive throwing (little leaguer's elbow).

Pulled elbow

In young children traction on the arm may pull the radial head beyond the annular ligament. There is pain and pseudo-paralysis. Function is restored by supinating the forearm when a click will be palpated as the radial head relocates. No immobilization is required.

Tennis elbow

The characteristic site of discomfort is in the region of the extensor muscle origin over the lateral epicondyle. In racquet players it may arise with the use of new equipment with a narrow handle.

SIGNS AND SYMPTOMS

There is pain at the lateral side of the elbow during use especially grasping with the hand since this requires active wrist extension. This pain can be reproduced by resisted extension of the wrist or passive flexion with the elbow extended. Tenderness is localized to the lateral epicondyle.

TREATMENT

Injection of local anaesthetic and steroid into the extensor origin is frequently successful. If this is coupled with rest and abstinence from the activity which caused the condition many cases will recover. Deep frictions and manipulation are indicated in resistant cases and the use of an epicondylitis clasp over the muscle bellies at the proximal forearm can be of help. Surgery is usually reserved for very persistent or recurrent symptoms. The common extensor origin is detached from the epicondylar ridge and allowed to slide distally.

Golfer's elbow

This can result from 'rotating out' during a snatch lift in weight lifting. It can also occur in golfers. The flexor origin from the front of the medial epicondyle is affected.

SIGNS AND SYMPTOMS

There is medial elbow pain on use which can be reproduced by resisted wrist flexion with the arm straight. Tenderness is localized to the front of the medial epicondyle.

TREATMENT

Rest, anti-inflammatory agents or local injection are effective measures as with tennis elbow.

DIFFERENTIAL DIAGNOSIS

The symptoms of tennis and golfer's elbow may be mimicked by cervical spine disease and this should be excluded in persistent cases particularly if the symptoms are bilateral. Similarly in tennis elbow posterior interosseous nerve entrapment may be a cause.

Olecranon bursitis

This condition has been described in karateka who break objects with the elbow. The olecranon bursa can also become inflamed in gout or infection.

SIGNS

On acute inflammation the bursa extends with fluid. Symptoms will settle if the causative activity is discontinued provided there is no infection. If there is chronic swelling and thickening of the bursa excision should be considered.

PAIN IN THE WRIST AND HAND

Acute frictional tenosynovitis

This is the result of repetitive and usually unaccustomed use of the wrist.

SIGNS AND SYMPTOMS

There is pain at the back of the wrist and thumb which affects the extensor tendons of the wrist. In the early stages crepitus is commonly elicited as the tendon moves in the inflamed sheath. This disappears when effusion develops within the tendon sheath.

TREATMENT

Splintage, in slight dorsiflexion, will ease symptoms. If this is coupled with anti-inflammatory drugs most cases will settle within 7–10 days. The movement which produces the symptoms should not be repeated until at least one week after the symptoms have settled. If this fails injection of depot steroid into the sheath is usually curative.

De Quervain's disease

This is a variety of tunnel syndrome which affects the sheath of the abductor pollicis longus and extensor pollicis brevis tendons over the radial styloid process.

SIGNS AND SYMPTOMS

Pain is felt at the back of the base of the thumb and over the radial styloid on using the thumb or wrist. Tenderness is maximal over the lateral aspect of the radial styloid where a swelling can be seen.

TREATMENT

The early acute condition can be treated as for acute frictional tenosynovitis but when the condition has become chronic slitting the sheath under local anaesthetic is successful in all cases.

FRACTURES AND DISLOCATIONS AROUND THE WRIST

Fractures of the scaphoid

This quiet fracture may cause problems if it remains unrecognized. Delayed and non-union, avascular necrosis and secondary degenerative arthritis of the wrist are all possible complications. They lead to pain and loss of wrist function. A scaphoid fracture should be suspected following even a minor injury, but the commonest cause is a fall on to the outstretched hand. Always be suspicious of the diagnosis of a 'sprained wrist'.

SIGNS AND SYMPTOMS

There will be pain over the radial side of the wrist after injury with tenderness in the anatomical snuffbox and pain on compression of the extended thumb. Even if symptoms are slight a fracture should be suspected.

DIAGNOSIS

Confirmation is by X-ray. Four views should be taken, antero-posterior, lateral and two oblique views, one in each of 45° pronation and supination. If there is no obvious fracture the patient should be treated as if he had a fracture and the wrist should be immobilized then X-rayed again 1 to 2 weeks later. A hairline fracture may then be seen due to the resorption around the fracture either in the waist or the distal or proximal poles of the bone. (Lesley & Dickson 1981). In a doubtful case the use of direct magnification radiography and scintigraphy can help establish the correct diagnosis.

TREATMENT

The forearm should be immobilized in a plaster of Paris cast which extends to include the thumb at its interphalangeal joint. This is maintained for a minimum period of 6 weeks before reassessment. Immobilization may be required for up to 12 weeks if union is slow. If the fracture is displaced even slightly primary internal fixation has been recommended since the incidence of non-union is much higher in this situation (Huene 1979).

NON-UNION

If the patient is pain free then no treatment is necessary. If there are painful symptoms internal fixation with bone grafting is indicated.

Avascular necrosis

This condition occurs after a fracture of the waist of the scaphoid and is due to the anatomical absence of appropriate blood supply to the proximal pole of the bone. It can be recognized on X-ray by 'increased density' as the surrounding viable bone becomes osteoporotic due to immobilization. It may lead to non-union although not inevitably.

Colle's fracture

In healthy sports people this fracture is caused by a heavy fall on to the outstretched hand. If displaced it produces a classical dinner fork deformity of the wrist.

TREATMENT

Such fractures must be reduced accurately and the length of the radius must be maintained. Reduction is held by plaster cast or more effectively by an external fixator. Union occurs in approximately 4 weeks and thereafter an intensive exercise programme must be followed to achieve return of function. There is not infrequently a little loss of full rotation in the forearm.

Epiphyseal injuries to the lower radius (juvenile Colle's fracture)

These are important injuries because occasionally they may affect the growth of the bone if the epiphyseal germinal layer is damaged. There is usually displacement of the epiphysis with an associated triangular fragment of the metaphysis immediately proximal to the epiphysis.

TREATMENT

If there is displacement, manipulation with plaster of Paris fixation is indicated.

INJURIES TO DIGITS
Dislocations and sprains of metacarpal phalangeal and interphalangeal joints

Most contact and combat sports carry the risk of digital injuries. Frequently these take the form of sprains of the digital collateral ligaments with associated pain and swelling. Provided there is stability, the affected digit may be strapped to its neighbour to allow the game to be completed. After the match basic treatment with ice, compression and anti-inflammatory medication can be started. 'Buddy' strapping should be used at sport for at least 3 months.

Digital dislocations may be reduced at the time of injury but only one attempt should be made. The player should be able to demonstrate movement of the joint after reduction if it has been successful. The injured digit is then taped to its neighbour. After the game X-rays should be taken not only to ensure complete reduction but also to exclude the possibility of an avulsion fracture of the base of the phalanx which might require open reduction and internal fixation. At the outset if there is obvious bony deformity or ligamentous instability the player should be advised to stop play and should then be assessed at an Accident and Emergency Department.

Gamekeeper's thumb

With forcible abduction at the metacarpo-phalangeal joint of the thumb the ulnar collateral ligament is overstressed and its distal attachment may become avulsed sometimes with a fragment of bone. The injury is prevented from healing by interposition of the adductor pollicis aponeurosis which if untreated will lead to instability of this joint.

TREATMENT

Open reduction and repair of the ligament or internal fixation of any avulsed fragment of bone stabilizes the joint.

Bennett's fracture dislocation

This is a common hand injury in boxing. The treatment is described in Chapter 13.

Metacarpal neck fractures

Unless there is marked displacement or angulation, conservative management in the form of simple analgesic is indicated. Manipulation or even open reduction may be necessary for gross deformities.

Mallet finger

This injury is most commonly caused by a ball striking the tip of the finger and producing forced flexion of the distal interphalangeal joint. The deformity is due to avulsion of the long extensor tendon from the distal phalanx with or without a fragment of bone. A plastic fingertip splint is applied to maintain reduction for 6 weeks.

Finger injuries in rock climbers

As the result of the stresses applied to the fingers in climbing, particularly in extreme rock climber rupture of the pulley of the proximal fibrous flexor sheath can lead to a bow string deformity of the flexor tendons across the base of the finger. Circumferential taping around the proximal phalanx may reduce the risk of this injury. In addition chronic inflammation at or close to the insertion of the tendon of flexor digitorum superficialis to the base of the middle phalanx (tenoperiostitis) can lead to flexion contracture of the proximal interphalangeal joint. This can be minimized by passive stretching after climbing activities and the use of anti-inflammatory drugs.

REFERENCES

Bannister G C, Wallace W A, Stableforth P G and Hutson M A 1989 The management of acute acromioclavicular dislocation. Journal of Bone and Joint Surgery 71B: 848–850

Binder A, De Silva M, Hazelman B L 1983 Soft tissue rheumatism (1), Hospital Update 9 3: 341–349

Bollen S R and Gunson C K 1990 Hand injuries in competition climbers. British Journal of Sports Medicine 24 1: 16–18

Cofield R H 1985 Rotator cuff disease of the shoulder. Journal of Bone and Joint Surgery 67A: 974–979

Ganel A, Israeli A, Engel J 1980 The early diagnosis of fractures of the carpal scaphoid bone. British Journal of Sports Medicine 14 4: 210–212

Hastings D E, Coughlin L P 1981 Recurrent subluxation in the humeral joint. American Journal of Sports Medicine 9: 352–359

Huene D R 1979 Primary internal fixation of carpal navicular fractures in the athlete. American Journal of Sports Medicine 7: 175–177

Helfet A J 1958 Coracoid transplantation for recurring dislocation of the shoulder. Journal of Bone and Joint Surgery 40B: 198–201

Lesley I J, Dickson R A 1981 The fractured carpal navicular. Natural history and factors influencing outcome. Journal of Bone and Joint Surgery 63B: 225–230

McLatchie G R, Fitzgerald B, Davies J E 1980 The medical implications of weight training and weight lifting. Medisport 2 3: 69–72

Neer C S, Welsh R P 1977 The shoulder in sport. Orthopaedic Clinics of North America 8: 583–591

Rowe C R and Zarins B 1981 Recurrent transient subluxation of the shoulder. Journal of Bone and Joint Surgery 63B: 863–867

Wolfgang G L 1974 Surgical repair of complete tears of the rotator cuff of the shoulder. Journal of Bone and Joint Surgery 56A: 14–16

24. Injuries to the pelvis, hip and thigh

GROIN PAIN

Symptoms relating to the groin are now being seen more frequently. Sports involved include soccer, handball, ice hockey, skiing, athletics, horse-riding and marathon running. The cause is either overuse or overloading of the muscles attached to the pubis. Often the pain is severe and may be associated with a limp. Its onset may be abrupt or insidious. There may also be radiation to the inner aspect of either thigh, to the perineum or to the lower abdomen. It is aggravated by coughing, sneezing or climbing stairs.

When there is an associated limp the patient has an antalgic gait and complains of a stiff tight feeling in the groin or adductor muscles (Coventry & Mitchell 1961).

The differential diagnosis includes stress fracture of the femoral neck, osteitis pubis, incipient inguinal/femoral hernia, urinary tract infection and ankylosing spondylitis (Gullmo et al 1984). In adolescence it is important to consider the possibility of slipped upper femoral ephiphysis which may lead to knee pain as well.

The more common overload problems affect the tendons of adductor longus, iliopsoas, rectus femoris and rectus abdominis (Renstrom & Peterson 1980).

HERNIAS

In young people inguinal/femoral hernias should be excluded as a cause of groin pain. A large number of symptomatic young people will have acquired hernias which may not be clinically apparent but which can be demonstrated by herniography (Gullmo et al 1984). After hernioplasty full activity can be restarted in about 6 weeks.

GROIN DISRUPTION

In recent years a syndrome of groin disruption has been recognized in male athletes rendered susceptible to the condition because of the embryonic descent of the testes.

The syndrome as described by Gilmore (1991) constitutes the following features:

1. A torn external oblique aponeurosis
2. Torn conjoined tendon
3. A dehiscence between the conjoined tendon and the inguinal ligament
4. The absence of a hernia sac.

CLINICAL FEATURES

The condition was originally recognized in professional soccer players but may occur in athletes, ice skaters, rugby players, racket games players, hockey players, dancers and karateka. The onset of symptoms is gradual with a history of a specific injury in only one-third of patients. The pain experienced prevented kicking a ball and was increased by external rotation or hyperextension. Sneezing, coughing, attempting to sprint, in fact any sudden change of movement, even getting out of bed led to further pain and discomfort. At presentation the athlete could localize his/her pain to the inguinal, adductor or perineal region.

On examination with the little finger inverting the scrotum in males, or by direct palpation in females the superficial inguinal ring on the affected side was dilated with tenderness and a cough impulse.

TREATMENT

In this syndrome surgical intervention appears to be very successful (>90% return to sport). The approach is as for an inguinal hernia with the aim of restoring the anatomy to normal. The following procedures are carried out:

1. Plication of the transversalis fascia as in the Shouldice hernia repair
2. Repair of the torn conjoined tendon
3. Approximation of the conjoined tendon to the inguinal ligament with nylon in darn fashion
4. Repair of the external oblique and reconstitution of the inguinal ring.

REHABILITATION

The procedure is usually performed as a day case or overnight stay. On the first postoperative day the patient is encouraged to stand erect and during the first week to walk slowly for up to 20 minutes 2–4 times daily according to discomfort.

In the second week jogging can begin and if tolerated running initiated.

By the third week most can run in straight lines and do sit-ups and adductor exercises. Swimming (not breast-stroke) is a useful adjunct to rehabilitation after the first week.

By 4 to 5 weeks kicking a ball, dancing techniques or whatever movement is specific to the particular sport may be attempted.

In our own unit we have treated 15 such players during the past year. Nine of them had groin disruption similar to that described above. Six patients (bilateral in one) had tiny indirect inguinal hernias and associated muscle and external ring disruption. We therefore believe that exploration of the groin is a logical avenue to take in patients with persistent symptoms in spite of appropriate physical therapy.

OSTEITIS PUBIS (OSTEOCHONDRITIS OF THE PUBIC ARCH), PUBIALGIA, PUBIC SYNDROME

This condition is most common in adolescence and young adults who take part in regular training. There is groin pain on exercise with tenderness over the lower part of the pubic bone. The diagnosis is confirmed by an X-ray which shows widening and fragmentation of the lower half of the pubic symphysis (Rispoli 1964). When these changes are noted the athlete must abandon the activity which is causing them. There is no known effect of treatment but slow spontaneous improvement is normal. The condition may also be associated with chronic pelvic instability which should be considered if there is also pain over one sacroiliac joint. This diagnosis can be confirmed by an X-ray of the pelvis standing on each leg in turn when upward movement of the pubis is seen when bearing weight on the affected side.

URINARY TRACT INFECTIONS, ANKYLOSING SPONDYLITIS

Both of these conditions are not common but should be excluded. In ankylosing spondylitis X-ray changes of osteitis pubis are often present but the specific history should arouse suspicion, particularly if there is a strong family history.

MUSCLE STRAINS
Adductor longus tendoperiostitis

This is a true overuse or overload injury frequently associated with adductor longus muscle strain.

SIGNS AND SYMPTOMS

There is chronic pain at the pubic symphysis with tenderness on palpation. Resisted adduction is painful. A true chronic adductor tear may appear as a mass on the medial side of the thigh when the patient attends for investigation of a possible soft tissue tumour.

Investigation is by pelvic X-rays and soft tissue radiography when ossification may be seen if chronic pain has persisted after an acute musculo-tendinous tear.

TREATMENT

Acute injuries to muscles in this region should receive local cooling with compression and elevation of the limb. The athlete should take high dose anti-inflammatory drugs for at least 5 days. As soon as he or she is free from pain the athlete can begin active movements without resistance which include progressive stretching. He can then progress to work against increased resistance but should reduce activities if the pain returns.

Chronic injuries may have to be rested for prolonged periods of time with persistent treatment until tenderness and painful movements have disappeared (Chapter 11, Physiotherapy and strapping in injury management).

Iliopsoas strain

This injury is seen in sports which involve repetitive or forced flexion of the hip such as football and Olympic weightlifting. Occasionally a sudden forceful injury may avulse a portion of the lesser trochanter or the lesser trochanteric epiphysis in the young adolescent.

SYMPTOMS AND SIGNS

There is pain in the medial aspect of the thigh over the insertion of the tendon into the lesser trochanter. Resisted hip flexion elicits the pain. An X-ray will confirm if there has been an avulsion of the lesser trochanter.

TREATMENT

Avulsion fractures should be treated surgically if they are significantly displaced. Otherwise the treatment is similar to adductor injuries.

Rectus abdominis strain

This injury is commonly produced by exercises involving excessive flexion such as sit-ups or leg raises and pain can be elicited by these movements. Tenderness is over the upper part of the pubic bone and over the lower tendon of rectus abdominis on the affected side. Treatment is as described previously but as with adductor longus tendonitis surgical exploration may be required in extremely persistent cases.

Quadriceps strain

The rectus femoris muscle can be strained or partly torn at its proximal musculo-tendonous junction during repetitive football shooting or sprinting.

SYMPTOMS AND SIGNS

There will be a palpable or visible gap at the proximal thigh depending on the severity of the injury. Resisted flexion of the hip and extension of the knee are painful and there may be local tenderness. An X-ray will show if the tendon of rectus femoris has avulsed in the anterior inferior iliac spine.

TREATMENT

Conservative measures are used for a complete tear. If there is an avulsion fracture surgery should be considered if the displacement is significant.

Quadriceps haematoma (dead leg, charley horse)

Intramuscular haematomata and tears due to direct blows are common in the quadriceps compartment. They can be so extensive as to produce considerable pain and swelling suggesting an underlying fracture. This swelling produces a transient neuropraxia and is referred to as a 'dead leg'. In the United States the injury is known as 'charley horse' (Ryan 1969).

TREATMENT

This is the same as for other muscle injuries but there is the added risk of myositis ossificans (ectopic ossification) which will prolong the recovery time.

SLIPPED UPPER FEMORAL EPIPHYSIS

This disorder is more common in boys. The usual age group affected is 12–15 years and it is a further cause of groin pain in young people. In some instances the onset of symptoms may be insidious with no history of any injury. It is thought to be due to hormonal imbalance which leads to weakening of the epiphyseal growth plate.

SYMPTOMS AND SIGNS

The onset may be sudden or chronic. When a sudden slip occurs there is severe pain mimicking a fracture of the femoral neck. However most cases are of gradual onset with intermittent pain in the groin and more important sometimes only in the lower thigh or the knee.

Clinical examination reveals reduced abduction and medial rotation with increased lateral rotation of the affected side. If acute displacement has occurred the leg will be shorter and lie in external rotation.

Confirmation is by antero-posterior *plus lateral* X-rays. Early changes will be seen only on the lateral X-ray with a normal AP appearance.

TREATMENT

When there are minor degrees of slip the epiphysis is not reduced but is internally fixed as it is. When gross displacement has occurred reduction by manipulation may jeopardize the blood supply to the capital epiphysis and an osteotomy of the trochanteric region or the neck of the femur may be necessary after which the osteotomy and epiphysis are internally fixed.

PROGNOSIS

After significant displacement despite optimum treatment the hip is unlikely ever to be normal and the risk of secondary osteoarthritis in early adult life is considerable if not inevitable.

STRESS FRACTURE OF THE NECK OF THE FEMUR

This results from cyclical overloading of the femoral neck. It occurs most commonly in long distance runners who are following a heavy schedule.

SYMPTOMS AND SIGNS

Initially pain occurs on activity but if the runner does not rest then pain becomes persistent. There may be few signs in the early stages but later there will be tenderness over the hip joint and pain on rotation.

X-rays taken early may be normal but at this stage diagnosis can be confirmed by scintigraphy. In the later stages the fracture will become visible and may begin to displace.

TREATMENT

In the early stages the fracture is likely to heal if the activity is stopped and stress on the hip relieved by crutch walking. Later if the fracture is very evident or there is some displacement, internal fixation is necessary.

OSTEOARTHROSIS OF THE HIP JOINT

Degenerative joint disease is associated with abnormal stress and with ageing. Changes in the large weight bearing joints are common from the third decade onwards (Lawrence et al 1966) and specific osteoarthrosis have been described in athletes (Oderken et al 1973, Brodeluis 1961). Most sports participants seem to be at no greater risk of developing osteoarthrosis of the hip joint than the general population provided the joint is put through a normal range of movement. However previously injured joints are thought to be more vulnerable to heavy loading (Fitzgerald & McLatchie 1980). Detailed follow up of marathon runners and gymnasts may disprove this. Athletes in whom osteoarthrosis has developed in the hip joint frequently show a predisposing cause such as mild acetabular dysplasia of congenital origin.

TREATMENT

Activities which produce great stress upon the hip joint must be avoided. For this reason sports activities may require to be changed in order to avoid weight bearing activities. It is important to maintain mobility in the hip joint by non-stressful exercises which put the joint through a full range of movement. If pain is troublesome anti-inflammatory drugs will be required and in later life progressive changes may require surgical treatment.

TROCHANTERIC BURSITIS

The trochanteric bursa separates the thickening of the fascia lata into which the gluteus maximus muscle is inserted from the lateral surface of the greater trochanter. Since the ilio-tibial tract passes backwards and forwards over the trochanter on flexion and extension of the hip the bursa can become painful and inflamed by overuse. A direct injury may cause a large haematoma—a haemobursa.

SYMPTOMS AND SIGNS

A post traumatic bursa is a large tender swelling over the greater trochanter. In overuse trochanteric bursitis there is pain and tenderness which may radiate to the lateral aspect of the thigh. Rotation of the hip may elicit pain as will flexion and extension.

TREATMENT

Post traumatic haemobursa should be treated by aspiration of blood followed by a compression dressing.

Overuse bursitis is treated conservatively with cold packs, anti-inflammatory drugs and selective rest. In chronic cases local injection of local anaesthetic and steroid is effective.

ILIO-TIBIAL BAND FRICTION SYNDROME

This is an overuse injury seen occasionally in cyclists and skiers but most commonly in long distance runners. The band is a thickening of the fascia lata of the thigh which extends from the anterior superior iliac spine to Gurdy's tubercle on the antero-lateral aspect of the proximal tibia. During flexion and extension of the knee the band or tract undergoes a degree of antero-posterior movement which may produce symptoms due to friction of the band against the lateral femoral condyle (Rennie 1975).

SYMPTOMS AND SIGNS

Symptoms are more common in men. Pain develops in the outer side of the knee joint superior to the lateral joint line and may radiate up or down (Fig. 24.1). Even pace running aggravates symptoms whereas activities such as badminton, squash, squatting or jumping are sometimes pain-free.

Tenderness is maximal over the prominence of the lateral femoral condyle. It should not be confused with a strain of the lateral ligament of the knee in which there will also be pain on varus stress of the knee.

TREATMENT

Training errors should first be corrected. The commonest cause is over-training and the runner should be persuaded to reduce his/her distances. Alteration of training regime is another possibility. Since intermittent activity is usually comfortable several sessions of interval running could be substituted for distance work. The running surface and footwear are also important. Running on grass or wearing a laterally wedged insole can provide relief. Combination treatment with anti-inflammatory drugs and cooling is effective for acute episodes and local steroid injection and short wave diathermy should be reserved for more chronic cases. For persistent symptoms attention should be directed to the anatomy and biomechanics of the foot since abnormality in this region can provoke this syndrome and can be cured by the prescription of an appropriate orthosis. If all such abnormalities have been corrected and symptoms persist then fasciotomy of the ilio-tibial band may cure the problem (Orava 1978, Noble 1979). The prevention of recurrence is by graded training and careful warm up including stretching.

POPLITEUS TENDONITIS

This is another cause of lateral knee pain produced by hyper-pronation of the foot in most instances. There is a point of tenderness over the lateral femoral condyle low down where the popliteus

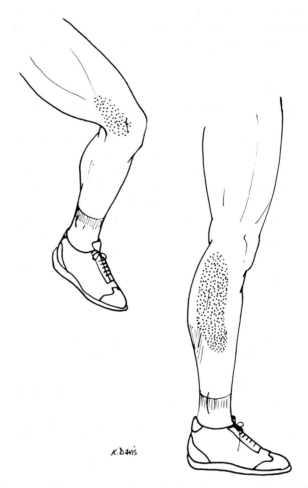

Fig. 24.1 Sites of friction in the ilio-tibial band friction syndrome (left) and the anterior compartment syndrome (right)

tendon is inserted after running around the lateral side of the knee.

Treatment is the same as for the ilio-tibial band friction syndrome, the most important aspect being correction of training errors and of biomechanical abnormalities in the foot.

HAMSTRING TEARS

These common injuries tend to be recurrent since they heal by scar tissue which does not stretch like supple normal muscle. The mainstay of treatment is early recognition and the prevention of further injury. Although muscles may be avulsed from their origins (see groin injury) the strain or tear most commonly occurs at the musculo-tendonous junction in either the upper or lower thigh (hamstring pull). Such injuries lead to haematoma formation as well as muscle injury.

TREATMENT

Minor pulls should be treated conservatively. The initial treatment is directed towards the haematoma and it is vital to prohibit the causative activity until complete healing has taken place which may take up to 6 weeks depending on the severity of the injury. As the haematoma resolves controlled stretching exercises will allow muscle length to be maintained and the scar developing to remain at a reasonably functional length. Such exercises can be more easily performed in water. A return to full normal function should be slowly progressive since if the player 'sprints' before the injury is healed there will inevitably be a recurrence of the problem.

Complete ruptures which are rare in the athlete should be treated surgically by repair.

REFERENCES

Brodeluis A 1961 Osteoarthritis of the talar joints in footballers and ballet dancers. Acta Orthopaedica Scandinavica 30: 309–314

Coventry M B, Mitchell W C 1961 Osteitis pubis. Journal of the American Medical Association 178 9: 898–905

Fitzgerald B, McLatchie G R 1980 Degenerative joint disease in weightlifters—fact or fiction? British Journal of Sports Medicine 14 283: 97–101

Gilmore O J A 1991 Ten years' experience of groin disruption—a previously unsolved problem in sportsmen. Rugby World Cup Medical Congress, Royal College of Physicians of Edinburgh

Gullmo A, Broome A, Smedburg S 1984 Herniography. Surgical Clinics of North America 64 2: 239

Lawrence J S, Bremner J M, Bier F 1966 Osteoarthrosis. Prevalence in the population and relationships between symptoms and X-ray changes. Annals of the Rheumatic Diseases 24: 1–23

Noble C A 1979 A treatment of ilio tibial band friction syndrome. British Journal of Sports Medicine 13 2: 51–54

Oderken J C, Chantraine A, Bernard A 1973 Arthrose et deviation axiale du genou chez les anciens joueurs de football. Journal Belge de Rheumatologie a de Medecine Physique 28: 74–85

Orava S 1978 Ilio tibial band friction syndrome in athletes—an uncommon exertion syndrome on the lateral side of the knee. British Journal of Sports Medicine 12 2: 69–73

Rennie J W 1975 The ilio tibial band friction syndrome. Journal of Bone and Joint Surgery 57A: 110–111

Renstrom P, Peterson L 1980 Groin injuries in athletes. British Journal of Sports Medicine 14 1: 30–36

Rispoli F P 1964 Schambeinsyndrom bei Fussballspielern. Zeitschrift fur Orthopaedie und ihre Grenzgebiete 99: 87

Ryan A J 1969 Quadriceps strain, rupture and charley horse. Medicine, Science and Sports 1: 106

25. Injuries to the knee and leg

The knee joint depends entirely on its associated ligaments and muscles for stability. It ranks second in frequency of injury after the ankle, most injuries being soft tissue in nature.

INJURIES TO THE EXTENSOR MECHANISM

The extensor mechanism is made up of the quadriceps femoris and its tendinous expansion which encloses the patella. It is inserted distally through the patellar tendon into the tibial tubercle.

Injury may occur at three levels: above the knee, through the patella and below the knee.

ABOVE THE KNEE INJURIES
Rupture of the rectus femoris

Usually the site of rupture is at the musculo-tendinous junction.

SIGNS AND SYMPTOMS

There is pain both at rest and on contraction of the muscle with tenderness and swelling. A characteristic lump is caused by the retracted muscle fibres (Fig. 25.1).

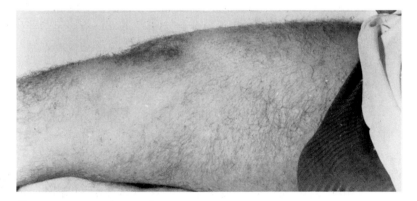

Fig. 25.1 Ruptured rectus femoris

TREATMENT

Conservative treatment as applied to all muscle injuries gives good results in general. If the musculo-tendinous injury is very extensive surgical repair may be indicated.

Rupture of the quadriceps tendon

This injury most commonly occurs in the over-fifties. In most instances it results from a forced flexion injury of the knee although can occur as a result of a vigorous extension of the knee against resistance.

SIGNS AND SYMPTOMS

Swelling occurs fairly rapidly at the site of injury but if carefully examined the gap in the tendon situated just above the patella can be palpated. There is loss of active extension in the knee.

TREATMENT

Since the proximal part of the quadriceps tendon retracts into the thigh surgical repair is mandatory. After operation immobilization in extension in a plaster cast is necessary for 6 weeks.

INJURIES AT THE LEVEL OF THE PATELLA

Fractures of the patella

Transverse fracture of the patella is an indirect injury caused by excessive contraction of the quadriceps muscle against resistance, e.g. badly miskicking a football.

Comminuted fractures result from a direct fall on to the patella.

SYMPTOMS AND SIGNS

There is pain localized to the patella, holding the knee in extension may be difficult or impossible and bearing weight is not possible. There is tenderness over the patella and a gap may be palpated in the bone.

TREATMENT

Undisplaced fractures can be treated conservatively but displaced fractures require surgical treatment either reduction and fixation or patellectomy in the most severely comminuted cases.

Stress fracture of the patella

Stress fractures of the patella develop within the first 2–3 weeks of intensive training. There is a history of unusual or increased exercise with pain in the patella on activity. Diagnosis is confirmed by bone scan in the early stages since X-ray confirmation may not be possible until 2–3 weeks after onset of symptoms.

TREATMENT

Protected weight bearing is required until there is no pain on walking. This usually takes 4–6 weeks after which a progressive increase in the load of the quadriceps mechanism can be applied.

Dislocation of the patella

In acute dislocation the displacement is usually laterally. This must inevitably be accompanied by rupture of the medial retinaculum and insertion of the vastus medialis component of the quadriceps mechanism. This must be allowed to heal satisfactorily or recurrent dislocation may ensue.

SYMPTOMS AND SIGNS

After the injury there is acute pain and the patella is seen to lie in a lateral position (Fig. 25.2).

TREATMENT

Reduction should be attempted but may require general anaesthetic. The knee must then be held in extension by means of a plaster cylinder for 4–6 weeks to allow the medial soft tissues to heal before recommencing an exercise programme for rehabilitation.

Recurrent dislocation may follow a totally treated acute traumatic dislocation but most commonly occurs in girls and young women. It is frequently associated with anatomical abnormalities such as genu valgum, genu recurvatum and patella alta. The first dislocation may occur spontaneously or with a minor injury. Repeated dislocations predispose to osteoarthrosis.

SYMPTOMS AND SIGNS

Incidents occur frequently without injury. When this occurs the knee may give way. The patella is noted to displace to the lateral side of the knee. Between episodes there are few symptoms but attempts to dislocate the patella laterally by pushing it laterally as the knee is flexed from the extended position produce apprehension in the patient.

TREATMENT

Several surgical procedures have been described to realign the quadriceps mechanism to prevent the recurrent dislocation.

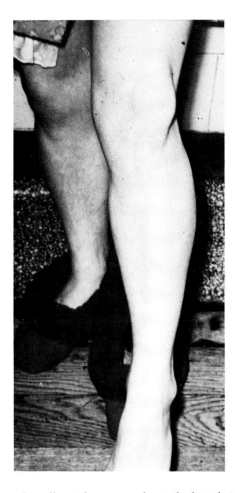

Fig. 25.2 Dislocated patella. Dislocation is also to the lateral side in recurrent cases

Anterior knee pain

This is an umbrella term used to describe pain which occurs in the front of the knee region in sports people for which there may be several causes.

By far the most common cause is pain arising from the patello-femoral joint formerly called chondromalacia patellae but other causes may be degeneration or injury to either the quadriceps or patellar tendon or the presence of a thickened plica within the knee which has been appreciated only since the advent of arthroscopy. In the older athlete or in those who have in the past suffered a fracture of the patella and the possibility of osteoarthrosis in the retropatellar region should be borne in mind.

Patello-femoral pain

This condition is still frequently referred to as chondromalacia patellae which is in reality a misnomer. It is an ill-understood condition affecting adolescents and young people, females more than males. Although the articular cartilage of the patella may undergo a spectrum of changes ranging from softening and blister formation through to surface flaking and extensive fibrillation these pathological changes bear no correlation to clinical symptoms. Indeed arthroscopy has shown that the patellar surface may be normal in some patients with significant pain. Although it may be provoked by an injury or overuse it is now thought that in many cases it is due to malalignment of the patello-femoral joint and quadriceps mechanism. In addition symptoms may arise secondary to an underlying deformity of the leg or foot which leads to altered mechanics proximally in the leg.

SYMPTOMS AND SIGNS

The patient complains of recurrent retropatellar pain and clicking often after exercise and prolonged sitting. It is usually worse on descending stairs. It may be related to unaccustomed or prolonged sporting activity. Acute episodes may be accompanied by swelling.

On examination occasionally a small effusion may be seen and there is usually wasting of vastus medialis muscle in longstanding cases. There is usually no restriction of full knee movement but retropatellar crepitus can be palpated on this movement. There is usually tenderness on the undersurface of the patella and the symptoms can be reproduced by compressing the patella against the underlying femur and moving it from side to side.

The alignment of the leg should be assessed together with any deformity of the corresponding foot.

TREATMENT AND PROGNOSIS

The outlook is generally good since the condition is usually self-limiting although it may be recurrent. The management includes the restriction of athletic activity during acute episodes coupled with static quadriceps exercises with the knee straight, progressing to exercises against a graded resistance within the range of 30° flexion to full extension (inner range exercises). The patient should be advised to avoid sitting with the knee in the flexed position for any length of time and to keep the knee moving as much as possible.

If pain persists arthroscopy is indicated to exclude other intra-articular pathology. Shaving of the patella has been advocated to debride softened articular cartilage but is mainly of value in the situation where there are mechanical symptoms due to a loose flap of articular cartilage. For more prolonged or severe symptoms a release of the lateral retinaculum followed by the above exercise programme may correct any minor malalignment and more extensive patello-femoral realignment procedures have been described although are rarely necessary. Patellectomy is reserved for knees in which there are major pathological changes in the patella.

LIGAMENT INJURIES

These are difficult problems, often complex both in diagnosis and treatment. Most happen when the knee is bent for this allows the capsule and collateral ligaments to relax and permit rotation. The classical injuries produced by a combination of rotation and valgus stress due to a lateral impact, such as occurred in a rugby or football tackle, and has been graphically described as 'total knee wipeout' or 'unhappy triad' (O'Donoghue 1976). There is a tear of variable degree of the medial collateral ligament and medial capsule, a tear of the anterior cruciate ligament and damage to the medial meniscus frequently a peripheral tear. When the impact force is to the medial side of the joint then the injury is to the fibular collateral ligament, the lateral capsule, the ilio-tibial band, the lateral meniscus and the anterior cruciate ligament. The extent of disruption depends on the impact force and degree of rotation. Obviously such lesions present major diagnostic problems. When a serious combination of injuries is suspected the patient must be transferred to hospital for assessment.

Collateral ligament injury

Valgus or varus forces can produce partial or complete rupture of the collateral ligament. The pitfall is in missing the complete rupture and treating the patient conservatively.

SYMPTOMS AND SIGNS

A partial tear is painful. There is swelling and local tenderness usually above the joint line over the epicondyle to which the ligament is attached proximally. Most importantly although there is pain, there is no abnormal laxity on stressing the ligament. Complete tears, by contrast, may be relatively painless with minimal swelling (because the joint capsule has been ruptured). Although abnormal laxity is present even this may be painless.

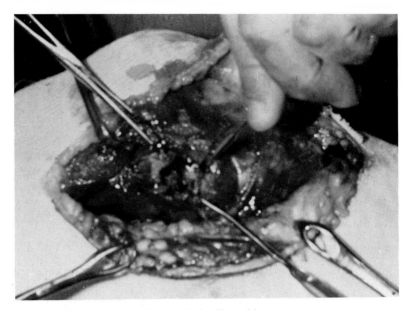

Fig. 25.3 Complete tear of the medial collateral ligament

TREATMENT

Partial tears should be treated conservatively by relieving the stress on the joint, if necessary by crutch walking. Physiotherapy treatment and an anti-inflammatory drug are useful to relieve pain and reduce swelling. Thereafter a rehabilitation programme of progressive exercises is instituted. Complete tears should in general be surgically repaired (Fig. 25.3). It is important to exclude the possibility of associated injury to the cruciate ligaments (Fig. 25.4). After repair immobilization in a plaster cast is required for 4–6 weeks after which a progressive programme of exercises is practised while the ligament repair is protected by some form of knee brace. This can usually be discarded around 12 weeks from the injury.

Cruciate ligament injury

Injury to these ligaments does not occur independently but is always associated with damage to other soft tissues in the knee.

Posterior cruciate ligament injury

This is fortunately the least common injury since even with repair the prognosis is less good and can lead to a fairly disabling type of

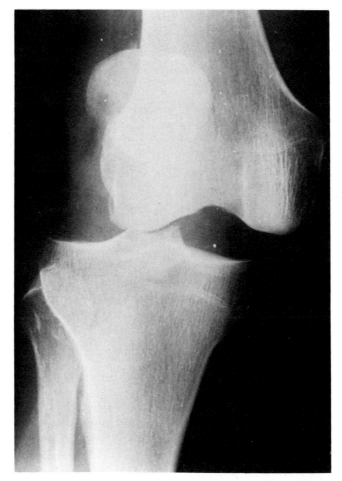

Fig. 25.4 Complete knee injury. There is cruciate and collateral ligament disruption

knee instability. It results from the tibia being driven backwards on the femur and usually also associated with rupture of the posterior capsule.

SYMPTOMS AND SIGNS

The classical sign is the presence of a backward sag of the tibia on the lower femur when the knee is flexed.

TREATMENT

Surgical repair is mandatory to achieve the best possible result. Immobilization in a plaster cast for a period of 6 weeks is then usually necessary followed by a programme of rehabilitation.

Anterior cruciate ligament injury

This is by far the most common type of injury and is usually associated with rupture of either the medial or lateral soft tissues (see above).

SIGNS AND SYMPTOMS

In addition to the signs of medial or lateral laxity, antero-posterior laxity can be assessed in extension by the Lachmann test and in flexion by the Drawer test both of which will indicate abnormal anterior movement of the tibia on the femur. Some degree of rotational instability of the tibia on the femur will also be found with the most severe injuries.

TREATMENT

Such complete tears represent a soft tissue emergency and should be surgically repaired. Attempts are usually made to repair the cruciate tear although there is some doubt as to whether this is necessary since the most important part of the repair is restoring the integrity of the capsule and collateral ligaments. After operation immobilization in a plaster cast for 4–6 weeks is necessary followed by an exercise programme.

It may be advisable for some form of protective brace to be worn long term.

RESULTS OF LIGAMENT REPAIR

Early operation within 2 weeks of injury gives the best results. Later repairs or any of the many reconstructive procedures described give an inferior outcome. It is therefore essential to be aware of the importance of early diagnosis and treatment of these severe injuries.

MENISCUS INJURIES

More than one third of all meniscus injuries occur in sport when a rotational force is applied to a partially flexed knee. Soccer alone accounts for 69% (Smillie 1970). Although meniscus injuries have traditionally been thought to be a common cause of knee pain it has become clear that not all produce symptoms. Arthroscopy has allowed increased accuracy of diagnosis and emphasized the errors of clinical diagnosis.

SYMPTOMS AND SIGNS

The player may present shortly after the incident with pain on the affected side of the knee, an effusion and a block to full extension.

However most commonly the acute episode subsides and only later does the player complain of recurrent pain usually located at the affected joint margin. Intermittent catching, locking or clicking may be reported leading to sudden changes in muscle tone in the leg such that the knee gives way. Between these incidents the knee may feel normal to the player.

In the acute situation the joint may be locked with inability to extend the knee beyond 20° together with some limitation to full flexion. A small effusion may be demonstrated and there will be tenderness over the corresponding joint line.

In the later stages the knee may be completely normal on physical examination apart from the presence of wasting of the quadriceps muscle and some slight tenderness over the affected joint line.

Types of tear

Vertical tears affect the substance of the meniscus or its peripheral attachment. They may be partial or complete. If partial it is usually the posterior horn that is most commonly affected. Complete tears produce the 'bucket handle' lesions of the meniscus. If this is present it may lie in the intercondylar area thus blocking full extension of the knee.

Horizontal tears classically occur in the older individual in whom there is some degenerative softening of the meniscus and a complaint of progressive joint line pain and discomfort with the knee tending to give way.

DIAGNOSIS

The diagnosis of such injuries can be confirmed by arthrography or arthroscopy.

TREATMENT

Some patients in whom meniscus tears are diagnosed settle without any treatment and unless symptoms are persistent or debilitating no treatment is necessary. This is particularly true of the horizontal tears of a degenerate nature.

When the patient complains of recurring episodes or has a locked joint the displaced or unstable portion of the meniscus should be excised. This will avoid further damage to the articular cartilage. This can be performed either at open operation or by arthroscopic techniques.

Usually only the torn fragment is excised to reduce the risk of post-operative osteoarthrosis, a well recognized complication of total meniscectomy.

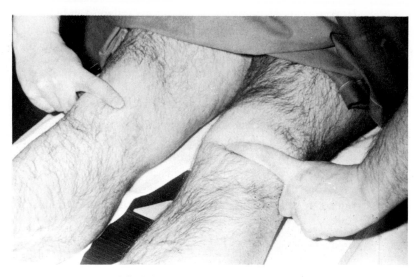

Fig. 25.5   Rupture of the left patellar tendon

Early arthroscopy and partial excision offers a speedy cure and is favoured for active sportsmen who can return to gentle training within days of the procedure. Open operation leads to a longer post-operative morbidity but may be preferable in certain circumstances if the arthroscopy is particularly difficult in achieving excision of all of the damaged area. It is most commonly used in patients with multiple complex tears.

Peripheral detachment of the meniscus can be treated by repair either at open operation or arthroscopically. Although not always successful it is worth attempting since it avoids the only alternative of total meniscectomy with its later complications.

Arthroscopic meniscectomy produces a shorter hospital stay and earlier return to full function. However, like all new surgical techniques its full effects and possible complications may not be known for some 10–20 years. Theoretically at least this technique may be associated with less degenerative joint disease.

BELOW THE KNEE

Rupture of the patellar tendon

This may be complete or partial resulting from a mechanism similar to that for rupture of the quadriceps tendon. This usually occurs at an earlier age (30 years) and unfortunately in some instances is the result of injudicious multiple injections of steroid into the patellar tendon region (see below).

Following injury the patient cannot extend the knee fully although may be able to extend the 45° by means of the medial and lateral retinacula which usually remain intact. A gap in the tendon may be felt below the patella if carefully examined (Fig. 25.5).

TREATMENT

Complete tears should be repaired surgically. Partial tears heal well if the diagnosis is made early and the limb is immobilized in a plaster cylinder for 4–6 weeks.

Patellar tendonitis (jumper's knee)

This may be acute or chronic. It is a frequent complaint of jumpers (high, long and triple) and basketball or netball players. It is usually due to a tear of a variable number of collagen fibres from the distal pole of the patella.

SYMPTOMS AND SIGNS

There is pain in the tendon on exercise. A local tender spot can be demonstrated at the distal pole of the patella. There is pain on holding the knee in extension against resistance.

TREATMENT

If symptoms are severe complete rest is indicated, either by crutch walking or a plaster cylinder. Many patients obtain relief with local physiotherapy treatment and anti-inflammatory drugs. Local steroid injection into the tender spot should be reserved for those cases which do not settle and should not be repeated in view of the risk of provoking complete rupture of the tendon (see above). A few tendons will require a surgical exploration usually with excision of the damaged area of tendon.

Osgood Schlatter's disease

This is a traction apophysitis of the tibial tubercle. It is caused by overuse and is seen most frequently in young footballers in their early teens.

SYMPTOMS AND SIGNS

The patient is a child or adolescent who complains of pain over the tibial tubercle during and after exercise. The tubercle is tender and swollen. There is pain on extending the knee against resistance.

The diagnosis is mainly made on clinical grounds although X-ray may show some fragmentation of the tibial tubercle.

TREATMENT

When pain is particularly troublesome rest is necessary to avoid the overuse situation. This may require the application of a plaster cylinder. It is important to explain to the parents of the child as well as the patient him or herself that the condition is self-limiting and will cure itself at skeletal maturity leaving a prominent tibial tubercle.

SHIN SPLINTS

This term describes pain usually experienced over the medial aspect of the shin although occasionally laterally and is commonly seen at the start of the season's training.

The three main causes of this syndrome are periostitis of tibialis posterior origin, stress fracture of the tibia or fibula and the compartment syndrome.

Periostitis

Classically this pain develops along the distal two-thirds of the tibial shaft on the medial side. Often the runner is a young novice, training on hard roads or in poor physical condition. Predisposing factors are malalignment problems such as excessive external rotation of the hip or hyperpronation of the foot. As a result of the overuse there is chronic traction of the posterior tibial muscle at its origin from the tibia and interosseous membrane which leads to reaction locally.

SYMPTOMS AND SIGNS

The pain gradually increases and eventually becomes so severe that it is present during and after running. Even walking may be painful. Careful examination will determine the tenderness over a length of the posterior border of the tibial shaft and may also reveal abnormalities of gait or malalignment of the foot.

Diagnosis can be confirmed by a bone scan which will show increased activity along the area of origin of the tibialis posterior muscle.

TREATMENT

Rest is essential initially in combination with anti-inflammatory drugs and local physiotherapy. When symptoms have settled the patient can return to running provided it is done prudently and gradually and on soft surfaces. Shoes which are worn should be replaced. If there is an underlying anatomical abnormality this should be compensated for with an orthosis. A poor running style should be corrected by proper coaching advice.

STRESS FRACTURE

This is due to cyclical stress loading which results in fatigue fracture of the bone. It occurs either at the junction of the upper and middle third of the tibia or the junction of the middle and lower thirds. (This phenomenon is also encountered in the lower fibula, neck of metatarsals and neck of femur.)

SYMPTOMS AND SIGNS

The pain is provoked by running and there will be well localized tenderness over the shaft of the tibia. X-ray diagnosis can only be made after 2–3 weeks when the changes due to healing become visible. The diagnosis can be established early by a bone scan.

TREATMENT

Rest is essential. If pain is present even on walking crutches should be used to relieve weight bearing until the bone becomes painless. At least 4 weeks should be allowed before commencing graduated training again although this will have to be modified in the light of any pain in response to exercise.

A general assessment should be made to exclude any other conditions which might have led to any abnormal reduction in bone strength, e.g. local disease, anorexia, metabolic causes.

COMPARTMENT SYNDROMES OF THE LEG

Compartment syndrome is the term used to describe the condition of increased pressure within the closed fascial compartments of the leg. In athletes this results in swelling of the muscles on activity and if severe may lead to muscle ischaemia. Since nerves and vessels run through such compartments they become compromised. This in turn leads to increased intramuscular oedema, further compression and ischaemia.

Although exercise is the most likely precipitating cause in athletes it may be precipitated by trauma to the muscle compartment. It may be acute or chronic.

The most commonly affected compartment is the anterior tibial compartment although involvement of the posterior and perineal compartment is not unknown.

Acute compartment syndrome

SYMPTOMS AND SIGNS

Most patients have undertaken unaccustomed exercise. Pain is usually experienced over the antero-lateral aspect of the leg and begins during activity. There is also paraesthesia in the second interdigital space of the foot. There is tenderness and usually a feeling of tightness on palpating the compartment and stretching the involved muscle exacerbates the pain. The pedal pulses are usually present since the compression leading to ischaemia affects the lower pressure capillaries and arterials only.

TREATMENT

The activity exciting the condition must be stopped and if there is no immediate recovery surgical decompression by fasciotomy should be carried out. Otherwise localized necrosis of the compartment muscles will occur with subsequent fibrosis and contraction. It has to be stressed that the acute syndrome is rare.

Chronic compartment syndrome

This is more common. Again the antero-lateral compartment is mostly affected and in 95% of patients the symptoms are bilateral (Reneman 1975).

SYMPTOMS AND SIGNS

The patient reports recurrent pain over the anterior tibial compartment. It is initiated by exercise and is described as cramping, tenseness or aching over the affected area. It is also brought on at specific running speeds or at a particular distance. Some sportsmen are obliged to stop the activity. In others a few minutes' rest is required before the activity can be continued.

Physical examination may confirm a fullness over the affected compartment with tenderness and weakness of dorsiflexion of the ankles and toes may be elicited, if examined when symptoms have been stimulated.

TREATMENT

The urgency is not so great as in the acute case. Fasciotomy is effective but many sportsmen will be prepared to alter their training patterns until symptoms settle. The differential diagnosis is from other forms of 'shin splints'. These causes must be considered and excluded.

ACHILLES TENDONITIS

The Achilles tendon does not have a synovial sheath but is enveloped in a paratenon which has a similar function. True acute Achilles tendonitis affects the paratenon primarily and not the tendon. However in severe or chronic cases the tendon itself may become involved as a result of adhesions between the paratenon and the tendon. In addition areas of mucoid degeneration within the tendon may lead to small ruptures with reactive nodularity which may produce secondary inflammatory changes in the paratenon.

The condition is common in middle and long distance runners but athletes engaged in football, volley ball, tennis, sprinting, jumping and ballet may also suffer from it.

Training errors and anatomical abnormalities can be the cause as can running shoes or boots with a high back. More recently following the vogue for long distance running young women have suffered from Achilles tendonitis. In daily life most of them wear shoes which maintain their feet in a degree of equinus which over a period of years effectively shortens the Achilles tendon. Thus when the woman takes up running the tendon is subject to increased stress in the more 'flat footed' position maintained by running shoes.

Training errors include excessive uphill running, wearing rigid shoes or training on hard surfaces.

Anatomical abnormalities such as talipes equinus, tight hamstrings or a tight gastrocnemius-soleus complex are other associated factors. Foot abnormalities such as a cavus deformity of hyperpronation may also be implicated.

SYMPTOMS AND SIGNS

Pain appears early during exercise but often subsides only to become more severe and unremitting after activity has stopped. Many patients report morning stiffness and pain which subsides during the day.

Clinical findings are varied. Often there is only diffuse tenderness along the line of the tendon. Sometimes there is crepitus and the presence of a localized nodule is usually indicative of a partial tear of the tendon and requires careful attention. There may also be abnormal gait patterns so the site of wear on the running shoes should be inspected. Anatomical or biomechanical disorders may be evident on examination.

TREATMENT

Both acute and chronic cases respond to cryotherapy and in only the most resistant cases is it necessary to resort to surgical intervention.

Abstinence from the activity which has caused the condition may be necessary for up to one month but relief can often be obtained by wearing heel raises (about 2 cm thick). This measure effectively places the foot in slight equinus and relieves the strain on the tendon. This may be provided by commercial heel pads such as 'Sorbothane' which also absorbs much of the force of heel strike. Anti-inflammatory medication should be given in acute cases and ice should be applied to the protected skin several times daily. Ultrasound may also give benefit in such patients.

Activities can continue in the form of swimming or cycling provided these do not lead to pain. This fulfils two functions. It maintains a degree of cardiovascular fitness important to the psyche of the injured player or runner and maintains proprioceptive activity in the ankle joint.

Steroid injection into the space between the paratenon and tendon in resistant subacute inflammation often helps but must be used with caution and not injected into the tendon. The use of steroid injection is contra-indicated in the presence of a nodule in view of its likely pathology.

PROGNOSIS

For patients treated in this manner half will return to full activity. A further 40% will be able to play sport but at a slightly reduced level and they may report occasional episodes of pain. Ten percent of patients will have persistent or recurrent problems. However only 5% will be unable to take part in sporting activity and perhaps require surgery, either stripping the tendon in chronic tendonitis or exploration of a partial tear.

ACHILLES TENDON RUPTURE

A healthy tendon will not spontaneously rupture. Spontaneous rupture results from the trauma of either an explosive contracture of the calf muscle or a forced stretch injury on a tendon which has become degenerate. It is most common in sports involving jumping or sudden changes of direction such as badminton and squash.

The tendon ruptures 2–5 cm above its insertion into the calcaneum where there is decreased vascularity leading to degeneration (Fig. 25.6). Early diagnosis and appropriate treatment are necessary for a successful return to sport.

SYMPTOMS AND SIGNS

The patient may report hearing a crack or maintaining that he was struck behind the heel. Pain is not always a clamant feature. Usually at the time of the rupture there is pain which gradually subsides and if the patient can walk he assumes there has been no major injury. In addition other tendons (tibialis posterior, long toe flexor and peronei) plantarflex the foot. Within a few hours there is

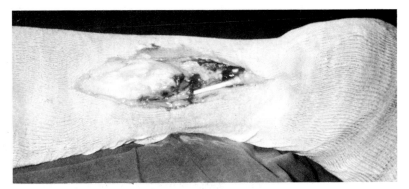

Fig. 25.6 Operative appearance of Achilles tendon rupture

marked swelling in the area which abolishes the gap in the tendon which may be visible immediately after injury and which renders palpation of the gap difficult. As a result up to 20% of Achilles tendon ruptures may be missed at the first examination.

However, clinical signs are always present. The patient may be unable to stand on tiptoe on the affected foot. There may still be a visible depression of the affected tendon when the patient lies prone (Fig. 25.7) and there is a palpable gap if looked for carefully even though swelling is present from the haematoma. Another useful observation is the absence of the normal plantar flexion appearance which the normal relaxed foot assumes. One further test involves pinching the relaxed calf muscle on the affected side. If there is no resultant reflex plantar flexion there is a rupture of the Achilles tendon.

TREATMENT

In high grade sportsmen best results are obtained by surgical repair. A suspected Achilles tendon rupture constitutes a soft tissue emergency and the patient should be referred to hospital as soon as possible. After surgical repair a plaster of Paris full length cast is applied with the foot in equinus. Cast immobilization is maintained for 6 weeks after surgery and progressive exercises commenced thereafter.

However there are significant local complications of this procedure and as an alternative, if the diagnosis is made within 48 hours of occurrence it is possible to treat such ruptures by plaster immobilization alone. The length of plaster immobilization will be somewhat longer (8 weeks) with a slightly slower rehabilitation but the results will be almost indistinguishable from the results of surgical repair when examined between 6 and 12 months later.

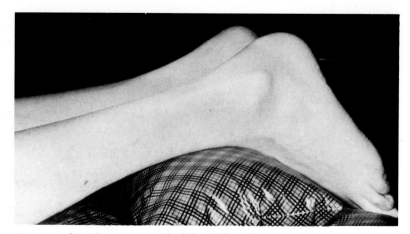

Fig. 25.7 Clinical appearance of a left Achilles tendon rupture. Note the depression in the tendon

REHABILITATION

When the cast is removed the patient begins to walk with a raised heel to relax the tendon. When normal heel toe gait is established the heel should be reduced gradually and active stretching and strengthening exercises of the calf muscle complex should begin. When these exercises can be performed without discomfort tiptoe walking can begin progressing to active plantar flexion against increasing resistance.

PROGNOSIS

Normal function can be recovered if treatment is early and an active rehabilitation programme is followed. One patient has won and retained a world karate championship title despite a traumatic rupture of the Achilles tendon.

Partial rupture

This condition is one of the forms of 'chronic tendonitis'. The definitive diagnosis can only be made at surgery. If there is suspicion of a partial tear the treatment is to remove the stress from the tendon which may include immobilization in a plaster cast with the foot in slight equinus for approximately 4 weeks. If this fails to relieve the symptoms the tendon should be explored surgically when degenerate material around the tear is excised and repair carried out. The effect of surgery is also to introduce a new blood supply to the area which will improve collagen turnover thus reducing degeneration.

REFERENCES

Aglietti P, Cerulli G 1979 Chondromalacia and recurrent subluxation of the patella: a study of malalignment with some indications for radiography. Italian Journal of Orthopaedic Traumatology 5: 187–201

Allen M J, Barnes M R 1986 Exercise pain in the lower leg. Journal of Bone and Joint Surgery 68B, 818–823

Carden D G, Noble J, Chalmers J, Lunn P, Ellis J 1987 Rupture of the calcaneal tendon. Journal of Bone and Joint Surgery 69B: 416–420

Dowd G S E, Bentley G 1986 Radiographic assessment in patellar instability and chondromalacia patellae. Journal of Bone and Joint Surgery 68B: 297–300

Gear M W L 1967 The late results of meniscectomy. British Journal of Surgery 54: 270–272

Lanzetta A, Meani E, Tinti G 1981 Injuries of the Achilles tendon in athletes: their causes and the indications for their treatment. Italian Journal of Sports Traumatology 3: 113–121

O'Donoghue D H 1976 Injuries of the knee. In: Treatment of injuries to athletes. 3rd edn. W B Saunders, Philadelphia, pp 563–579

Ogilvie-Harris D J, Jackson R W 1984 Arthroscopic treatment of chondromalacia patellae. Journal of Bone and Joint Surgery 66B: 660–665

Orava S, Osterback L, Hurme M 1986 Surgical treatment of patellar tendon pain in athletes. British Journal of Sports Medicine 20 4: 167–169

Reneman R S 1975 The anterior and the lateral compartmental syndrome of the leg due to intensive use of muscles. Clinical Orthopaedics 113: 69–74

Scott G A, Jolly B L, Henning C E 1986 Combined posterior incision and arthroscopic intra-articular repair of the meniscus. Journal of Bone and Joint Surgery 68A: 847–861

Simpson D A, Thomas N P, Aichroth P M 1986 Open and closed meniscectomy. A comparative analysis. Journal of Bone and Joint Surgery 68B: 301–304

Smillie I S 1970 Injuries of the knee joint. Churchill Livingstone, Edinburgh

26. Injuries to the ankle and foot

LATERAL LIGAMENT INJURY

Injury to the lateral ligament of the ankle resulting from an inversion injury is common both in sport and life in general. Every day in the United Kingdom 5 000 people sustain this injury.

The lateral ligament is made up of three bands, the common origin of which is the tip of the fibula. The anterior and posterior bands (the talo-fibular ligaments) both insert into the talus. The middle band (the calcaneo-fibula ligament) passes vertically from the fibula to the calcaneum.

Mechanism of injury

A combination of inversion and plantar flexion causes initial damage to the anterior talo-fibular ligaments. As the deforming force increases the other membranes of the ligament complex are stretched or torn. The extent ranges from partial tears to complete ligamentous disruption. In the most severe injuries there is often stretching of the anterior part of the inferior tibio-fibular ligament as well.

SYMPTOMS AND SIGNS

The patient will give a history of a twisting injury as described above. There is local bruising and swelling with tenderness on palpation over the lateral ligament complex and frequently also extending on to the tip of the lateral malleolus and the inferior part of the tibio-fibular ligament anteriorly.

DIAGNOSIS

Radiology is necessary to exclude a fracture and is of value in assessing whether there is instability of the joint. Stress films, comparing both ankles can be performed under local anaesthetic and may demonstrate talar tilt of greater than 30° or marked forward shift of the talus within the mortice when the heel is pushed forward (anterior drawer test). Both of these findings suggest complete rupture. Arthrography or tenography of the peroneal tendon may also be performed to assist in the assessment of the degree of injury.

TREATMENT

Treatment should be considered under three grades of severity

Grade 1: Ligament strain without instability.

Grade 2: Incomplete tear with mild instability.

Grade 3: Complete tear with marked instability.

In grades 1 and 2 the prognosis is good. Treatment should therefore be directed against the pain and swelling. In young fit people high dose anti-inflammatory drugs permit an earlier return to sport than the use of strapping alone. Early active movements within the limitations of pain should always be encouraged. Grade 3 tears should also be treated conservatively. The standard treatment is the application of a below knee plaster cast for 6 weeks after which gentle mobility exercises can be started. A better alternative in the athlete is the application of a cast brace which allows flexion and extension at the ankle but prevents inversion and eversion. The cast brace can be removed after 4 weeks and active rehabilitation can then continue. The results of the technique are encouraging. It allows fitness to be maintained during the recovery period and reduces the incidence of post inversion instability by maintaining muscle function at a better level and also reducing the loss of ankle proprioception caused by immobilization.

REHABILITATION

Patients with inversion injuries should be actively encouraged to exercise as soon as they have relief from pain. This prevents proprioceptive loss in the joint and recurrent injury. A wobble-board is a valuable aid to this, the intensity of exercise being adjusted to the degree of pain. Other exercises include a gentle full range of ankle movement within the limits of pain and rotating movements of the foot which move all the joints of the foot and ankle. As recovery progresses heel raises, hopping and progressive resistance exercises with weights can be introduced.

The use of strapping has been shown to be effective in reducing the incidence of these injuries both primary and recurrent.

'POTT'S' FRACTURES

Fractures of the malleoli require hospital treatment. The modern approach to treatment is fairly aggressive and whenever possible unstable fractures are internally fixed to allow early mobility although avoiding weight bearing. This reduces the osteoporosis, muscle wasting and joint stiffness associated with immobilization and allows earlier return of normal function. In addition whenever possible stable undisplaced fractures of the lateral malleolus should not be immobilized but should be treated in a fashion similar to injuries of the lateral ligament.

HINDFOOT DISORDERS

Plantar fasciitis (policeman's heel, heel spur syndrome)

This is a common condition of runners (especially in the older age group) who have recently increased their mileage. It is due to an avulsion strain of the short plantar muscles at their origin from the calcaneum which in turn is often due to the excess stress applied to this area during running if tight calf muscles do not allow full dorsiflexion of the ankle.

SYMPTOMS AND SIGNS

The patient complains of pain on the underside of the heel, worse on getting up in the morning when beginning to put weight on the foot. The pain then diminishes but may gradually return after a long run. On examination there is tenderness on the medial aspect of the heel.

An X-ray may show a calcaneal spur but this bears no relationship to the condition.

TREATMENT

Treatment involves stretching the gastrocnemius muscle and Achilles tendon complex. In some cases shortening here may be the sole cause. If the complex is vigorously stretched less tension is placed on the proximal origin of the plantar fascia. The exercises should be performed twice daily. A Sorbothane heel pad will relieve the pain of heel strike.

Oral anti-inflammatory drugs should be prescribed when the patient first presents. If symptoms persist over several weeks then a local injection of local anaesthetic and depot steroid into the tender area usually cures the condition.

STRESS FRACTURES

These may develop in the calcaneum. They should be suspected from the history and the clinical finding of tenderness over the calcaneum. Radiography or bone scan is used to confirm the diagnosis.

BURSITIS (PUMP BUMP)

Two bursae in association with the Achilles tendon may become inflamed. One is subcutaneous, and the other lies between the lower end of the Achilles tendon and the bare area of the calcaneum. Inflammation of the former is usually due to friction from footwear and inflammation of the latter from overuse. Occasionally the subcutaneous bursa may arise because of an abnormally prominent calcaneum.

SYMPTOMS AND SIGNS

Subcutaneous bursitis is easy to diagnose because of its superficial situation when swelling and tenderness are present often with inflammation. There may also be an unusually prominent bump palpable on the calcaneum.

A deep bursitis is less easy to palpate but tenderness is felt deep to the Achilles tendon on both sides.

TREATMENT

For a subcutaneous bursa the source of friction must be removed and anti-inflammatory drugs prescribed. Surgical treatment may be required if the condition becomes chronic particularly if it is in relation to a calcaneal bump.

A deep bursa may also respond to reduction in exercise together with anti-inflammatory treatment but failing this an injection of steroid is usually curative.

MIDFOOT DISORDERS

Tendonitis and tenosynovitis

The foot is frequently affected by overuse. Often there is combined pathology such as ligamentous strain of one or more of the joints of the foot accompanied by a strain or inflammation of the tendon attachment. The posterior tibial tendon at its insertion into the navicular bone or the peroneus longus tendon where it passes under the cuboid bone are commonly affected sites.

SYMPTOMS AND SIGNS

There is pain on activity and on passive stretching of the involved tendon. There is also tenderness over the tendon and occasionally crepitus can be elicited. There may be deformities of the foot which are contributing to the condition.

RADIOLOGY

There may be bony abnormalities in the foot which may have a bearing on the production of symptoms. Occasionally calcification may be seen in the affected tendon.

TREATMENT

Oral anti-inflammatory drugs and the use of an orthotic device combined with reduction in activity are standard methods which produce good results. Strapping can also be used to prevent excessive movement. Few patients require surgery.

TARSAL TUNNEL SYNDROME

This condition manifested by pain in the medial side of the foot and parasthesiae in the forefoot and toes is caused by compression of the posterior tibial nerve or its distal branches usually within the medial retinaculum behind the medial malleolus or as it passes into the sole of the foot. It can be produced by wearing ill fitting shoes but most commonly is secondary to some malalignment of the foot.

SYMPTOMS AND SIGNS

There may be severe forefoot pain or parasthesiae and if the shoes are examined there may be excess padding leading to pressure. A foot deformity may be seen. Tinel's sign can be elicited by compressing the affected area. The condition can be confirmed and the level of the compression determined by nerve conduction tests.

TREATMENT

If the cause is straightforward then removal of the stimulating factor may allow symptoms to settle in 4–6 weeks and can be assisted by using a heel raise, wedged on the medial side to place the heel in a more neutral position. The running shoes must be examined and areas of pressure identified. Unsuitable shoes should be discarded. An orthosis will be required to control any foot deformity to prevent recurrence.

FLATFOOT

In this condition the apex of the arch of the foot collapses inwards. It may be associated with orthopaedic problems like external tibial rotation, genu valgum or a varus forefoot. Alternatively it may be simply related to ligamentous laxity in the subtalar or midtarsal joints or a short Achilles tendon.

SYMPTOMS AND SIGNS

Symptoms result from repeated episodes of overuse. The main complaint is of pain in the midfoot although secondary forefoot deformities may result in pain under the metatarsal heads.

TREATMENT

If the Achilles tendon is short stretching exercises will help. If there is hyperpronation of the foot an orthosis with medial wedge is indicated. In all cases the correct footwear is important and a shoe with adequate cushioning, especially where the foot is rigid, provides protection and relief. Exercises to strengthen leg and foot muscles to control the foot arches will help prevent recurrence.

FOREFOOT CONDITIONS

Metatarsalgia is the term used to describe pain under the metatarsal heads for which there are several possible causes—foot strain, plantar interdigital neuroma, stress fracture, Freiberg's disease, and sesamoiditis.

Foot strain

Overuse may produce pain in the region of the metatarsal heads if some foot deformity is present (see below). It is probably related to stretching of the ligaments and muscles running across the forefoot which maintain the 'transverse arch'.

SYMPTOMS AND SIGNS

Pain comes on during walking, running and ceases with rest. There may be generalized tenderness around the metatarsal heads. There will usually be some primary foot deformity.

TREATMENT

Local physiotherapy and foot exercises will relieve the symptoms. An orthosis may be required to prevent recurrence if a significant foot deformity is present.

Plantar interdigital neuroma

A neuroma may develop on any of the plantar digital nerves and is usually found at the bifurcation on the clefts. Classically (Morton's metatarsalgia) the neuroma is in the third or fourth interdigital cleft.

SYMPTOMS AND SIGNS

There is pain and tingling in the forefoot which is usually localized to the appropriate cleft. There is well localized tenderness over the neuroma which may be palpated if large enough. Pain is also stimulated by compressing the metatarsal heads from side to side.

TREATMENT

Protective padding to relieve compression should be tried initially. If symptoms fail to resolve the condition the neuroma is surgically excised.

Stress fracture

Stress or 'March' fractures affect the necks of the long (second or third) metatarsals.

SYMPTOMS AND SIGNS

There is pain and tenderness over the second or third metatarsal shafts which later becomes thickened due to callous formation during healing.

The diagnosis is confirmed in the early stages by bone scan or later on X-ray when the callous becomes radiologically visible.

TREATMENT

The only effective treatment for stress fractures is rest from the activity which produced it and from any other that produces pain. If pain is troublesome on everyday walking it may be necessary to apply a plaster shoe for 2 weeks.

Freiberg's disease

This is one of the pressure osteochondritis conditions which affects the head of the second metatarsal in adolescence. The pathology is avascular necrosis of the intra-articular part of the head of the metatarsal which develops a flat deformity due to collapse of bone. Occasionally a piece may separate (osteochondritis dissicans). Spontaneous healing usually occurs (unless a fragment has separated) although the deformity persists.

SYMPTOMS AND SIGNS

A young adolescent, often female, presents with a painful second metatarso-phalangeal joint which is swollen and tender to touch.

X-ray confirms a flattened and often enlarged metatarsal head with a widened joint space.

TREATMENT

Treatment consists of a protective doughnut padding and decreased activity. If this fails and symptoms are significant surgical treatment may be required in the form of metatarsal head excision.

Sesamoiditis

Pain under the metatarso-phalangeal joint of the great toe may be due to sesamoiditis; its pathology is usually chondromalacia.

Adhesive doughnut pads will permit symptoms to resolve by relieving pressure whilst running continues. If there are persistent symptoms excision of the affected sesamoid may be necessary if injection of steroid has proved to be unsuccessful.

MISCELLANEOUS CAUSES OF METATARSALGIA

The following conditions can all lead to the development of pain with callous formation under the metatarsal heads:
- Claw toe in which there is flexion at both interphalangeal joints
- Hammer toe in which the metatarso-phalangeal joint is extended, the proximal interphalangeal joint flexed and the distal interphalangeal joint extended.

Hallux valgus

If this is producing symptoms and the protective padding has not helped there may be a need for operative correction of the under-lying deformity.

MISCELLANEOUS CAUSES OF FOOT PAIN

Subungal haematoma

Haematomata under the nails are common in runners, (runners toe). When acute, immediate pain relief can be achieved by puncturing the nail overlying the haematoma with a sterile needle. Long term prevention depends on the use of adequate footwear.

Ingrown toenail

Athletes usually wait until infection has set in before presenting with this condition. The infection is treated under local anaes-thetic by avulsing the nail. Advice should be given on footwear and nail hygiene thereafter.

If there is recurrence then nail bed ablation will be required, either the margin of the affected site or if the condition is bilateral and extensive, the entire nail bed — usually achieved using phenol.

Blisters

They usually result from new or illfitting footwear. Once estab-lished the blister should be punctured under sterile conditions and the area should then be protected with adhesive strapping over a dry dressing. The skin of the blister should not be excised but should be left in place as a dressing.

If recurrently troublesome they can be prevented by greasing the feet with baby oil or petroleum jelly.

FOOT ALIGNMENT

It has become increasingly obvious that many painful conditions of the lower limb may result from the abnormal stresses applied during exercise when malalignment of the foot leads to an abnormal gait pattern (trochanteric bursitis, ilio-tibial band syndrome, anterior knee pain, shin splints).

The deformities which must be sought are excessive valgus or varus in the hindfoot and pronation or supination of the forefoot.

Such malalignments can usually be compensated for or controlled by a suitable orthosis although some of the more severe, especially those in the hindfoot, may require surgical treatment.

FOOTWEAR

It is evident that many foot problems are related to poorly fitting shoes. This single fact is so important for successful training that we suggest that serious sports people (and indeed most people who take exercise) have their feet measured in length and width at a specialist sports footwear store.

In general terms the heel counter should be firm to prevent lateral movement. The heel tab should not extend so far as to cause friction over the Achilles tendon. It is also important that there is cushioning in the heel and the sole is flexible. A rigid sole may lead to Achilles tendon strain. There should be approximately 1 cm of clearance between the great toe and the front of the shoe with no rough edges inside.

When examining a patient with lower limb problems the doctor must inspect the footwear, either running shoes or soccer/rugby boots. Is there excessive wear? Is the shoe too rigid? The solution to the patient's problem often lies in simple corrective measures.

REFERENCES

Cass J R, Morrey B F 1984 Ankle instability: current concepts, diagnosis and treatment. Mayo Clinic Proceedings 59: 165–70

Hutson M A, Jackson J P 1982 Injuries to the lateral ligament of the ankle: assessment and treatment. British Journal of Sports Medicine 16 4: 245–249

McLatchie G R, Allister C, Hamilton G, Colquhoun I, McEwen C, McGregor H, Pickvance M J 1985 Variable schedules of ibuprofen for ankle sprains. British Journal of Sports Medicine 19 4

Ruth C J 1961 Surgical treatment of injuries to the collateral ligaments of the ankle. Journal of Bone and Joint Surgery 43A: 220–239

Tait G R, Tuck J S 1987 Surgical or phenol ablation of the nail bed for ingrowing toenails: a randomised controlled trial. Journal of the Royal College of Surgeons of Edinburgh 32: 358–360.

Index

Abdominal injuries, 280
 diagnosis, 280–281
 management, 281
 prevention, 281–282
 types, 276–277
Above knee injuries, 318–319
Acclimatization, 109–110
Achilles tendon rupture, 334–336
 partial, 336
 rehabilitation/prognosis, 336
 symptoms/signs, 334–335
 treatment, 335–336
Achilles tendonitis, 332–334
 symptoms/signs, 333
 treatment/prognosis, 333–334
Acromioclavicular joint, injuries, 286,
 293–294
Adductor longus tendoperiostitis, 310–311
Adenosine triphosphate (ATP), muscle
 contraction, 56–57
Aerial sports, injuries, 175–176
Ageing
 and exercise, 27–28
 fitness gap, 28
Aikido, injuries, 166
Airway
 maintenance, 203–204
 warming (AW), in hypothermia, 185–186
Altitude, acclimatization, 109–110
Amenorrhoea, 50, 107, 483
Amnesia, post-traumatic (PTA), 256, 257,
 259–260
Anabolic steroids, 84–85
Angina, 104
Ankle
 injuries, 291–292
 lateral ligament injury, 338–339
 grades, 339
 protection, 101–102
 strapping, 131–132
Ankylosing spondylitis, 310
Anterior cruciate ligament injury, 326
Anti-inflammatory agents, topical, 146–149
 action mode, 146–147
 reasons for use, 147–148
 see also NSAIDs
Arm protection, 98–99
Arthrography, 227
Arthroscopy, knee, 286

Asthma, 27
 cold-air-associated, 196
 exercise-induced, 27, 104–105
Athlete's heart syndrome, 105–106
Automatism, post-traumatic amnesia,
 259–260
Avascular necrosis, scaphoid fractures, 304
Axial loading, cervical injury, 267–268
Axonal injury, diffuse, 256

Badminton injuries, 171–172
Bankhart's operation, 296
Barotrauma, pulmonary, sub-aqua diving,
 173
Bath University, Diploma course, 36
Below knee injuries, 328–336
Bends, sub-aqua diving, 173
Bennett's fracture dislocation, 158, 306
Biceps
 rupture, 300–301
 tendonitis, 300
Bicipital syndromes, 300–301
Birmingham University, sports sciences,
 37–38
Black eye, 240
Blisters, 150
Blood vessels, major, rupture, 280
Blowout fracture, eyes, 240, 241, 250–251
Blunt injuries, thorax/abdomen, 276
Blunt trauma
 cardiac, 278–279
 eye, 240–244
Body fat content, 46–47
Body weight, strength development, 60
Boxing, 157
 ear injuries, 163
 eye injuries, 162–163
 facial injuries, 162–163
 hand injuries, 158–159, 160
 head injuries, 159–162
 injury prevention, 163–164
 knockout rules, 159
 nasal injuries, 163
 subdural/extradural haemorrhage, 160
Brain damage
 pathology, 255–256
 primary, 256
 secondary, 257–258

Brain damage (contd)
    sequelae, 257–259
Brain swelling, 257
Breach of the peace, competitors, 15–16
Breast
    injuries, 278
    lumps, 227–228
Breathing, checking in emergencies, 204
Bristow-Helfet procedure, 296
Bronchitis, 27
Brucellosis, 121
Bubonic plague, prevalence, 120–121
Burns, 150
    chemical, eyes, 245–246, 249
    physical, eyes, 246
Bursitis, 152–153

Caecal-slap syndrome, 177
Caffeine, as stimulant, 88
Calcaneum, stress fractures, 340
Carbohydrates, dietary, 80–81
Cardiac arrest, resuscitation, 205, 206
Cardiac contusions, 279
Cardiac rupture, 278–279
Cardiac trauma
    blunt, 278–279
    penetrating, 279
Cardiopulmonary resuscitation, 204–206
Cardiovascular diseases
    cold effects, 196
    prevention, exercise, 23
    sports participation, 104
    sports-related, 105–106
Cauliflower ear, 163
Cerebral abscess, 257
Cerebral contusions, 256
Cerebrospinal fluid (CSF), leakage, 257
Cervical injury
    clinical presentation, 269–270
    conscious patient, 269–270
    mechanisms, 265–268
    posture, 270
    risk sports, 268–269
    unconscious patient, 270
Cervical sprain, acute, 273–274
Changing rooms, infection transmission,
        114, 118–119
Charley horse, 312
Cheating, control of, 18
    governing bodies guidelines, 18–19
Chemical burns, eyes, 245–246, 249
Chest injury, emergency care, 209–210
Children, facial injuries, 235–237
    prevention, 235–237
Chondromalacia, 345
    patellae, 283
Choroid, rupture, 242, 243
Chronic fatigue syndrome, 112
Circulation, in emergencies, 204

Civil law suits, 9–10
Claw toe, 345
Clostridium tetani, 117
Cold applications, soft tissue injury,
        134–137
Cold injury, 179, 182–198
    local, 179, 188–193, 198
        after-effects, 194–195
        prevention, 195
        muscle tears, 195–196
        non-freezing (NFCI), 193–194, 195–197,
            198
        systemic, 179–187, 197–198
        see also various types
Collateral ligament injury, knee, 323–324,
        325
Colles' fracture, 287–288, 305
    juvenile, 305
Combat sports, injuries/sudden death,
        157–165
Communication, and emergency care, 200
Compartment syndrome, leg, 331–332
    acute, 331–332
    chronic, 332
Competitions, medical cover, 200
Competitors
    breach of the peace, 15–16
    disqualifying medical conditions, 40–41
    duties, 8–12
        to organizers, 11–12
        to other competitors, 8–11
        to spectators, 11
    general medical advice, 103
    human requirements, 4–5
    medical evaluation, 41
    pre-existing disease, advice, 103–105
    safe prescribing, 90–91, 110
    see also Participation
Computerized tomography (CT) scans, 226,
        227
Conjunctivitis, cold-induced, 195
Consciousness, Glasgow coma scale, 262
Contact sports, injuries, 168–171
Contusions
    cardiac, 279
    thoracic, 277
Coordination, restoration, post-injury, 128
Corneal abrasions, 242, 249
Coronary heart disease, and exercise, 24–25
Cricothyrotomy, 207–209
    tube insertion technique, 219–220
Criminal assaults, and the law, 8–9, 10–11
Cruciate ligament injury, 290, 324–326
Cryotherapy (cryokinetics), 136
Cyst formation, soft tissue injuries, 153

De Quervain's disease, 303
Dead leg, 312
Deceleration injuries, thorax/abdomen, 276

Dehydration
  risks, 83–84
  side-effects, 87
Dental injuries, 230, 231–234
  examination, 231–234
Detraining, 59
Diabetes mellitus
  and exercise, 26
  and sports, 105
Diaphragm, rupture, 280
Diarrhoea, 106, 176, 177
  see also Travellers' diarrhaea
Diathermy
  microwave, 129
  short-wave, 129
Diet in sport, 79–92
Digits
  dislocations, 305–306
  injuries, 305–307
  sprains, 305
  see also Fingers; Thumb
Diphtheria, immunization, 108
Diploma in Sports Medicine (Royal Medical
      Colleges, Scotland), 33–36
  regulations, 34–35
  syllabus, 35–36
Disc injuries, 274
Diving injuries, 175
  sub-aqua diving, 172–174
Donway traction splint, 215
Drug abuse, 88–89, 110
Drugs, emergency, 201–202
Dysmenorrhoea, strenuous exercise effects,
  49

Ear injuries, boxing, 163
Elbow
  injuries, 287
  painful, 301–302
  pulled, 301
Elective patients, investigations, 223
Emergency care, 199–221
  ABC management, 203–204, 205
  advanced life support, 204–210
  and communication, 200
  patient lifting, 215, 218
  personal equipment, 201
Emergency drugs, 201–202
  administration route, 202
Encephalopathy, traumatic, 160–162
Endurance
  aerobic, testing, 70–72
  anaerobic, testing, 74–75
  definition, 70
  restoration, post-injury, 128
  testing, 70–74
  training, aerobic, 61–62
Environmental injury, 142, 178–180
Epilepsy, and sports, 105

Ergometers, cycle, 70, 74
Erysipelas, scrumpox, 116
Ethics of practice, World Medical
      Association, 38–39
Exercise
  and age progression, 27–28
  body function effects, 21–22
  cardiovascular disease prevention, 23
  and coronary heart disease, 24–25
  glucose hepatic output, 81
  health benefits, 29
  and hypertension, 23
  and lifestyle, 21–22
  and metabolic disease, 26
  osteoporosis, prevention/management of,
    26–27
  and peripheral vascular disease, 22, 23,
    25–26
  post-infarction rehabilitation, 25
  pregnancy, 50–51
  psychological wellbeing, 28
  tolerance tests, 22
  vigorous/habitual, 25
Eye injuries
  assessment, 247–249
    in casualty department, 247–249
    on field, 247
    hospital examination, 247–249
  blowout fracture, 240, 241, 250–251
  blunt trauma, 240–244
  boxing, 162–163
  chemical burns, 245–246, 249
  epidemiology, 239
  foreign bodies, 245, 246, 249
  penetrating, 244–245, 251
  physical burns, 246
  prevention, 252–254
  rehabilitation after, 252
  risk of, 239
  specialist referral, 249
  treatment, 249–251
  types, 239–246
Eye protection, 95, 97, 252–254
  dangers of, 95

Facial injuries, 229
  anatomical aspects, 229–230
  in boxing, 162–163
  in children, 235–237
Familial cold urticaria, 187
Fat, dietary, 79–80
Femoral epiphysis
  slipped, 288
  upper, slipped, 312–313
Femur neck, stress fracture, 313
Fencing
  fatalities, 167–168
  injuries, 166–168

Fingers
    injuries, rock climbers, 306–307
    mallet, 306
    see also Frostbite
Fitness assessment
    laboratory, 66–77
    pre-test procedures, 68
    purpose/intention of tests, 69
    tests and equipment, 69–75
Fitness gap, ageing, 28
Flatfoot, 342–343
Flexibility
    restoration, post-injury, 127
    testing, 70
Fluid balance, hypothermia, 182–183
Fluid replacement, 83–84, 107
Foot
    alignment, 346
    blisters, 345
    protection, 101–102
    strain, metatarsalgia, 343
    see also Frostbite
Footwear, 346
Forefoot disorders, 343–345
Foreign bodies, eye, 245, 246, 249
Foul play, 263
    rugby injuries, 170
    soccer injuries, 169, 170
    see also Violence
Fractures, splinting, 215
Frostbite, 179, 188–193, 198
    bleb formation, 189–190
    precipitating factors, 188
    thawing, 188–193
        excessive heat effects, 189, 192–193
Frostnip, 188
Fungal infections, 150–151

Gamekeeper's thumb, 306
Gastrointestinal disease, sports-related, 106
Gastrointestinal symptoms, in running
        events, 176–177
Giardiasis, 118
Glasgow coma scale, 262
Glasgow University, sports sciences/sports
        medicine, 38
Glenohumeral joint
    dislocation, 286
    injuries, 294
    recurrent subluxation, 296–297
Glenoid labrum detatchment, 295
Gluconeogenesis, 81
Glycogen loading, 85–87
    advantages/disadvantages, 86–87
    dietary technique, 85–86
Glycogen sparing effect, 21
Glycogen uptake, dietary carbohydrates,
        80–81
Golfer's elbow, 302

Grappling sports, injuries, 166
Groin
    disruption, 308–310
        clinical features, 309
        treatment/rehabilitation, 309–310
    pain, 308
    protection, 99, 101
Gumshields, 96–97
    dangers of, 97
Gymnasts, female, injuries, 51
Gynaecological problems, sports-related,
        107

Haemarthrosis, and arthroscopy, 290
Haematomas, 149–150
    intracranial, 257, 260
    peri-orbital, 240
    quadriceps, 312
    subungual, 345
    thoracic, 277
Haematuria
    sports, 177–178
    traumatic, 178
Haemoglobin, mean concentration, women
        in sport, 48
Haemorrhage, control, 210–211, 212
Haemothorax, 279
Hallux valgus, 345
Hammer toe, 345
Hamstring tears, 316–317
Hand
    injuries, boxing, 158–159, 160
    pain, 303
    protection, 98–99
    strapping, 133–134, 136, 137
Head, protection, 93–95, 96, 263
Head injuries, 255–264
    boxing, 159–162
        chronic sequelae, 160–162
        death, 160
    hospital admission, 261–262
    infection, 247, 261–262
    management, 259–262
        warning card, 42
    guidelines, 260, 261
    prevention, 263
    psychological/intellectual functioning,
        257, 258
    recurrent, sequelae, 257–259
    return to sport, 262–263
    soccer, 169
Headgear, 263
    dangers of, 94–95
Heart disease, congenital, mortality in sport,
        157
    see also Hypertrophic cardiomyopathy
        (HCM)
Heart rate
    and training, 61, 62, 63, 64

Heart rate (*contd*)
  and VO$_2$max, 70–72
Heat
  acclimatization, 109
  collapse, treatment, 179
  treatment, soft tissue injury,
      128–129
Heel spur syndrome, 340
Helmets
  dangers of, 94–95
  design of, 93–94
Henry Moore's University at
      Liverpool, sports sciences, 37
Hepatitis B infections, 118,
      121–122
Hernias, inguinal/femoral, 308
Herpes gladiatorum, 112, 113, 115
Herpes simplex, scrumpox, 113,
      116
Hillsborough disaster, 13, 15
Hindfoot
  bursitis (pump bump), 341
  disorders, 340–341
Hip
  injuries, 288
  osteoarthrosis, 313–314
  posterior dislocation, 288
Hippocrates manoeuvre, 295
HIV infection, 118, 122–123
  consensus statement, 122
Hockey, field, injuries, 170–171
Hyperextension, cervical injury,
      266
Hyperflexion, cervical injury,
      265–266
Hyperprolactinaemia, 50
Hypertension, 104
  and exercise, 23
Hypertrophic cardiomyopathy
      (HCM), 106, 157
Hyphaema, 242–243, 244, 255
  sequelae, 243
Hypoglycaemia, exercise-induced,
      26
Hypotension, postexertional, 22
Hypothermia, 178–179, 179,
      182–187, 197–198
  classification, 183–184
  death
    after rescue, 187
    and revival, 185
  fluid balance, 182–183
  late effects, 187
  rewarming methods, 185–186
  symptoms and signs, 184–185

Ice
  physical effects, 134
  soft tissue injury, 134–137

Ilio-tibial band friction syndrome, 315, 316
Iliopsoas strain, 311
Immediate care, 199–221
  tetraplegia, 272–273
Immersion injury, 180, 196–197
Immunization, 108–109, 123–124
Impetigo, scrumpox, 116
Indoor sports, 1, 4
Infections
  changing-room-associated, 114, 118–119
  soft tissue injuries, 153
  sports-related, 107, 112–125
    prevention, 123–125
  and travel abroad, 119–121
  water-sports-related, 118
Influenza virus, cardiac muscle effects, 119
Infra-red heat, 128–129
Infraspinatus muscle, 293
Infraspinatus tendonitis, 297–298
Ingrown toenail, 345
Injuries
  classification, 142–144
  and consent/risks, 6–7
  on the field, investigations, 222–223
  incidence, 140, 141
  investigations, 222–228
  legal aspects, 8–11
  legal categories, 10–11
  and negligence, 11
  sites, 142, 143, 145
  types, 140–142
  women in sport, 51–52
Injury clinics
  establishment, 43–44
  guidelines, 44
Instantaneous power, testing, 74–75
Interphalangeal joints, dislocations/
      sprains, 305–306
Interval training, 62
Intra-oral examination, 231–234
Intracranial haematomas, 257, 260
Intubation, endotracheal, 206–207
Investigations
  elective patients, 223
  on the field injuries, 222–223
  injuries, 222–228
  practice standards, 223, 224
  see also Laboratory investigations
Iridodialysis, 242
Iron deficiency, women in sport, 48
Isokinetics/isometrics, strength
      development, 60

Joggers' nephritis, 106, 107
Joint injuries
  closed, 283
  examination, 284–286
  history, 284
  open, 283

Joint injuries (*contd*)
  see also individual joints
Jump, standard vertical, 75
Jumper's knee, 329

Karate, injuries, 164–165
  prevention, 164–165
Knee
  anterior pain, 321–322
  collateral ligament injury,
    323–324, 325
  effusion, 289–290
  extensor mechanism injuries,
    318
  injuries, 289–291
  jumper's, 329
  ligament injuries, 323–326
    repair results, 326
  meniscal tears, 290
  stability assessment, 291
  strapping, 132–133, 134, 135
  see also Above knee; Below knee;
    Patella
Kocher's manoeuvre, 295

Labial injuries, tooth fragments,
    232, 233
Laboratory investigations, 223, 225
Lactate
  blood accumulation onset test
    (OBLA), 73
  endurance testing, 72–74
Laryngeal mask airway, 207
Lassa fever, 120
Law
  and injury, 8–11
  self-defence, 10
Le Fort fractures, 229
Leg
  compartment syndromes,
    331–332
  protection, 100–101
Legionella micdadei, 118
Leisure time activities, and
    infections, 121–123
Life support, advanced, 204–210
Lifestyle, and exercise, 21–22
Lifting the patient, 215, 218
Ligament injuries, 150–151
  knee, 323–326
Lipoproteins, high density (HDL),
    exercise effects, 21, 23
Lochgoilhead fever, 118
Log-rolling
  cervical injury, 269
  team, 272
  technique, 215, 216–217,
    270–272

London Sports Medicine Institute
    (LSMI), general practitioner
    courses, 36
Long-distance runners, menstrual
    disorders, 50
Loughborough University, sports
    sciences, 37
Low back pain, 274
Lower limb
  injuries, running events, 176
  ischaemia, exercise testing, 22
  see also various anatomical parts

Magnetic resonance imaging (MRI),
    227
Malaria, 120
  prophylaxis, 124
Malleoli, fractures, 339–340
Mallet finger, 306
Mandible
  fractures, boxing, 163
  injuries, 230
March fractures, 344
March haemoglobinuria, 106, 178
Massage, for soft tissue injury, 130
Maxilla, injuries, 229
Maximal oxygen uptake test
    (VO$_2$ max), 70–72
Medical cover, competitions, 200
Medical problems, general,
    103–111
Melker emergency cricothyrotomy
    catheter set, 207–208
  tube insertion technique,
    219–220
Menarche delay, sports-related, 49
Meningitis, 257
Meniscus injuries, 290, 326–328
  tear types, 327
Menstrual cycle, and athletic
    performance, 49
Menstruation disorders, 47, 50–51,
    107
Metabolic disease, and exercise, 26
Metacarpal joints, dislocations/
    sprains, 305–306
Metacarpal neck fractures, 306
Metatarsalgia, 343–345
Metatarsals, stress fracture, 344
Methandienone, 84
Midfoot disorders, 341–343
Minerals
  dietary, 83
  replacement, during training,
    83–84
Misuse of Drugs Regulations
    (1985), 201
Morton's metatarsalgia, 343
Mountain sickness, 110

Mouth protection, 96–97, 236–237
Muscle
  injury, 149
  strains, 310–312
  tears, cold-related, 195–196
Musculoskeletal disorders, amenorrhoea,
    483
Myocardial infarction, 104
  post-infarction rehabilitation, 25
Myoglobinuria, exercise, 178
Myositis ossificans (traumatica), 153–154,
    227, 312

Nasal injuries, boxing, 163
Neck protection, 97, 98
Negligence, and injury, 11
Nervous system, cold effects, 197
Neuromas, plantar interdigital, 343–344
Nitrogen narcosis, 173
Nottingham University, 36
NSAIDs
  mortality/self-poisoning, 146
  oral/topical combination therapy, 146
  role, 145
  side-effects, 146
  use recommendations, 148–149
  see also Anti-inflammatory agents, topical
Nucleus pulposus, herniation, 274
Nutrition, women in sport, 47–48

Obesity, exercise and diet, 26
Objectivity, of performance tests, 76–77
Obstructive airways disease, management,
    exercise, 27
Oesophagus, rupture, 280
Olecranon bursitis, 302
Oligomenorrhoea, 50
Orbit, fracture, 240, 250
Organizers, duties, 12–13
Orofacial injuries, 229–238
  clinical examination, 230–234
Osgood Schlatter's disease, 329–330
Osteitis pubis, 310
Osteoarthrosis, hip, 313–314
Osteoblastic sarcoma, 227
Osteochondritis, pressure, 344
Osteoporosis
  prevention/management, exercise, 26–27
  in vegetarians, 48
  women in sport, 48, 50
Otorrhoea, 257
Outdoor sports, 1–3, 5
  see also various sports

Overseas travel, 107–110
  infections, 119–121
Overuse injuries, 142
Oxygenation, emergency, 206

Pangamic acid (vitamin B_{15}), 82–83
Parachuting, injuries, 175–176
Paramedics, 33
Participation
  influencing factors, 3
  risks, 3–4, 6–7
  socio-economic aspects, 3, 6
  statistics, 1–6
  see also Competitors
Patella
  dislocation, 320–321
  fractures, 289, 319
  recurrent dislocation, 320
    associated anomalies, 320
  stress fracture, 319–320
Patellar tendon, rupture, 328–329
Patellar tendonitis (jumper's knee),
    329
Patello-femoral pain, 322–323
Penetrating injuries
  eye, 244–245, 251
  heart, 279
  thorax/abdomen, 276
Performance assessment
  laboratory, 67–77
  objective, 67
  statistical criteria, 75–77
  subjective, 67
  use of results, 77
Periostitis, tibialis posterior, 330
Peripheral vascular disease, and
    exercise, 22, 23, 25–26
Peritendonitis, 152
Peroneal tenography, 227
Phalangeal joints, dislocations/
    sprains, 305–306
Pharyngotracheal lumen airway
    (PTLA), 207
Physical burns, eyes, 246
Physical inactivity, effects, 21
Physical Work Capacity (PWC)
    Test, 72
Plantar fasciitis, 340
Plantar interdigital neuromas, 343–344
Pneumothorax, 279
  tension, 209–210
Policeman's heel, 340
Popliteus tendonitis, 315–316
Portex chest drainage set, 209
Post-traumatic amnesia (PTA), 256, 257,
    259–260
  automatism, 259–260
Post-traumatic syndrome, 258–259, 263
Posterior cruciate ligament injury, 324–325

Posture, cervical injury, 270
Pott's fracture, 339–340
Power, instantaneous, testing, 74–75
Pre-existing disease, advice, 103–105
Pregnancy, exercise, 50–51
Premenstrual tension, 49
Prescribing
    banned substances, 90
    permissible agents, 90–91
    safe, 90–91, 110
Prostaglandins, inhibition, NSAIDs, 145
Protective equipment, 93–102
    see also various types and anatomical
        areas
Protein, dietary, 79
Puberty, female/male, 46–47
Pubialgia, 310
Pubic arch, osteochondritis, 310
Pubic syndrome, 310
Public order, requirements, 14–16
Pugilist's nose, 163
Pulmonary injuries, 279
Pulmonary oedema, high altitude, 196
Pump bump, 341
Punch drunkenness, 160–162
Putti-Platt procedure, 296

Quadriceps
    haematoma, 312
    strain, 312
    tendon rupture, 319

Racket sports, injuries, 171–172
Radiology
    injuries, 225–228
    protocol, 225
    soft tissues, 226
Radius, lower, epiphyseal injuries, 305
Raynaud's phenomenon, 196
Records, injury investigations, 223, 224
Recreation, informal, 1, 3
Rectus abdominis strain, 311
Rectus femoris, rupture, 318–319
Rehabilitation, after eye injuries, 252
Reliabilty, of performance tests, 76
Renal function, abnormalities,
        sports-related, 106–107
Resistance
    skill-specific, strength development,
        60–61
    variable, and strength development, 60
Respiratory disorders
    cold effects, 196
    and sports participation, 104–105
Respiratory infections, travel-related, 120
Resuscitation, cardiac arrest, 205, 206
Rhinorrhoea, 257
Rib fractures, 277

Rock climbers, finger injuries, 306–307
Rotator cuff, 293
    impingement, strengthening exercises,
        299, 300
    lesions, 297–300
    rupture, 298–299
Rugby football injuries, 169–170
    prevention, 170
Runners, long-distance, menstrual
        disorders, 50
Runners' high, 28
Running events, injuries during, 176–178

Safety, guidelines for governing bodies,
        18–19
Sager splint, 215
St Andrews University, sports sciences, 37
Scaphoid, fractures, 288, 303–304
    avascular necrosis, 304
Scapular fractures, 277–278
Scintigraphy, 226
Scrub typhus, 120
Scrumpox, 112, 113, 115–116
    infective agents, 116
Self-defence law, 10
Sesamoiditis, 344–345
Shin splints, 330–332
Shock, 210
    haemorrhagic, 210–211, 212
Shoulder
    anterior dislocation, 294–295
    frozen (pericapsulitis), 300
    injuries, 286–287
    movements, rotator cuff, 293
    recurrent dislocation, 295–296
    unstable, 296–297
Shoulder cuff
    impingement, 283
    tendon injuries, 286–287
Side positioning, in unconsciousness,
        214–215, 216–218
Snow blindness, 246
Soccer injuries, 168–169
Society of Apothecaries of London, 36
Soft tissue injuries
    acute, treatment, 137–138
    card, 43
    chronic, treatment, 138
    complications, 153–154
    elective care, 234–235
    immediate care, 234
    intra-articular, 285–286
        imaging, 286
    pathophysiology, 144, 145
    radiology, 226
    rehabilitation, 126–128
    treatment, 144–149, 234–235
        techniques, 128–137
Spearing, cervical injury, 267

Specificity, of performance tests, 75–76
Spectators
  duties, 12
  human requirements, 5
  injury risk/consent, 7
  statistics, 1, 2
  sudden death in, 157
Speed
  definition, 70
  testing, 70
  training, anaerobic, 61
Spinal injuries, 211, 213–214
  causes, 265
  incidence, 265
  prognosis, 272
Spinex card, spinal cord injury, 211, 214
Spleen, delayed rupture, 281
Sport, social opportunity/implacations, 56
Sport selection
  age factors, 55–56
  influencing factors, 54–56
Sporting activity, statistics
  participators, 1–6
  spectators, 1, 2
Sports Council (England), London NMSI,
    36, 40
Sports Council (Scotland), medical training
    initiatives, 39–40
Sports medicine
  definition, 32
  practitioners, 32–33
  training, 33–38
Sports science courses, 37–38
Sprains, 150–151
Squash
  injuries, 171–172
  sudden death, 172
Sterile packs, 124
Sternal fractures, 277–278
Stitch, 106
Strains, 151
Strapping
  objectives, 130–131
  soft tissue injury, 130–134, 135, 136, 137
Strength
  definition, 69
  restoration, post-injury, 127–128
  testing, 69
Strength development
  body weight, 60
  free weights, 59–60
  isokinetics, 60
  isometrics, 60
  three-set system, 59–60
Sub-aqua diving, injuries, 172–174
Subscapularis muscle, 293
Sudden immersion injury, 180, 196–197
Sunderland University, Sports medicine
    courses, 36–37
Supervitamins, 82–83

Supraspinatus muscle, 293
Swimming
  hazards, 174
  marathon, injuries, 174
Swimming pool burns, eyes, 245–246, 249

Tarsal tunnel syndrome, 342
Team doctors, 40–43
  communication with players/officials,
    42–43
  match/competition attendance, 41–42
Teeth
  avulsed/dislocated, 235
  injuries, 230, 231–234
Tendonitis, 152
  acute, 297–298
  chronic, 298
  midfoot, 341–342
  see also named tendons
Tendons, injuries, 152
Tendovaginitis, 152
Tennis elbow, 283, 301–302
Tenography, peroneal, 227
Tenosynovitis
  acute frictional, 303
  midfoot, 341–342
Tension pneumothorax, 209–210
Teres minor, 293
Testicular cancer, 228
Tetanus
  immunization, 108
  sports-related, 117
Tetraplegia
  immediate care, 272–273
  on-field prognosis, 272
  prevention, 273
Thal-Quick chest tube set, 209
Thigh protection, 100, 101
Thoracic injuries
  deep, 278–279
  management, 279–280
  prevention, 281–282
  superficial, 277–278
  types, 276–277
Thrower's elbow, 301
Thumb, fracture dislocation, 158, 306
Tibia, stress fracture, 331
Tibialis posterior, periostitis, 330
Tinea barbae, scrumpox, 116
Tinel's sign, 342
Toenail, ingrown, 345
Training effect, 21
Training for sport, 55–56
  cycle, 58
  detraining, 59
  duration, 58
  fluid/mineral replacement, 83–84
  frequency, 57–58
  intensity, 58

Training for sport (*contd*)
  overload, 57
  phases, 57–65
  purpose, 56
  rest and recovery, 59
  specificity, 56–57
  strength development, 59–61
  training load, 57
Training, sports medicine
  Bath University, 36
  London Sports Medicine Institute, 36
  Nottingham University, 36
  Royal Medical Colleges, Scotland,
      33–36
  Society of Apothecaries (London), 36
  Sunderland University, 36–37
Traumatic injuries, 142
Travel abroad, 107–110
  acclimatization, 109–110
  immunizations, 108–109
  infections, 119–121
  sterile packs, 124
Travellers' diarrhoea, 106, 113,
      119–120
Treadmills, 70
Trench foot (NFCI), 193–194, 198
  risk factors, 194
Trochanteric bursitis, 314
Tuberculosis, 120
Typhoid, vaccination, 109
Typhus, 120

Ultrasonography, 226
Ultrasound therapy, soft tissue injury,
      129–130
Unconscious patients, side positioning,
      214–215, 216–218
Urinary tract infections, 310
Urticaria, familial cold, 187

Validity, of performance tests, 75
Vegetarians
  amenorrhoea, 50
  osteoporosis, 48
Violence, in sport, 5–6
  see also Foul play
Viral haemorrhagic fevers, 120
Visual acuity testing, eye injuries, 247–248
Vitamin A, 81
Vitamin B_{15} (pangamic acid), 82–83
Vitamin B complex, 82–83
Vitamin C, 82
Vitamin D, 81–82
Vitamin E, 82
Vitamins, dietary, 81–83
Vygon chest drainage set, 209

Water skiing, injuries, 172
Water sports
  infections, 118
  injuries, 172–175
Weight gain, 88
Weight loss, 87–88
  and training, 64, 65
Well-being and health, training for, 62–65
Women in sport, 46–53
  injury, 51–52
  iron deficiency, 48
  menarche delay, 49
  nutrition, 47–48
  osteoporosis, 48, 50
  sexing, 48
  training response, 47
World Medical Association, Ethics of
      practice, 38–39
Wound infections, sports-related, 117–118
Wrestling, injuries, 166, 167, 168
Wrist
  fractures/dislocations, 303–305
  injuries, 287–288
  pain, 303